Forensic Approaches to Death, Disaster and Abuse

edited by
Marc Oxenham
The Australian National University

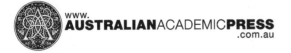

www.
AUSTRALIANACADEMIC**PRESS**
.com.au

First published in 2008 from a completed manuscript presented to
Australian Academic Press
32 Jeays Street
Bowen Hills Qld 4006
Australia
www.australianacademicpress.com.au

National Library of Australia cataloguing-in-publication data:

> Oxenham, Marc.
>
> Forensic approaches to death, disaster and abuse / editor, Marc Oxenham.
>
> 1st ed.
>
> 9781875378906 (pbk.)
>
> Forensic sciences.
> Forensic anthropology.
> Criminal investigation.
>
> 363.25

Editing and typesetting by Australian Academic Press, Brisbane.

Contents

(continued over)

Contents (continued)

Contents (continued)

The Forensic Sciences, Anthropology and Investigations Into Abuse and the Loss of Life

Marc Oxenham

Mention the word forensics and most people will conjure up images of popular television shows such as CSI, where you will find Gil Grissom pondering a crime scene, or Bones, where you find Temperance Brennan reading the clues trapped in grisly human remains. That CSI (Las Vegas version) won the 2004 Saturn award, and was nominated for the same award in 2005, from the Academy of Science Fiction, Fantasy & Horror Films, United States, underlines the fact that these popular depictions of forensic investigations, particularly many of the gadgets and techniques employed, often stray into the realms of total fantasy. In contrast to such forms of forensic entertainment, and considering the Asia–Pacific region only, the devastating affects of the Asian (Boxing Day) Tsunami in late December 2004 where almost 230,000 people died (UN Office of the Envoy for Tsunami Recovery, n.d.), the terrible aftermath of the Bali bombings in October 2002 killing 202 including 38 Indonesians and 88 Australians (AFP, n.d.), and the senseless killings, tortures and rapes in the Solomon islands between 1998 and 2003 (Amnesty International, 2004), bring home the realities of both natural and human engineered death, destruction and abuse.

Popular, and somewhat unrealistic, portrayals of what forensic science is all about, as well as the recent spate of real human disasters, have no doubt fuelled much public and government awareness in the forensic sciences. The glamour and perceived infallibility of forensic experts and what they can do (never what they cannot achieve) has had a major influence on the court system in recent years, so much so that it has been coined 'the CSI effect' (see Toobin, 2007). The general interest has also spilled into the education sector, with an influx of students interested in enrolling in forensic courses. An increase in the popularity of such courses, which have been taught in many tertiary institutions for years, albeit without a particularly high profile, has been met by a multiplication in Australia-wide university offerings. A perusal of Hobsons' online *Good Universities Guides* (2007) shows 26 Australian tertiary institutions currently offering 69 academic qualifications in the form of various certificates, diplomas, bachelors, masters and doctoral degrees in various subdisciplines of the forensic sciences (Table 1). Many of the qualifications listed in Table 1 are quite specialised, particularly those relating to forensic medicine, psychology, chemistry and computing, while others are poorly represented in the academic curricula: forensic archaeology and anthropology are good examples.

One of the chief motivations behind the development of this edited book was a desire to bring together as many of the disparate forensic subdisciplines as possible into a single volume in order to: (a) show where and how they articulate with each other; and (b) introduce the role and importance of forensic anthropology and archaeology; under (c) the umbrella of a specific theme: forensic approaches to death, disaster and abuse. The genesis of this project extends back to late 2003 when Michael Westaway, an Executive Officer at the Willandra Lakes World Heritage Area and PhD candidate at the ANU, approached me to jointly organise and convene a 2-day conference and series of workshops titled *Forensic Anthropology for Australian Field Conditions and Beyond*, held between March 5 and 6, 2004, at the National Museum of Australia. This conference turned out to be extremely popular and made me realise how much interest there was in such issues in Australia generally. At around the same time, late 2003, I became involved in teaching forensic anthropology and archaeology at the Canberra Institute of Technology (CIT) as part of their Bachelor of Applied Science (Forensic Investigation). The success of the aforementioned conference and my CIT teaching led me to develop a major in forensic anthropology at the Australian National University as part of the program in expanding the School of Archaeology and Anthropology's interests into human skeletal biology, both past and present. The ANU now offers Australia's only, to my knowledge, Master of Arts — Forensic Anthropology.

Like many people, I am not immune to the lure of analysing clues or evidence in the form of human remains and associated archaeological artefacts to reconstruct aspects of the lives of those once living: putting flesh back on their bones! Broad research and curricular interests have led me to become involved with diagnosing disease and trauma in ancient skeletal material (Oxenham, Walters Nguyen, & Nguyen, 2001; Oxenham, Nguyen, & Nguyen, 2005; Oxenham, Matsumura, & Nishimoto, 2006; Oxenham, 2006); determining what people ate in the past and other aspects of their subsistence and adaptive behaviours by looking at their oral health (Oxenham, Locher, Nguyen, & Nguyen, 2002; Oxenham, Nguyen, & Nguyen, 2006; Oxenham & Matsumura, 2008; Bower, Yasutomo, Oxenham, Nguyen, & Nguyen, 2006); the history of human skeletal research in South-East Asia (Tayles & Oxenham, 2006); human and comparative anatomy (Oxenham & Whitworth, 2006: Chapter 6) and, more recently, investigating more abstract aspects of human behaviour by examining and interpreting burial or mortuary practices — particularly aspects of childhood (Oxenham, Matsumura, Domett, Nguyen, Nguyen et al., in press) — and Australian mortuary practices (Oxenham et al., in press: Chapter 4). With this background in biological anthropology and archaeology, including consulting experience relating to the identification of human remains both in the United States and Australia, I have been particularly keen to develop and promote, primarily through the auspices of tertiary education and curricular development, the forensic sciences generally and their articulation and relationship to forensic anthropology and archaeology in particular.

In facilitating this aim I have been keen to place the substantive contributions to forensic investigations available through archaeological and osteological techniques

Table 1

Australian Tertiary Institutions Offering Qualifications in Forensic Disciplines

Institution	Degree
Australian National University	Master of Arts: Forensic Anthropology
	Graduate Diploma: Forensic Anthropology
Bond University	Master of Psychology: Forensic
	Master of Forensic Science
	Bachelor of Forensic Science
Canberra Institute of Technology	Bachelor of Applied Science: Forensic Investigation
	Diploma of Public Safety: Forensic Investigations
	Advanced Diploma of Computer Forensics
	Advanced Diploma of Applied Science: Forensic Investigation
	Advanced Diploma of Computer Forensics
Charles Sturt University	Bachelor of Biotechnology: Medical/Forensic
Curtain University of Technology	Master of Internet Security and Forensics
	Master of Forensic Sexology
	Postgraduate Diploma of Forensic Sexology
	Bachelor of Science: Forensic and Analytical Chemistry
Deakin University	Doctor of Psychology: Forensic
	Bachelor of Forensic Science
Edith Cowan University	Postgraduate Certificate in Forensic Mental Health Nursing
	Graduate Certificate in Nursing: Forensic
	Bachelor of Forensic Investigation
	Bachelor of Science: Environmental Forensics
	Bachelor of Science: Forensic and Biomolecular Science
Flinders University	Graduate Diploma of Forensic Science: DNA Technology
	Bachelor of Technology: Forensic and Analytical Chemistry
Griffith University	Doctor of Psychology: Forensic
	Master of Forensic Psychology
	Master of Forensic Mental Health
	Master of Science: Forensic Science
	Bachelor of Forensic Science/Bachelor of Arts: Criminology and Criminal Justice
	Bachelor of Forensic Science
	Graduate Certificate in Forensic Mental Health
James Cook University	Master of Forensic Mental Health
	Postgraduate Diploma of Forensic Psychology
	Postgraduate Certificate in Forensic Psychology
	Graduate Diploma of Forensic Mental Health
	Graduate Certificate in Forensic Mental Health
La Trobe University	Postgraduate Diploma of Forensic Science
Monash University	Master of Forensic Medicine
	Graduate Diploma of Forensic Medicine
	Graduate Diploma of Forensic Pathology
	Graduate Certificate in Forensic Medicine
	Graduate Certificate in Forensic Studies: Construction and Engineering
	Graduate Certificate in Forensic Behavioural Science
	Graduate Certificate in Forensic Studies: Accounting
Murdoch University	Postgraduate Diploma of Environmental Forensics
	Bachelor of Science: Forensic Biology and Toxicology
Swinburne University of Technology	Certificate IV in Forensic Science
TAFE, NSW, Hunter Institute	Diploma of Laboratory Technology: Chem. and Foren. Testing
TAFE, NSW, South West. Syd. Inst.	Diploma of Laboratory Technology: Chem. and Foren. Testing
Victoria University	Master of Social Science: Forensic and Crime Studies
	Bachelor of Science: Medical, Forensic and Analyt. Chemistry
University of Adelaide	Graduate Diploma of Forensic Odontology
University of Canberra	Bachelor of Forensic Studies/Bachelor of Laws
	Bachelor of Forensic Studies
University of South Australia	Master of Psychology: Forensic
University of Melbourne	Master of Criminology: Forensic Psychology
	Graduate Diploma of Forensic Odontology
	Graduate Certificate in Criminology: Forensic Disability
	Graduate Certificate in Business Forensics
University of New South Wales	Master of Psychology: Forensic
University of Technology, Sydney	Bachelor of Science: Applied Chemistry: Foren. Sci. (Hons)
	Bachelor of Science: Biomedical Science: Forensic Biology
	Bachelor of Science: Environmental Forensics
University of Western Australia	Master of Forensic Science
	Graduate Diploma of Forensic Science
	Graduate Diploma of Forensic Science: Odontology
University of Western Sydney	Master of Psychology: Forensic Psychology
	Bachelor of Science: Forensic Science
University of Wollongong	Master of Forensic Accounting

into a much broader context. At the Australian National University I have been determined to develop a Major and Master of Arts in Forensic Anthropology that situates the contributions of many forensic subdisciplines within the general framework of anthropological and archaeological approaches. My first problem was the lack of any appropriate broad spectrum text(s) that had been written with such a purpose in mind. Numerous excellent specialist texts that deal with issues of forensic archaeology and anthropology have been written in recent years, and examples include: William Haglund and Marcella Sorg's (1997) *Forensic Taphonomy: The Post-mortem Fate of Human Remains*, and their subsequent (2002) volume, *Advances in Forensic Taphonomy: Method, Theory, and Archaeological Perspectives*; John Clement and David Ranson's (1998) *Craniofacial Identification in Forensic Medicine*; Margaret Cox and Simon Mays' (2000) *Human Osteology in Archaeology and Forensic Science*; and Zvonka Zupanic-Slavic's (2004) *New Method of Identifying Family Related Skulls: Forensic Medicine, Anthropology, Epigenetics*. Many of these texts are (and rightly so) technical, specialist, and seek to present specific methodological approaches to particular forensic problems.

This book, on the other hand, does not set out to provide a competing specialist resource, but rather aims to assemble in one place the approaches of various forensic scientists and practitioners in a readily accessible form to the public and academics alike. To be sure, forensic science is a vast discipline and is beyond the scope of any single volume to summarise in any useful form, which is why the intention of this text is to draw together experts in a range of forensic specialties that intersect at investigations of death, disaster and abuse, particularly as these are, or have been, relevant in the Asia–Pacific region (with the occasional international excursions where necessary). This will provide a context in which to understand how these various approaches and processes in forensic investigations contribute to a successful outcome (often measured in terms of a conviction) and also, importantly, inform each other on the way to this goal. A further endeavour of this book is to explore advances in the techniques and approaches of the various subdisciplines involved in death and abuse, particularly in the Asia–Pacific context.

The book has been arranged into four sections covering broadly related aspects of forensic investigations of death, disaster and abuse. In some cases, chapters can be used as a handy field guide, in others as background for more in-depth study, while others will provide both the specialist and interested reader with insights into how, and on what basis, forensic investigations are run. The first section focuses on forensic archaeology and begins (Chapter 2) with Ian Hanson's insights into international forensic archaeological investigations. Ian starts with a review of the history and development of forensic archaeology as a distinct subdiscipline in national and international forensic investigations, and then goes on to discuss the role and benefits of forensic archaeological participation in international investigations, essentially those involving death and burial on a large scale. Ian makes the important point that as evidence recoverable by way of forensic archaeological techniques may be of use in both humanitarian and criminal investigative contexts, evidence recovery must be maximised regardless of context or perceived immediate need. Moreover, maximising evidence recovery can contribute to other associated issues, including maintenance of human rights, repatriation of remains, atrocity deterrents and countering the activities of historical revisionists. Ian also reviews the application of archaeological methods and techniques to forensic settings, as well as discussing forensic archaeology as a forensic science as opposed to the sometimes more subjective or heavily inferential nature of some archaeological interpretations in nonmedico–legal contexts. Ian concludes with an examination of how forensic archaeology articulates with what are always multidisciplinary forensic investigations.

Mark Tibbett, in Chapter 3, examines perhaps the most important factor involved in the interpretation of archaeologically derived evidence: taphonomic processes. Following a review of decomposition processes in general, including generally recognised decomposition stages, Mark goes on to a consideration of factors most important in influencing the decomposition of a cadaver over time. Both biological aspects of the deceased (including height, weight, sex, and so on) as well as their clothing have a marked affect on the rate and nature of decomposition, with artificial clothing fibres providing a measure of preservation. With respect to the burial site itself, soil type (texture, chemistry and faunal/floral content) appears to have an extremely important influence on the decomposition trajectory, while variations in temperature (extreme cold aids in preservation) and moisture (arid environments also aid preservation by way of desiccation of the corpse) are important environmental variables to consider when determining the postmortem interval. Mark provides significant insights into a relatively underresearched aspect of forensic science. His call for more experimental research into forensic taphonomy is well taken.

In Chapter 4, Tom Knight, Michael Westaway and I review the ethnographic, historical and archaeological evidence for Aboriginal burial practices. The aim of this chapter is to describe various forms of Aboriginal Australian body disposal that have occurred in the distant and more recent past. Given that homicide rates are not particularly high in Australia, and that clandestine burial of murder victims even rarer, in most cases recovered human remains will turn out to be either historic and/or Aboriginal and of no forensic interest. A range of Aboriginal burial practices are discussed with an emphasis on the types of burial situations that will preserve remains into modern times. In general, Aboriginal body disposal methods included cremation, ground burial, tree burial or various forms and storage of remains in relatively inaccessible caves and crevasses. Drawing heavily on ethnohistoric sources, Tom, Michael and I have highlighted the manner in which the deceased were dealt with in a way that will provide clues as to the identity and nature (Aboriginal or recent clandestine) of the remains. Some mortuary practices naturally enhance preservation of the corpse, such as ground burial in certain situations and mummification and cave stowage in others, and can be readily identified as Aboriginal. Other disposal methods, particularly the burial and inclusion of European artefacts, can cause problems in the ultimate identification of remains as archaeological and/or historic, or recent and thus forensically relevant. Anyone armed with this review of Aboriginal mortuary practices should be in a much better informed position to take appropriate measures on the discovery of human remains, whatever the circumstances of discovery.

In Chapter 5, Tim Anson and Michael Trimbal take us back to the international stage with their firsthand account of the role of forensic anthropologists in mass grave investigations. They make the point that while crimes resulting in the loss of life on massive scales are not new, investigations and punishment of such acts of mass violence at a coordinated international level is a relatively recent phenomenon. Tim and Michael provide a practical and procedurally oriented approach to the excavation of mass graves, using their recent experiences in Iraq as a framework. They stress the need for a team approach to such investigations, with the inclusion of personnel covering a broad range of specialist skills and abilities; from heavy plant operators to logistics managers, not to mention forensic anthropologists and archaeologists. While specific operational procedures in mass grave investigations will vary from site to site and jurisdiction to jurisdiction, the basic and fundamentally important aspects of such investigations have now been relatively standardised. Towards the close of their chapter they explore the issue of interpretation of mass graves. Potentially different victim profiles may throw light on the actions and nature of the mass homicide perpetrators. For instance, execution style may be reconstructed, which could lead to inferences regarding the type of executioner, such as secret police versus regular army personnel. Tim and Michael provide a relevant, contemporary, if somewhat topical, context for their overview.

This section is concluded with Chapter 6, where Richard Barwick and I present a basic guide to the identification of human remains in Australia. The remains of animals similar in size and mass to humans, such as sheep and kangaroos, can easily be confused with human skeletonised material. Richard and I provide illustrations of the more commonly preserved bones (i.e., limbs, pelvis and vertebrae) of an adult human, sheep and kangaroo. The chapter is structured to enable a direct comparison of any given bone between these three organisms: for example, the thigh bone (femur) of a human, sheep and kangaroo are illustrated together and the chief differences and similarities pointed out in the text. The aim of this chapter is to provide a quick and easy to use field guide for the layperson or nonspecialist interested in differentiating between human and other commonly encountered animal bones.

Section 2 focuses on the contributions from forensic anthropology where the chief emphasis is on the various aspects and techniques of human identification. Denise Donlon, in Chapter 7, introduces this section with a review of forensic anthropology in Australia followed by illustrative case studies of incidents in which she has been involved over the past 15 years. Denise notes an increase in the number of cases involving forensic anthropology over this same period and attributes this to an increasing awareness of the contribution and role of this subdiscipline. To maintain and, ideally, further promote forensic anthropology in medico–legal investigations there is a need to ensure the highest quality of professionalism and technical skill. Denise notes a situation where a mistake in sex estimation of skeletonised remains held up the successful resolution of a case by 17 years! The case studies outlined by Denise are particularly useful in highlighting the range of problems and variability in conditions and approach encountered by forensic anthropologists in the field and laboratory. Further, her focus on the types of agencies requiring forensic anthropological consultants, geographic locations, nature of cases, condition of remains, and appearances in court provide a useful and relevant structural context in which to discuss the role of the forensic anthropologist.

In Chapter 8 Richard Wright describes the use of morphometric approaches to human identification in the context of a computer program, CRANID, which he has developed and refined over several years. Richard argues that advances in multivariate statistical approaches and more sophisticated approaches to morphometric analysis of the human skull mean that such techniques have great value in determining human ancestry. Further, morphometric techniques continue to have value in the face of problems with DNA survival in many instances and where the need for a quick determination of identity (and perhaps a cheap one) is of greater importance. Richard's chapter covers both the basics of determining ancestry using linear measurements of the human skull and successfully answers several important criticisms of this approach. Details on how to use the program to achieve accurate results are given, as well as information on how to obtain this 'freeware'. Finally, Richard illustrates the applications of CRANID in the areas of forensic anthropology, repatriation and even archaeological research.

Hallie Buckley and Kelly Whittle examine, in Chapter 9, one of the more disturbing aspects of forensic investigations: child abuse. Their focus is on the identification of abuse in skeletonised remains and they detail insights to be gained through analysis of both fractures and periosteal reactions. Child abuse is more common in younger children, aged between birth and 3 years, as this is a developmental period characterised by limited mobility and reduced defensive abilities. The authors outline a number of apparent 'telltale' fractures such as bilateral rib trauma, metaphyseal fractures and multiple and/or complex skull fractures. Similarly, periosteal reactions, that can be observed radiologically or in dry bone, can give insights into periods of trauma that may be indicative of abuse. Hallie and Kelly stress, however, that periosteal reactions are part of the developmental biology of bone in children under 6 months old, whereas a range of infectious diseases can produce subperiosteal reactions as well. Clearly, a detailed understanding and familiarity with both trauma and bone biology is a requisite of anyone involved in interpreting child abuse in skeletonised material. The key point is that trauma, whether in the form of fractures or periosteal reactions, needs to be assessed in terms of its patterning (distribution in the body) and timing (differential traumatic events). While abuse may be a one-off event, it usually occurs over a period of time leading to more than one traumatic event in different stages of healing. The abhorrence with which the community receives cases of child abuse, and the complexity associated with interpreting its presence in skeletonised remains, will place considerable pressure on consulting forensic anthropologists and other medically trained personnel where such behaviour is suspected.

In Chapter 10, Carl Stephan, Ronn Taylor and Jane Taylor review the history, development and methods of facial approximation and skull-face superimposition with a focus on the Australian scene. Superimposition, the methods of which date back to the late 19th century, has been successfully (as measured in hundreds of cases) used in Australia since the 1960s, with the use of video techniques beginning in the 1970s. The technique, which essentially involves superimposing a fleshed image of a known individual on the bony framework of an unknown skull and assessing the fit, has been found to be very accurate and reliable, particularly if both frontal and lateral imaging is used (using images of the front and side of the face and head). However, and despite the high level of accuracy, Carl and colleagues note that the technique has seldom been used for the positive identification of human remains. The other technique reviewed by Carl, Ronn and Jane is that of facial approximation. Some readers will be familiar with the publicity this technique received in the 1983 feature film *Gorky Park* and more recently in computer-generated facial approximations in popular crime shows such as *Bones*. Less extensively used in Australia, only 20 reconstructions are reported by Carl and colleagues over the past 30 years and only four of these contributed to a positive identification. While the technique can involve different media such as drawing, computer generated images and sculpture, the latter method seems most popular and is extensively reviewed in this chapter.

While the underlying principle of the technique is that there is a correlation between one's soft tissues and the underlying bony substrate, emphasis varies between reconstruction of the underlying musculature and a focus on soft tissue depths at various anatomical landmarks. As with superimposition, testing of the accuracy and reliability of facial approximation has been formally carried out, albeit with less satisfactory results.

Judith Littleton, in Chapter 11, discusses the basic analytical tasks of any physical anthropologist: determination of sex, age-at-death, ancestry, and stature. However, any sense of human identification security a forensic anthropologist working in the Asia–Pacific region may have will be tested in this chapter. Judith notes that despite a marked increase in forensic anthropological texts, the focus of published research remains on North American populations and situations. Her discussion addresses problems, and at times solutions, to determination of ancestry, sex, age-at-death, and stature in the Asia–Pacific region, particularly in Australia/Papua New Guinea and New Zealand. With respect to ancestry, or 'race', the biggest problems concern the enormous range of morphological variation in Asia and the Pacific coupled with limited and/or difficult to access literature on the topic. For instance, catch all terms such as Mongoloid have no practical or morphological discriminatory relevance in the forensic anthropology of this region. The same issues are apparent when it comes to sexing human remains, with sexual dimorphism being population specific and the most commonly available sexing criteria being based on North American or European samples. All biological anthropologists with any familiarity with Australian remains are aware of the specific issues associated with determining the sex of Australian Aboriginal crania. Age-at-death estimation is often seen as being immune from the regional or population-based problems associated with sex estimation. Nonetheless, commonly used epiphyseal fusion and tooth development/eruption standards need to be used with extreme caution in this part of the world. Asian and Australian (regardless of ancestral background) dental development and eruption schedules can vary considerably from those published by Massler et al. (1941) and Ubelaker (1999), for example. Stature is another important biovariable often estimated by forensic anthropologists and has proven an important identifying characteristic in mass grave excavations recently. As with other biological characteristics, it varies by region, ancestry, sex, diet, health and environment. While Judith points to a robust literature examining stature among various populations in the Asia-Pacific region, she also highlights some important deficits, particularly in terms of stature estimation of Aboriginal Australians. This chapter is an important resource and point of departure for anyone associated with forensic reconstructions of identity in this part of the globe, and with forensic anthropological investigations generally.

Chapter 12 concludes this section with Donald Pate's discussion of the observation that we are what we eat. The chemical composition of our tissues can provide clues as to our geographic origin and even aspects of our residential mobility though life. Analyses of isotopes, different varieties of particular elements, have been commonly carried out in order to determine the diet and subsistence orientations of past individuals or populations. Donald uses such research as a springboard into discussions of how stable isotopic studies can shed light on where an individual may have grown up, where or whether or not he/she spent their adult life in another locality (were they a migrant?) and even where they had been living in the past several weeks or months! Different human tissues have varying turnover rates that allow for the determination of geographic residence at various stages of life. The fastest turnover is in fingernails and hair, with the latter proving more useful for the most recent and shortest time periods. Different teeth, on the other hand, due to their differential development during childhood, provide access to information on where the individual grew up or even what the individual ate as a child. Skeletal tissues, on the other hand, provide an averaged summary, generally of the past decade, of dietary and locational information. Donald points out that these tried and tested techniques are commonly used in archaeology but are relatively untapped in forensic situations; a situation doubtless soon to dramatically change.

The third section of this book deals with forensic aspects of the determination of the time, manner, and cause of death. In Chapter 13, David Ranson introduces this section with a discussion on perhaps one of the most diverse and complex jobs that involve investigations of death: the coroner. This is the largest chapter in the book as it has the additional aim of reviewing important aspects of death, disaster and abuse not treated as separate chapters: for example, disaster victim identification, forensic odontology and DNA identification. David notes the important role the coroner has in the way a community manages death, even though relatively few deaths are actually investigated by the coroner. After reviewing the historical development of the coroner over the past thousand years, David focuses on the operation of the modern office of the coroner by reviewing the duties, functions and personnel: specialist coronial clerks, the police, bereavement services, medical services (particularly the pathologist), death investigation coordination and even exhumation where necessary. David also reviews the nature and importance of human identification as a function of the coroner's office. Here, a range of identification techniques (visual, fingerprinting, molecular, pathology, radiology, anthropology) are summarised along with a detailed discussion of one of the most important identification techniques (particularly in mass disasters): forensic odontology (identification using dental remains). This chapter is particularly important in drawing together the disparate and specialised roles, functions, duties, investigative and analytical techniques of modern forensic investigations into death.

Ian Dadour and Michele Harvey review in Chapter 14 the forensic entomology literature, highlighting the diversity of ways insects and arthropods have been employed in forensic investigations. Ian and Michele look at three broad categories of forensic entomological application: urban, stored product, and medico-legal applications. Urban applications can include litigation between individuals or community groups and those involved in activities leading to an increase in nuisance insect populations (for example, operation of an abattoir). Other situations may involve litigation and/or financial loss due to the structural damage caused by termites. An example of a stored product application may involve litigation in connection with insect infestation of commercial foodstuffs. Medico–legal implications are perhaps the broadest and most commonly encountered in terms of forensic entomology. Much attention has been focused on determination of the postmortem interval (PMI), particularly with respect to different insect colonisation sequences with varying geographic and climatic conditions. Advances in determining these sequences more accurately has been furthered by way of sophisticated genetic identification technologies. More recent research has also successfully addressed issues such as cause and manner of death: identification of gunshot residues and various drugs in feeding insects, for instance. Clearly new technologies continue to open new investigative channels for forensic applications involving insects and arthropods.

In Chapter 15, Shari Forbes investigates a comparatively underresearched approach to determining the postmortem interval (PMI): the chemistry of decomposition and preservation. Investigations into the chemical process involved in this topic will improve the evidential data recoverable in incidents involving disasters and death on whatever scale and in whatever manner these occur. For instance, Shari notes that the PMI can be assessed using amino acid signatures generated during the decomposition process. Moreover, the chemical products of decomposition can affect the surrounding environment, visually apparent by way of vegetative changes, and thus signal the presence of human remains; while odours associated with protein decomposition can be detected by cadaver dogs. Other aspects of decomposition chemistry can be employed in interpreting soil samples from beneath or around cadavers to determine the rate of decomposition and ultimately an estimation of the PMI, or even the identity of a burial site that contains no other evidence (artefactual or biological) of a crime. Decomposition and preservation chemistry is a relatively new area in the forensic tool kit and promises to be an important future component of forensic investigations into death.

In Chapter 16, Walter Wood draws on over 30 years of experience as a forensic anthropology consultant who has been involved in consulting on fatal crocodile attacks in northern Australia. After summarising relevant aspects of the biology and behaviour of fresh and saltwater crocodiles, Walter goes on to review the fatal attacks on humans over the past 30 years with a series of case studies illustrating important aspects of the process and timing of the modification and decomposition of human tissue. The manner in which crocodiles process and consume human victims and the biology of their digestive system result in an extremely rapid destruction of ingested material, and the tropical climate where crocodiles are found facilitates further rapid decomposition of noningested human material. Understandably, identification of crocodile attack victims can be difficult, although success has been achieved using standard forensic anthropological techniques such as finger printing of keratin-rich skin and, to an extent, DNA analysis. Walter's work is relevant in terms of time, cause and manner of death, as well as in relation to the issues concerning human identification explored in Section 2.

The final section of this volume deals with more legal, ethical and procedural issues in forensic investigations of death, disaster and abuse. James Robertson begins this segment, in Chapter 17, with a discussion of the role of the Australian Federal Police (AFP) in investigations of deceased people and their remains. It may come as a surprise to many that the significant contribution by the AFP in dealing with the aftermath of major terrorist attacks and natural disasters involving Australian and neighbouring country casualties is a relatively recent occurrence. This is due to the youth of the organisation, established in 1979, and relatively recent changes in the nature of international terrorism. James provides a detailed and comprehensive overview of the AFP, which has a pivotal role both nationally and internationally in a range of areas that include, but are not limited to, the identification of deceased people in isolated cases through to large-scale natural disasters and human-engineered death. Moreover, the AFP is the Interpol hub for Australia. It operates through its international officer liaison network and, in more specific and targeted situations, its international deployment group (AFP involvement in restoring law and order in the Solomon Islands being a case in point). Recent extensive experience following the Bali bombings and Asian Tsunami has meant that the AFP is recognised regionally as an important source of expertise and training in situations of mass casualty management and victim identification. While the AFP may be one of the first on the scene, such as in the Bali bombings, often forensic investigations operate within zones of compromised security where initial deployment by defence forces is necessary (an example being the initial Solomon Islands response by Australia). This highlights the often neglected point that investigations into mass disasters, particularly terrorist-initiated, can involve considerable risk to the forensic investigative team (an issue also raised in Chapter 7). This chapter is invaluable in providing the procedural and collaborative context in which responses to, and investigations into, mass fatalities involving Australians and/or of South-East Asian neighbours operate.

In Chapter 18 Tom Faunce highlights the types of conflicts (ethical, moral, legal and so forth) medical practitioners may have to face when dealing with patients implicated or involved in forensic investigations into death, disaster and abuse, particularly those involving or associated with terrorist attacks. Tom then goes on to explore the way the issues surrounding ethics and medical professionalism may be influenced or compromised by recent technological developments, particularly in the rapidly developing area of nanotechnology. Apart from the improvement in clandestine surveillance capabilities, nanotechnology has the potential to revolutionise the day to day processing of forensic evidence, both by requiring much smaller sample sizes and by increasing the sensitivity of existing forensic explorative and analytical techniques. In terms of biosecurity, Tom suggests that future academic collaboration and the sharing of data and research outcomes may be restricted, given the potential risks associated with easy public availability of some forms of research — development of new viruses, for instance. Further, while nanotechnology has the potential to produce more sophisticated warning systems (biotoxin nano-sensors built into clothing for example) and thus aid in the detection and nullification of bioterrorist attacks, the same nanostructures themselves may pose unknown health risks to the very people they are ostensibly protecting. In the second part of this chapter Tom discusses his experiences in an intensive care unit in Melbourne during the Bali Bombings. The discussion of the types and forms of injuries encountered in such incidents associated with deliberate delayed bomb blasts, lead into discussion of the potential for bioterrorists to employ secondary hazards, such as radiation and/or biological agents, in such cases. Nanotechnology has the potential to assist in the quick and large scale assessment of secondary risks in situations of human engineered mass disaster.

Christine Phillips, in Chapter 19, discusses forms of what are generally institutionalised, or at least normalised, abuse that can affect the lives and well being of prisoners and detainees. The two chief types of such abuse include: (a) state sanctioned acts of violence (failures of commission) with the aim of extracting information (torture), and (b) failures to protect the health of, or provide adequate health care to, prisoners (failures of omission). Christine reviews various international conventions ostensibly designed to protect prisoners and detainees from these categories of abuse; conventions often reinterpreted by governments in times of national or international crisis or simply ignored, particularly with respect to torture. For instance, it is estimated that electro-shock devices have been employed for the purposes of torture in over 87 countries in the past decade or so. In contrast to the more publically visible abuses, especially by way of recent and spectacular exposés of state complicit torture, Christine discusses important failures of omission and the main ways in which prisoners can be afforded protection. Perhaps the most important, and least accomplished, method is preventing people entering prison in the first place. The appalling increase in the proportion of Aboriginal Australians in custody over recent years is illustrative of such failure. Other mechanisms include the adoption, in practice and not only on paper, of internationally recognised and sanctioned standards such as the provision of adequate levels of health care, including psychiatric and psychological, for prisoners; and mechanisms by which the system can be monitored. The treatment of prisoners and detainees is a controversial topic, with ethics and international standards often in conflict with the perceived and immediate requirements (political and/or economic interests) of the state in times of crisis. Christine provides a valuable and even-handed treatment of this difficult topic in her chapter.

In the final chapter, 20, Maciej Henneberg draws on his considerable national and international experience in discussing the role of the expert witness. Maciej begins with a discussion of legal systems in general, highlighting the differences between civil and criminal law as well as inquisitorial versus adversarial systems (as used in Australia). Following this is an overview of the functioning and nature of the tiered court structure in Australia: Magistrate, District and Supreme courts. Given that forensic archaeologists and anthropologists are more likely to be called as expert witnesses in criminal cases, this forms the focus of the remainder of the discussion. In particular, Maciej discusses the nature of evidence, the role and duties of the expert witness with respect to evidence examination, report preparation, pretrial conferences, and admissibility of evidence hearings, committal hearings and trial appearances. In addition to outlining the entire process from initial approaches to a witness, through the expectations and responsibilities of expert witnesses, to the specific, if somewhat ritualised, behaviour expected in a court of law, Maciej frequently illustrates the discussion with advice based on his extensive experience as an expert witness in many jurisdictions over more than a quarter of a century. He emphasises that regardless of which party approached an expert witness, the role of the expert witness is to provide facts and objective opinion and not to support one side or the other; advocacy of any form also needs to be avoided. Interestingly, Maciej notes the pressures expert witnesses can be placed under to provide absolute statements where, in reality, only statements of varying levels of probability can be made. In the interests of justice, as well as your own future career as an expert witness, bowing to such pressure needs to be avoided. This chapter provides a refreshingly straightforward and painless introduction to the Australian court and legal system, as well as an indispensable and thorough guide to anyone contemplating providing their specialists skills, knowledge and experience as an expert witness.

As with any edited volume there have been some omissions, cancellations, reorganisations and compromises in content and coverage. However, I believe this is the first book to focus on forensic approaches to death, disaster and abuse in the Asia–Pacific region, and certainly the first to draw on such a breadth of the subdisciplines in the forensic sciences. While this book is not definitive it will, I hope, contribute to a greater understanding of the main issues, problems, solutions, debates, controversies and everyday practical approaches to the practice of forensic science in our region in the context of the theme death, disaster and abuse.

References

Australian Federal Police. (n.d.). Retrieved May 1, 2007, from http://www.afp.gov.au/international/operations/previous_operations/bali_bombings_2002

Amnesty International. (2004). Solomon Islands: women confronting violence. (AI index: ASA 43/001/2004)

Bower, N.W., Yasutomo, Y., Oxenham, M.F., Nguyen, L.C., & Nguyen, K.T. (2006). Preliminary reconstruction of diet at a Neolithic site in Vietnam using stable isotope and Ba/Sr analyses. *Bulletin of the Indo-Pacific Prehistory Association, 26*, 79–85.

Clement, J.G., & Ranson, D.L. (Eds.). (1998). *Craniofacial identification in forensic medicine*. London: Arnold.

Cox, M., & Mays, S. (Eds.). (2000). *Human osteology in archaeology and forensic science*. London: GMM.

Good universities guides. (2007). Retrieved May 1, 2007, from http://www.thegoodguides.com.au/site

Haglund, W.D, & Sorg, M.H. (Eds.). (1997). *Forensic taphonomy: The post-mortem fate of human remains*. Boca Raton: CRC Press.

Haglund, W.D., & Sorg, M.H. (Eds.). (2002). *Advances in forensic taphonomy: Method, theory, and archaeological perspectives*. Boca Raton: CRC Press.

Massler, M., Schour, I., & Poncher, H. (1941). Developmental pattern of the child as reflected in the calcification pattern of the teeth. *American Journal of Diseases of Children, 62*, 33–67.

Oxenham, M.F. (2006). Biological responses to change in prehistoric Vietnam. *Asian Perspectives, 45*, 212–239.

Oxenham, M.F., Walters I., Nguyen L.C., & Nguyen, K.T. (2001). Case studies in ancient trauma: Mid-holocene through metal periods in northern Vietnam. In M. Henneberg & J. Kilgariff (Eds.), *The causes and effects of biological variation* (pp. 83–102). Australasian Society for Human Biology: University of Adelaide.

Oxenham, M.F., Locher, C., Nguyen, L.C., & Nguyen, K.T. (2002). Identification of *Areca catechu* (betel nut) residues on the dentitions of Bronze Age inhabitants of Nui Nap, northern Vietnam. *The Journal of Archaeological Science, 29*, 909–915.

Oxenham, M.F., Nguyen, K.T., & Nguyen, L.C. (2005). Skeletal evidence for the emergence of infectious disease in bronze and iron age northern Vietnam. *American Journal of Physical Anthropology, 126*, 359–376.

Oxenham, M.F., Matsumura, H., & Nishimoto, T. (2006). Diffuse idiopathic skeletal hyperostosis in late Jomon Hokkaido, Japan. *International Journal of Osteoarchaeology, 16*, 34–46.

Oxenham, M.F., Nguyen, L.C., & Nguyen, K.T. (2006). The oral health consequences of the adoption and intensification of agriculture in Southeast Asia. In M. Oxenham & N. Tayles (Eds.), *Bioarchaeology of Southeast Asia* (pp. 263–289). Cambridge: Cambridge University Press.

Oxenham, M.F., & Whitworth, J. (2006). Frequency, location, morphology and aetiology of osseous mandibular condylar concavities. *International Journal of Osteoarchaeology, 16*, 517–527.

Oxenham, M.F., Matsumura, H., Domett, K., Nguyen, K.T., Nguyen, L.C., Nguyen, et al. (in press). Childhood in late Neolithic Vietnam: Bio-mortuary insights into an ambiguous life stage. In K Bacvarov (Ed.), *Babies reborn: Infant/child burials in pre- and protohistory* (B.A.R. International Series). Oxford: Archaeopress.

Oxenham, M.F., & Matsumura, H. (2008). Oral and physiological health in cold adapted peoples: Northeast Asia, Hokkaido. *American Journal of Physical Anthropology, 135*, 64–74.

Tayles, N, & Oxenham, M.F. (2006). Southeast Asian bioarchaeology: Past and present. In M. Oxenham & N. Tayles (Eds.), *Bioarchaeology of southeast Asia* (pp. 1–30). Cambridge: Cambridge University Press.

Toobin, J. (2007, May 7). The CSI effect: The truth about forensic science. *The New Yorker*.

Ubelaker, D.H. (1999). *Human skeletal remains: Excavation, analysis, interpretation*. Washington: Taraxacum.

UN Office of the Envoy for Tsunami Recovery (n.d.). Retrieved May 1, 2007, from http://www. tsunamispecialenvoy.org/country/humantoll.asp

Zupanic-Slavic, Z. (2004). *New method of identifying family related skulls: Forensic medicine, anthropology, epigenetics.* New York: Springer Wien.

Forensic Archaeology

2

Forensic Archaeology: Approaches to International Investigations

Ian Hanson

Forensic archaeology has been extensively defined and considered as a specific emerging discipline (e.g., Connor & Scott, 2001; Hunter & Cox, 2005; Hunter, Roberts, & Martin, 1996). Some of its applications internationally have been specifically described, namely the excavation of mass graves (Hanson, 2004; Haglund & Sorg, 2002; Haglund, Connor, & Scott, 2001; Wright, Hanson, & Sterenberg, 2005), alongside a wider nonspecific literature describing human rights investigations (e.g., Akhavan, 1996; Freund, 1979; Stover, 1995; Stover & Peress, 1998). International investigations include genocide, war crimes, crimes against humanity, mass disaster victim recovery, and repatriation of war dead. This chapter seeks to set the current and future potential for forensic archaeology in the context of international investigations.

Development of Forensic Archaeology in International Investigations

In the last 10 years archaeologists have grown to become one of the key coordinators for the investigation of mass death scenes, and forensic archaeology has made great advances in firmly rooting itself as a successful and separate forensic science. The precursors to this evolution can be traced back to several taproots feeding the new discipline. These have been the application and development of the scientific application of archaeological principles and methods, physical anthropology, archaeological management, crime scene investigation principles, and human rights investigation.

With the development of international laws in the 19th to 20th centuries, the rise of bodies to proscribe, administer and adjudicate these laws, increasing public appreciation of the law, monitoring of its implementation by NGOs and international organisations, and changes in perspective on humanitarian intervention and state sovereignty, there have developed vehicles and an international will to investigate abuses of international and national law. It should perhaps be remembered that the first attempt at international tribunals to investigate war crimes were by the Allies against Germans and Turks after the treaties of Sèvres and Versailles at the end of World War I; this was not achieved, and the world waited until Nuremberg, and the trials in the Pacific[1] for tribunals to try cases of war crimes (Bass, 2000; Sob, 1998).

The development of systematic approaches to excavation progressed at the end of the 19th century and into the 20th century in North America and Europe, allowing methodologies for finding, recovering and analysing the buried dead to evolve. The connection between forensic investigation and the benefits of an archaeological approach to mass grave investigation were first noted by Sir Sydney Smith, the New Zealand pathologist, who saw 'something of the worries of an archaeologist' when excavating a mass grave under the floor of a house in Egypt in 1924 (Smith, 1959: 71–73). World War II saw the first investigations of war crimes by pathologist led teams. Surprisingly, it was the Nazi investigation in 1943 of Soviet murders of thousands of Polish officers in 1940 at Katyn, Ukraine that introduced the use of international scientific teams to war crimes investigations. Though an exercise in antisoviet propaganda (as was the subsequent soviet investigation of the massacres that blamed, unsurprisingly, the Nazis) it demonstrated through mass grave excavation, autopsy and analysis of bullets and shell cases that the soviets had carried out mass killings three years earlier (Margry, 1996). Work by the British pathologist Keith Mant investigating Nazi war crimes in 1945–1948 involved developing systematic excavation methods to recover the clandestine burials of UK servicemen murdered in Germany (Mant, 1950). He also introduced ideas about site formation processes, decay, taphonomy and autopsy of decomposed remains to war crimes investigations (Mant, 1987). The work of Emeritus Professor of Anthropology at Sydney University, Richard Wright, and the Australian War Crimes Prosecutions team, applied archaeological excavation and crime scene investigation principles during excavations of WWII mass graves in Ukraine in 1990–1991 (Wright, 1995).

Following ideas for using human remains for human identification with foundations in 19th century America (Davis, 1992), the use of techniques of physical anthropology to recover and identify the dead developed in the Korean War. Developing from this, the work of Clyde Snow and others in applying physical anthropology techniques to forensic work (e.g., see Snow, 1970) led to the setting up of teams to investigate human rights abuses in Argentina from 1984 and then Guatemala from 1991. Members of these teams subsequently took part in investigations in the Balkans and elsewhere. In the last 20 years physical anthropological research that can assist in identifications has spread widely (Iscan, 1988, 2001).

During the 1990s the development of teams to investigate human rights abuses continued with Physicians for Human Rights (PHR) undertaking excavations in Rwanda and Former Yugoslavia for the new War Crimes Tribunals (Simmons & Haglund, 2005). At this time a consensus developed globally that scientific teams could undertake such work. In the 1990s teams developed to work on human rights cases in most South and Central American countries, as well as for the United Nations Tribunal's work in the Balkans, and investigations were undertaken in many countries including Africa and Asia. This coincided with a change in perception in the realms of media, science, law and criminal investigation of the value of the physical remnants of atrocities as evidence. The term 'mass grave' took on a new meaning in the public consciousness as the physical manifestation of crimes and deaths, interest sometimes stretching back generations. The International Tribunal for the Former Yugoslavia (ICTY) teamworked from 1996 to 2001 in Bosnia and Croatia. Here, archaeologists and anthropologists from human rights, academic and professional archaeological backgrounds around the world combined their skills with other scientists and scene of crime investigators to develop procedures for locating, excavating and managing mass graves. The importance of managing evidential integrity and maintaining chain of custody (which can be defined as the systematic physical documentation demonstrating the seizure, custody, control, transfer, analysis, storage, alterations to, and disposition of, physical and other evidence) were emphasised, as was the systematic autopsy of victims in mortuaries set up for this purpose. The development by the International Committee of the Red Cross (ICRC), PHR and International Commission for Missing Persons (IC-MP) of mechanisms to identify victims with mass ante-mortem data gathering operations and DNA testing, showed the way forward in a complete approach to investigating atrocity crimes internationally.

Excavation of mass graves and memorialisation of the dead have also been undertaken frequently in the past by noninternational scientific or law enforcement agencies. These may be national medical teams, volunteers, international aid or human rights agencies. In Cambodia and Rwanda, the remains of the dead have been preserved in memorials to genocide. The Nanjing Memorial Museum, China encloses mass graves from the 1937 massacre. Communities have excavated graves in search of their relatives (e.g., Iraq 2003) especially when there no international assistance is available. Graves accidentally discovered by construction have been excavated in Sri Lanka and Cyprus.

Investigations into atrocities have continued in the 21st century, with UN Tribunals and Special Courts set up for Sierra Leone, East Timor and Cambodia. Forensic archaeological input has continued in human rights investigations for local, national and international organisations worldwide, including South and Central America, the Balkans, East Timor, Spain, Cambodia, Afghanistan, Iraq, Kuwait, Cyprus and DR Congo (see Anson and Trimble, Chapter 5, for a discussion of investigation mass graves and the role of the biological anthropologist). Archaeologists continue to assist and advise in the repatriation of war dead from the United States, the United Kingdom and Australia.[2] Archaeologists have increasingly found a complementary role for their forensic skills internationally in search, location and recovery in mass disasters, including 9/11 and the Asian tsunami, undertaking searches, excavating graves and debris, and sieving material for fragmentary remains.

How Can Forensic Archaeology Benefit International Investigations?

There are several key roles for forensic archaeology in international investigations, including the search, location, confirmation, and survey of death scenes, such as mass graves, surface scatters and execution sites; the excavation, recording, and recovery of evidence and remains; assisting in the control and protection of evidence in chain of custody; and the analysis of evidence.

These roles provide data for such investigative priorities as: demonstrating or refuting that a crime has occurred; identification of the dead; identification of ethnic, religious or cultural groups; determining of cause of death; where the dead are from; whether the dead have been moved after death; reconstruction of the crime scene;

the perpetrators actions and evidence of perpetrator identity. These factors enable successful criminal prosecution and identification of victims to take place.

Historically, many international investigations have taken place from a humanitarian standpoint, the emphasis being on repatriation of the missing. It should now be remembered, however, evidence initially thought to be only of interest for humanitarian identification may, in the future, be of interest to a criminal investigation — conflicts end, priorities of judiciaries change, as do regimes and governments (e.g., Guatemala or South Africa in the 1990s). The requirements for evidence may not be known at the time of recovery and analysis, and because of this, maximum evidence recovery, high standards of evidential integrity and the ability to store and control evidence in secure facilities are required to mitigate for this change in evidential need. Maximum evidence recovery also aids in identifying victims — more evidence will provide more chance of identification — for example, careful crime scene reconstruction will provide strong evidence to corroborate witness statements of events concerning where victims were last seen.

There are several outcomes from the collection and analysis of evidence and the recovery of remains that have been described (Haglund, 2002; Juhl, 2004): prosecution of perpetrators, identification of the dead, repatriation of remains and closure for families, upholding human rights, deterrence of further atrocities. Moreover, prevention of historical revisionism must be discussed.

The physical artefacts recovered from atrocities, mass graves and other crime scenes provide the material evidence of past events. The ongoing debate of whether the Armenian massacres in World War I were genocide (Dadrian, 1997; McCarthy, 1996), and revisionist arguments about the holocaust are in part fuelled by the lack of physical evidence, in the form of documents or remains. Recent release by the German government of documents listing the executed and their numbers from concentration camps provide the evidence to refute revisionist histories of the holocaust (Hawley, 2006). The massacres at Srebrenica in Bosnia 1995 and the numbers involved were debated variously as propaganda, estimate, and fact until the tally of bodies excavated, and admissions by perpetrators in the courts at ICTY, began to provide the factual evidence. Physical evidence helps to dispel conjecture and conspiracy about events and provides a historical record as well as evidence for identification and criminal prosecution. In this sense the role and responsibility of investigators and scientists in these cases is greater than that on domestic murder investigations.

Archaeologists use systematic excavation processes to help achieve these outcomes through maximum evidence recovery from atrocity crime scenes allowing for criminal prosecution and humanitarian identification.

The Application of Archaeological Methodology and Techniques

Morse, Crusoe and Smith first described forensic archaeology as a concept in 1976; the archaeological techniques that could be used in assisting law enforcement agencies in domestic settings have been further described in the last 30 years (Bass, 1978; Hunter, Roberts, & Martin, 1996; Spennemann & Franke, 1994). This progress has been possible because archaeologists have transferred the scientific organisation of research and rescue archaeology (that of a multidisciplinary and systematic approach to field investigation) to a forensic setting.

Archaeological techniques of survey, excavation, evidence recognition, recovery, conservation, and analysis have been shown to add new approaches to specific types of crime and disaster scene analysis. Internationally, the archaeological investigation of mass graves has been developed and discussed (Duric & Tuller, 2006; Haglund, 2002; Haglund et al., 2001; Hanson, 2004; Skinner, 1987; Wright et al., 2005). The main consideration for archaeological approaches to such investigations is the recognition of a process that can be systematically applied to all sites. In comparison with domestic murder cases, the scale and complexity of such sites, and therefore the complexity of management and organisation of the teams, has led to protocols to normalise field investigations. Published procedures for this work have been lacking, with teams having to rely on the Minnesota protocols (UN, 1995), which were published to provide a framework for investigating human rights abuses but are limited in terms of archaeological methodology. Detailed protocols discussing procedures and methods are now being published (Cox, Flavel, Hanson, Laver, & Wessling, 2007). The process can be broken down into several stages.

Mission Planning

This includes the costing, organisation, management, and preparation for site investigations. Without proper organisation of a team's activities and planning for field investigations, time, money, resources, and personnel will be wasted. Archaeologists can determine a great deal of information about a site and its history from desktop studies. The political pressures of international investigations require efficiency and successful results from fieldwork as a return on the investment made to retrieve physical evidence and remains.[3]

Search and Location

The key principle to successfully search for and locate sites is to pinpoint anomalies to examine. Many investigations have wasted time and money searching wide areas because basic methods of searching were not followed. Site location requires using techniques to pinpoint specific areas on the ground within a wider area of interest, using physical examination, observation and remote sensing of anomalies to 'zoom in' on specific points of interest. For example, graves from the Srebrenica massacre were located by soil disturbance observed on archived aerial imagery; reconnaissance visits to the locations then pinpointed the sites on the ground by observing vegetation change and soil disturbance.

Confirmation

Once anomalies have been pinpointed they need to be tested to confirm they are relevant to an investigation. Surface scatters of remains or artefacts are more straightforward to examine. Mass graves need to be proved by testing to confirm presence of multiple human remains. The main methods of doing this are probing, trenching and surface stripping, which are discussed in some detail in Wright et al. (2005).

Recovery

This refers to the identification, definition, recording, and retrieval of evidence and remains from an identified surface or burial site. Evaluations for the presence of ordnance, and other health and safety concerns, may be needed in investigations in war zones. Many gravesites are also sites of execution or disturbance subsequent to burial and there may be shell cases, clothing or remains on the ground surface. Recovery should be controlled in a systematic way within a defined three-dimensional space. Stratigraphic excavation (for definitions see Hanson, 2004; Harris, 1979; Harris, Brown, & Brown, 1993) provides a universal framework for archaeologists to understand, justify, describe and record site formation processes, the archaeological sequence of events, and to maximise evidence recovery. For each archaeological context, or piece of evidence, a sequence of procedures can ensure suitable standards of recovery, recording, and interpretation, including: the cleaning, photography, logging, recording, excavation, sampling, recovery, packaging, and secure storage in a systematic chain of custody. Evidence to be considered should include all surface finds, the structure of graves (sides and bases), artifacts, and human remains.

Identification, Analysis, Preservation and Conservation

These aspects of buried evidence are areas in which archaeologists have great experience. There is no point excavating graves and recovering evidence and human remains if the wide range of environmental, trace, physical, archaeological, and forensic evidence is not recognised and preserved for use in courts and for identification.

The main skills that archaeologists employ in these phases of investigation are:

- the recognition of disturbed soil
- soil removal and safety issues of soil stability
- familiarity with the usefulness and pitfalls of heavy earth-moving machinery
- finding and recovering objects in soil (often quite tiny and fragile objects that need conservation)
- recording the location of objects in 2D and 3D, and representing them in plans and computerised images
- recognising when to use other experts, such as soil scientists and dating expertise
- managing large teams of people, with disparate experience and disparate egos, and managing them under stress (Wright et al., 2005).

These archaeological techniques are important contributors for successful identification of the dead, crime scene reconstruction, and criminal evidence determination in international investigations and presentation of such evidence in reports and courts.

Forensic Archaeology and Crime Scene Investigation

There is a natural symmetry between investigation of archaeological features and crime scene investigation that has been recognised and developed in international investigations in the Balkans and Iraq, with archaeologists adapting their discipline to the stringent legal requirements of crime scene and chain of custody protocols. Archaeologists and crime scene investigators have the following in common:

- search and location techniques
- use evidence to build interpretation of events
- the ability to reconstruct past time lines
- use logical deduction based on observation

- reconstruct a sequence of events
- use teamwork, and understand the importance of different specialists in a team
- the ability to recognise evidence
- the ability to perform recovery and control of evidence
- record events and evidence in detail
- spatial awareness
- structured survey, planning, reporting, and presentation of interpreted findings.

In the same way that archaeologists on forensic cases need to adapt to the discipline of evidence custody and control, crime scene investigators need to understand the structure and context of buried evidence. The most straightforward way to depict this is to imagine a grave as a subterranean room. As with any room where a crime takes place, evidence is left on the floor and walls, and routes leading to and from the scene. Bodies in a grave lie on surfaces and seal trace evidence beneath. The backfilled soil of the grave can be seen as a 'roof', sealing and protecting the buried remains and evidence. The long-term survival of evidence varies from environment to environment: after five years of burial in clays of Bosnia, bodies still retained soft tissue as well as documents and photographs aiding identification. Arid sites in Iraq retain the same documents after twenty years, but soft tissue can disappear in months. Treating the grave as a room that can be entered and searched allows appropriate understanding of methods to be used that do not destroy the room structure that would cause loss of trace and other evidence, as well as loss of context. A crime scene within a house would not approached by pulling down the walls and roof of the house to get to the body and the evidence, neither should a grave unless necessary.

Archaeologists and crime scene investigators are both detectives (traditionally separated in their focus of interest by time since events took place) and identifiers of physical evidence and its context. Archaeologists working in international investigations have used their knowledge of the structure of soil strata and anthropogenic deposits and features to increase the appreciation by crime scene investigators of the potential of archaeology as a forensic tool, and this has also filtered through to domestic murder investigations.

Forensic Archaeology as Forensic Science

Forensic archaeology is now organising itself under a series of laws and principles that can be applied to demonstrate it satisfies the requirements for forensic science in courts and legal systems of the United Kingdom and United States. Science as evidence in forensic cases must use methods that can be tested for accuracy and error rate, and have been discussed, accepted and peer reviewed in the scientific community, and is valid for an enquiry (Keily, 2001).[4] Barker (1987) has described excavation as an unrepeatable experiment, in that excavation destroys that which it analyses. It shares this trait with crime scene investigation — evidence once removed can never be replaced (Gerberth, 1996) — and as such there is great responsibility for the excavator and CSI to deliver accurate retrieval of evidence and documented interpretation.

Archaeology as a discipline has always been described in mixed terms of art and science, and archaeologists and archaeological bodies have always been vague about the exact requirements in standards of fieldwork. Such vagueness is not acceptable for forensic work, and archaeologists are now debating which methods destroy evidence or maximise its recovery and thus have a suitable forensic application as part of a methodological toolkit. Archaeology has always drawn on techniques, methodologies and scientific approaches of other disciplines to improve all aspects of its investigations. This principle is equally applied in its forensic approaches to provide flexibility, and a range of methodologies have now been consolidated as suitable for death investigation, recognising: (a) that anything at a scene may be of evidential value until proved otherwise, (b) excavation is destruction (techniques should maximise evidence recognition and recovery, and techniques that cannot determine rates of evidential loss should not be used), (c) the laws of stratigraphy define rules governing the sequencing of deposits to assist in identifying the sequence of events, and (d) stratigraphic excavation and recording provides evidence and context in three dimensions, and can be presented in a standard form using the Harris Matrix to provide a verifiable record.

Other principles can provide a focus to maximise consideration for evidence distribution and identification. The principle of the forensic landscape describes the fact that perpetrators and victims of crimes will move between crime scenes across the landscape creating a linked system of evidential sites of interest to an investigation. For example during the Srebrenica massacres, victims were captured in ambush sites, were held by roads until transported in requisitioned vehicles, moved to holding buildings such as warehouses and gyms, moved to execution sites, buried, dug up two months later and reburied in different locations, moved by excavator and truck. This left evidence that can be recovered, and links that can be identified and analysed between sites, vehicles, victims, weapons and perpetrators. Realising that a crime scene is not an isolated scene can allow approaches to identifying evidence to reconstruct events to be developed; this has led to several successful prosecutions at ICTY concerning Srebrenica.

Multidisciplinary International Investigations

A variety of experts are often required in a team to provide the highest standard of evidence location and recovery at large forensic excavations. This is due to the size of the operation and the variety of evidence types and the sampling and analysis required. It is also due to the complete approach to investigation advocated that requires evidence recovery and analysis, prosecution, identification of the dead and repatriation. For example, among experts used in one investigation for ICTY were anthropologists, aerial imagery analysts, archaeologists, pathologists, investigators, geophysicists, crime scene examiners, logisticians, radiographers, palynologists, engineers, ordnance disposal officers, surveyors, mortuary technicians, soil scientists, ante-mortem data collectors, photographers, data entry specialists, crime scene managers, mechanics, machine operators and drivers, ballistics experts, DNA analysts, lawyers, communication analysts, document analysts, administration support, and project managers.

The role of the archaeologist has become central to the analysis of mass grave crime scenes. Working with crime scene managers, they can assist in:

- location, assessment and confirmation of ground anomalies
- management of archaeological scenes
- dealing with the complexity of intermingled and entwined human remains

- proper evidence identification, recording, collection, processing, analysis, conservation, packaging, storage and transport of evidence and remains
- specialist equipment procurement, use and maintenance
- liaison with communities/families/authorities
- production of descriptive reports, plans, and images for agencies and courts.

It is an oxymoron that archaeologists combine an exact expertise in archaeological methods with a general understanding in other areas, recognising the indispensable roles of other experts in providing investigative competence. For example, anthropologists in resolving skeletal commingling and identifying trauma, crime scene managers in controlling chain of custody, or soil scientists in suitable sampling and analysis. Archaeologists by profession should be used to recognise the limitations of their own expertise while understanding when to use and cooperate with other experts.

Considerations for international investigations include:

Scale. These can be very large sites, with hundreds of bodies, and may need a lot of time, resources, and money to excavate to standard where evidence can be used by a court.

Management. They require expert management of personnel, time, costs, and resources.

Logistics. The requirements to provide equipment, transport, and shelter to maintain the team, and to package and store evidence and the dead need to be considered.

Site integrity/security. Scenes and personnel may need protection in volatile environments of politically unstable regions and war zones.

Chain of custody. Crime scene examiners may need to deal with hundreds of pieces of evidence to the same standards.

What links these considerations are cost, time and resources — they are interdependent. Investigations are often undertaken with limited resources of one sort or another, or without consideration for the above. This introduces the risk that the ability to locate, recover, preserve, and analyse evidence, and identify the missing may be compromised or made more difficult in the long term. Criminal investigations such as those undertaken by the International Tribunals are always more time consuming and expensive, as the full processes of legal proceedings are undertaken. The gravity of cases against dictators charged with genocide and other international crimes, and the historical and cultural importance of uncovering and recording these events seems to demand a global investment. Many investigations, however, lack adequate resources to be able to guarantee fulfilment of the optimal outcomes of the investigation as described in the section addressing the benefits of forensic archaeology in international investigations.

Conclusion and the Future

What archaeologists and anthropologists have helped to develop in the last twenty years is a series of practical approaches to deal with the physical evidence of atrocity crimes, and to find and identify the missing. As many of the scenes involved are mass graves and execution sites it has logically become the remit of archaeologists to search for, locate, excavate, recover, record, and analyse scattered and buried remains and evidence.

It has also become clear that because of the complexity of these cases, the only way to recover the maximum amount of evidence and ensure proper recovery of human remains from mass graves is to use a multidisciplinary approach. This provides the answers for investigators, courts, families, communities, the media and the public, to questions that are asked concerning these crimes: to determine who has been killed, how they were killed, by whom they were killed, when they were killed, where they were killed, and why they were killed.

Examples of genocide (such as Bosnia and Rwanda), human rights violations (such as in Iraq and Kosovo) and mass disaster (like the Asian tsunami) act to demonstrate how the multidisciplinary approach to archaeological investigations (applying tried and tested principles of the scientific analysis, techniques and methodologies, site assessment, logistics, and management) have brought forensic archaeology to a recognised position as one of the prime tools for international death scene analysis. It has combined with other areas of expertise to build a process that leads from the scene to repatriation of the dead and conviction of perpetrators.

New types of evidence that can be recovered from and link scenes (such as pollen used in Bosnia to determine the movement of remains and soil) are being recognised. The development of methods of retrieval of buried evidence demonstrates that tool marks and trace evidence can survive in buried environments and can be recovered. The ever increasing range of evidence that can be recovered requires specialists and needs detailed processes and management principles to control sites. This costs in both money and resources and takes time; few organisations can afford to do this. Will the international community be willing to pay for such complex investigations, or will they be undertaken with what resources are available and perhaps partially answer the questions asked above, and only partly satisfy the intended outcomes of investigation such as prevention and revisionism? It is difficult to argue that criminal accountability and the need to establish an effective International Criminal Court (ICC) to deter future war criminals should take precedence over the immediate suffering of, for example, northern Ugandans benefiting from a ceasefire in their civil war because of a prosecution amnesty. On the other hand, it is inconceivable that those directly responsible for these unspeakable crimes should escape being held accountable. The answer is probably that some investigations will be supported if there is an international political will and others will be ignored if there is not. This is a pattern seen in the past that may extend to the future.

Endnotes

1 Australian military courts conducted 296 trials for war crimes between 1945 and 1951 under the War Crimes Act 1945. Trials were conducted in eight venues — Labuan, Wewak, Morotai, Rabaul, Darwin, Singapore, Hong Kong, and Manus Island (National Archives of Australia, 2003).

2 United States Government policy is to repatriate all war dead, and the team at JPAC CIL excavate plane crashes and other sites, recovering remains each year. Excavations on Saipan have recovered and repatriated Japanese war dead (Russell, 2001).

3   The ICTY forensic field team and temporary mortuary 1997–2001 cost some $2,000,000 to $3,000,000 a year to run to locate, excavate and undertake postmortems on victims of the wars in Bosnia and Croatia.

4   The cases in United States law centred on the US Supreme Court hearing of *Daubert v. Merrell Dow Pharmaceuticals* is most often cited in defining these requirements.

References

Akhavan, P. (1996). The international criminal tribunal for Rwanda: The politics and pragmatics of punishment. *American Journal of International Law, 90*, 501–510.

Barker, P. (1987). *Techniques of archaeological excavation*. London: Batsford.

Bass, G.J. (2000). *Stay the hand of vengeance: The politics of war crimes tribunals*. Princeton, NJ: Princeton University Press.

Bass, W. (1978). Exhumation: The method could make the difference. *FBI Law Enforcement Bulletin, 47*, 6–11.

Connor, M., & Scott, D.D. (2001). Paradigms and perpetrators. *Journal of Historical Archaeology, 35*, 1–6.

Cox, M., Flavel, A., Hanson, I., Laver, J., & Wessling, R. (Eds.). (2007). *The scientific excavation and analysis of mass graves*. Cambridge: Cambridge University Press.

Davis, J. (1992). Forensic archaeology. *Archaeological Reviews from Cambridge, 11*, 152–156.

Duric, M., & Tuller, H. (2006). Keeping the pieces together: comparison of mass grave excavation methodology. *Forensic Science International, 27*, 192–200.

Freund, M.L. (1979, May). The law and human rights in Argentina. *Worldview*, pp. 37–41.

Gerberth, V. (1996). *Practical homicide investigation*. Baton Raton, FL: CRC Press.

Haglund, W.D. (2002). Recent mass graves, an introduction. In W.D. Haglund & M.H. Sorg (Eds.), *Advances in forensic taphonomy* (pp. 243–261). Boca Raton, FL: CRC Press.

Haglund, W.D., Connor, M., & Scott, D.D. (2001). The archaeology of contemporary mass graves. *Journal of Historical Archaeology, 35*, 57–69.

Hanson, I. (2004). The importance of stratigraphy in forensic investigation. In K. Pye & D.J. Croft (Eds.), *Forensic geoscience: Principles, techniques and applications* (Vol. 232, pp. 39–47). London: Geological Society, Special Publications.

Harris, E. (1979). *Principles of archaeological stratigraphy*. London: Academic Press.

Harris, E.C., Brown, M.R., & Brown, G.J. (1993). *Practices of archaeological stratigraphy*. London: Academic Press.

Hawley, C. (2006, April 19). Germany agrees to open holocaust archive. *Der Spiegel*. Retrieved January 19, 2007, from http://www.spiegel.de/international/0,1518,411983,00.html

Hunter, J.R., Roberts, C.A., & Martin, A. (1996). *Studies in crime: An introduction to forensic archaeology*. London: Routledge.

Hunter, J.R., & Cox, M. (2005). *Forensic archaeology: Advances in theory and practice*. London: Routledge.

Iscan, M.Y. (1988). Rise of forensic anthropology. *American Journal of Physical Anthropology, 31*, 203–229.

Iscan, M.Y. (2001). Global forensic anthropology in the 21st century. *Forensic Science International, 117*, 1–6.

Juhl, K. (2004). *The contribution by (forensic) archaeologists to human rights investigations of mass graves*. *AmS-Nett* 5, Stavanger: Museum of Archaeology.

Keily, T.F. (2001). *Forensic evidence: Science and the criminal law*. Boca Raton, FL: CRC Press.

Mant, A.K. (1950). *A study in exhumation data*. Unpublished doctoral dissertation, University of London, London.

Mant, A.K. (1987). Knowledge acquired from post war exhumations. In A. Boddington, A.N. Garland & R.C. Janaway (Eds.), *Death, decay and reconstruction: Approaches to archaeology and forensic science* (pp. 65–80). Manchester: Manchester University Press.

Margry, K. (1996). The massacre at Katyn. *After the Battle, 92*, 1–33.

Morse, D., Crusoe, D., & Smith, H.G. (1976). Forensic archaeology. *Journal of Forensic Science, 21,* 323–332.

National Archives of Australia. (2003). *Factsheet 61.* Retrieved August 20, 2006, from http://www.naa.gov.au/fsheets/FS61.html

Russell, S. (2001). Dealing with human remains, an approach from the northern Marianas. *Cultural Resource Management, 24,* 23–24.

Simmons, T., & Haglund, W.D. (2005). Anthropology in a forensic context. In J.R. Hunter & M. Cox (Eds.), *Forensic archaeology: Advances in theory and practice.* London: Routledge.

Skinner, M. (1987). Planning the archaeological recovery of evidence from recent mass graves. *Forensic Science International 34,* 267–287.

Smith, Sir S. (1959). *Mostly murder: An autobiography.* London: Harrap.

Snow, C., Gatliff, B.P., & McWilliams, K.R. (1970). Reconstruction of facial features from the skull: An evaluation of its usefulness in forensic anthropology. *American Journal of Physical Anthropology, 33,* 221–228.

Sob, P. (1998). The dynamics of international criminal tribunals. *Nordic Journal of International Law, 67,* 139–163.

Spennemann, D.H., & Franke, B. (1995). *Archaeological techniques for exhumations: A unique data source for crime scene investigations. Forensic Science International, 74,* 5–15.

Stover, E. (1995). In the shadow of Nuremberg: Pursuing war criminals in the former Yugoslavia and Rwanda. *Medicine and Global Survival 2&3,* 140–147.

Stover, E., & Peress, G. (1998). *The grave: Srebrenica and Vukovar.* New York: Scala.

United Nations. (1995). *Guidelines for the conduct of United Nations inquiries into allegations of massacres.* New York: UN Office of Legal Affairs.

Wright, R. (1995). Investigating war crimes: The archaeological evidence. *The Sydney Papers, 7,* 39–44.

Wright, R., Hanson, I., & Sterenberg, J. (2005). The archaeology of mass graves. In J.R. Hunter & M. Cox (Eds). *Forensic archaeology: Advances in theory and practice* (pp. 137–158). London: Routledge.

3

CHAPTER

The Basics of Forensic Taphonomy: Understanding Cadaver Decomposition in Terrestrial Gravesites

Mark Tibbett

Clandestine graves are a common way to dispose of human (or animal) remains. Burials provide an easy disposal route for cadavers and perpetrators of crimes rely on the decomposition of corpses to hinder identification and obfuscate estimates of time since death or burial.

The burial environment is a complex and dynamic system of interdependent chemical, physical and biological processes. These processes influence, and are influenced by, the inclusion of a body and its subsequent decay. Experimental studies of the decomposition of human cadavers under controlled conditions have rarely been carried out (Mann, Bass, & Meadows, 1990). Field studies, occasionally using human bodies, (Mant, 1950, 1953; Rodriguez & Bass, 1983, 1985) but more commonly animal surrogates, have been undertaken (Mann et al., 1990; Micozzi, 1985; Payne & King, 1968; Turner & Wiltshire, 1999). However, knowledge of the decomposition processes and the influence of the burial environment from such studies are limited.

Mant (1950, 1953) studied 150 exhumations in Germany, and described the decay processes that take place under a number of burial conditions. Although Mant (1987) concluded that there was little difference in taphonomic change between burial environments, the observations were qualitative rather than quantitative. No thorough investigation of the burial environment or decayed tissue was undertaken. Rodriguez and Bass (1983, 1985) examined the decomposition of adult human cadavers but did not take into account different soil types that may be more important than previously thought (Carter, Yellowlees, & Tibbett, 2007).

The terrestrial environment has been much studied as a decomposition environment for materials of little forensic value such as leaf litter or dead roots (Cadisch & Giller, 1999); and only in recent years have studies been conducted with mammalian tissues and cadavers from both ecological and forensic standpoints (see Carter et al., 2007).

The primary goals of forensic taphonomy are to estimate postmortem interval, and postburial interval as well as assist in the determination of the cause and manner of death (Haglund & Sorg, 1997; Vass, Barshick, Sega, Caton, Skeen et al., 2002). In addition, taphonomic processes have been used to aid in the search and location of clandestine graves (e.g., Hunter, 1994). These goals are reached through the study of the internal (autolysis, putrefaction) and external (decay) processes of cadaver decomposition and the factors that influence them, such as temperature and moisture.

In order to undertake a study in forensic taphonomy it is necessary to understand the fundamental decomposition processes associated with a cadaver: autolysis, putrefaction and decay.

Postmortem Decomposition

Following the cessation of the heart, oxygen is no longer distributed to cells and their metabolic byproducts (including CO_2) are no longer removed (see also Forbes, Chapter 15, for a discussion of the chemistry of decomposition and preservation). This starts to kill the cells of the body almost immediately. The rate of cell death varies across tissue types: for example, the brain dies within minutes whereas skin cells can be cultured two days after death. After the termination of aerobic metabolism and the destruction of cells by enzymatic digestion (i.e., autolysis) starts to occur (Dent, Forbes, & Stuart, 2004). Autolysis can begin within minutes after death (Vass et al., 2002) and can be significantly affected by temperature and moisture (Gill-King, 1997). At this time, optimal conditions are created for anaerobic microorganisms originating from the gastrointestinal tract and respiratory system. These organisms multiply within the cadaver, transforming carbohydrates, lipids and proteins into acids and gases that result in colour change, odour and bloating of the cadaver. This process is known as putrefaction. Autolysis and putrefaction will dominate cadaver decomposition until the skin loses integrity, which results in the reintroduction of oxygen to the system. This reestablishes aerobic metabolism and designates the beginning of the decay process (Micozzi, 1986). Decay typically represents the period of most rapid breakdown due to the loss of cadaveric moisture and the activity of decomposer organisms such as arthropods, vertebrate scavengers and the soil microbiota (e.g., bacteria, fungi, and microarthropods).

The decomposition process initially occurs independently of microbial action and microbes play a greater role in the later stages of breakdown. The degradation of tissue types normally proceeds in the following order: (a) intestines, stomach, organs of digestion, heart, blood; (b) air passages and lungs; (c) kidneys and bladder; (d) brain and nervous tissue; (e) skeletal muscles; (f) connective tissues, hair and integument (Gill-King, 1997).

Identifiable Stages of Cadaver Decomposition

Immediately after death the body goes through changes that offer evidence to allow postmortem estimates to be made. These changes include *algor mortis*, *livor mortis* and *rigor mortis* that occur in the first few hours following death. *Algor mortis* (Latin: *algor*, meaning 'coolness'; and *mortis*, meaning 'death') is the reduction in body temperature following death as it equilibrates with ambient temperature. The rate of cooling can be used to estimate postmortem interval but this may be ineffective in hot climates. Postmortem lividity or *livor mortis* occurs soon after the cessation of the heart as a result of the settling of blood in capillaries due to gravitational pooling (Geberth, 1996). This causes a purple-red discolouration of the skin that begins between 20 minutes to 10 hours after death. Maximum lividity occurs within 6 to 12 hours and is concomitant with a loss of usual skin colour from the upper surfaces of the body. Rigor mortis, perhaps the most well known postmortem change, occurs as a result of a chemical process that causes the muscles and joints to become immobile and rigid. This can affect the entire body in 24 hours and has usually passed with 48 hours. Further details of these processes can be found in Forbes (2007a, 2007b).

After these preliminary changes, cadaver decomposition can be divided into five (or more) stages from a fresh corpse to a clean skeleton. The stages that follow are based on those suggested by Payne and King (1968) but are by no means definitive and represent identifiable stages with characteristics distinct from other stages. These stages exist on a continuum of decomposition that follow a sigmoidal pattern of decay (Carter et al., 2007):

(a) *fresh*: initial discoloration over a period that covers immediate postmortem changes described above

(b) *inflated (or bloated)*: at which time anaerobic gases cause swelling, particularly to the abdomen and scrotum

(c) *deflation* and *decomposition*: once the skin ruptures there are visible signs of faunal activity and blood and body liquors escape, along with a strong odour — this is the most rapid phase of decomposition and soft tissue loss

(d) *disintegration*: the cadaver loses its integrity, bones appear and parts of the cadaver may disconnect

(e) *skeletonisation*: the final stages of soft tissue decay with remaining skin and hair slowly decomposing. This stage may take longer than the others as only the most recalcitrant parts of the cadaver are left (for a more detailed discussion see Carter & Tibbett, 2006).

Considering the Cadaver

The decomposition of any material in the environment is affected by the nature of the material (e.g., Cadisch & Giller, 1997). This holds true for cadavers and gravesites. Specific aspects of human physiology have been shown to have an important bearing on the rate of decomposition. These include the age, height, weight, sex, and fitness level of the individual in life. Integrating these into scientific principles, it seems the surface area of the cadaver (per unit mass) and the amount of fatty tissue may be the underlying controlling factors but clear experimental evidence for this is lacking.

Clothing can have a major effect on the rate of decomposition as this can prevent easy access by external decomposer organisms, particularly invertebrates. The type of material used in clothing, from hats to shoes, can also have a profound effect. Artificial fibres are far more resistant to breakdown in the environment than natural fibres, providing long-term protection of the cadaver (for more detailed discussion see Janaway, 2007). Also important is the integrity of the cadaver. Puncture wounds to the skin or dismemberment can have a profound influence on the progress through the stages above, particularly in the *inflation* stage.

Considering the Burial Site

Soil (into which cadavers are buried or left on its surface) is a complex and heterogeneous environment that offers a range of conditions that can affect decomposition of cadavers. These can vary by the type of soil as described by pedologists (see Fitzpatrick, 2007) and have a range of eclectic physical, chemical and biological characteristics (Dawson, Campbell, Hillier, & Brewer, 2007). Examples of some basic characteristics of the burial environment that might affect the rate of cadaver decomposition include the following: (a) *physical texture*: whether the soil is sandy, silty or clayey can profoundly affect the rate of decomposition by limiting the movement of gasses and water to and from the cadaver; (b) *chemistry*: the pH or how acid or alkaline the soil is may affect decomposition; and (c) *biological activity*: a soil with an active faunal population may have the capacity to decompose soft tissue more quickly.

There is little experimental evidence to support the above statements from the forensic literature but the general principles are known from the decomposition of other materials in the soil science and ecological literature (Brady, 1990; Cadisch & Giller, 1997; Carter & Tibbett, 2006; Carter et al., 2007). There is clearly a need for experimental forensic taphonomy to provide rigorously tested information to practitioners and the courts in order to better understand the effect of burial site on decomposition rate.

One of the few aspects of taphonomy where some experimental work exists concerns the effect of soil pH on soft tissue decomposition. An experimental study was carried out with two types of soil. One soil type, called a Rendzina, was known for its alkaline pH while the other type, called a Podsol, was known for its acidity. The rate of decomposition of skeletal mammalian muscle tissue (1.5 g — cuboid) was measured along with any changes to the soil pH. The methods used followed those described previously (Tibbett, Carter, Haslam, Major, & Haslam, 2004) and organic lamb (*Ovis aries*) was used as an analogue for human tissue.

The results of this study have led to some interesting findings for forensic taphonomy (Figures 3.1 and 3.2). First, it confirmed what had previously been reported: that soil pH increases in the presence of a decomposing cadaver and that this is caused by the soft tissue decomposition; probably due to the release of ammonium (Hopkins et al., 2000). Second, that the basal soil pH has a profound effect on the change caused by soft tissue decomposition. In an already alkaline soil it does not change by much, whereas in an acidic soil, pH can rise by over three units (1000 times more alkaline). Third, the decomposition dynamics were quite different between the two soils. Between 2 and 3 weeks the muscle tissue in the acidic Podsol had decomposed twice as fast as in the alkaline Rendzina. By the end of the experiment (6 weeks), the Podsol had completely decomposed the muscle tissue where there was still a residual amount in the Rendzina soil. From this type of study one might conclude that the type of soil may have a more important role to play in post-mortem interval and postburial interval estimates than previously recognised.

Considering the Burial Environment

There are two main environmental factors that control the rate of cadaver decomposition and these are temperature and moisture (Carter, Yellowlees, & Tibbett,

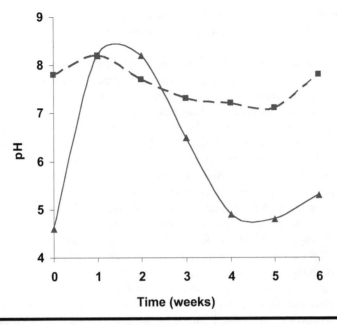

Figure 3.1
The effect of burial of mammalian muscle tissue (*Ovis aries*) on soil pH in an acid soil (triangles and unbroken line; Podsol: pH 4.6) and an alkaline soil (squares with dashed line) (Rendzina: pH 7.8). Note the greatly contrasting starting pH and the relationship of this to the size of temporal changes (Haslam & Tibbett, unpublished data).

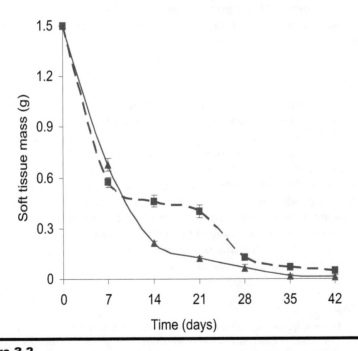

Figure 3.2
The rate of soft tissue mass loss (decomposition) of mammalian muscle tissue (*Ovis aries*) when buried in two soils on contrasting pH. The two soils were an acidic soil (triangles and unbroken line; Podsol: pH 4.6) and an alkaline soil (squares with dashed line; Rendzina: pH 7.8; Haslam & Tibbett, unpublished data).

2007). Both tend to vary seasonally and can have a significant impact on postmortem interval and postburial interval, and time estimates must therefore account for these environmental factors.

The range of the moisture content of soil can extend form fully saturated, where all the pores in the soil are filled with water, to extreme desiccation where only small amounts of moisture remains tightly locked away in soil a few tiny pores. At these extreme ends of the moisture gradient cadaver decomposition is strongly restricted. In soils that are fully saturated or extremely wet such as peat bogs, decomposition is restricted by the degrading pathways being limited to anaerobic metabolism that is far more inefficient than aerobic metabolism. In arid environments, such as tropical or polar deserts, decomposition is restricted through the desiccation and ultimately mummification of the soft tissue (Bereuter, Lorbeer, Reiter, Saidler, & Unterdorfer, 1996; Galloway, 1997; Galloway, Birkby, Jones, Henry, & Parks, 1989). Between these two extremes, little is known about the effect of moisture in the burial environment.

Extremes of temperature can also slow cadaver decomposition. Most obviously, freezing can preserve cadavers for thousands of years, including those of humans and mammoths. Extremely hot conditions can cause either very rapid decomposition if the soil is wet, or very slow decomposition (after desiccation) if the soil is dry. The effect of temperature on decomposition is better understood than moisture, and this has been used to develop methods of estimating postmortem interval from decomposed human remains using accumulated degree-days (the sum of average daily temperature; Megyesi, 2005; Vass et al., 1992). Controlled experimental work has shown that the relationship between temperature and the decomposition of soft tissue is not linear over a $20°$ temperature range ($2\ °C$ to $22\ °C$; Carter & Tibbett, 2006). This was possibly because the lowest incubation temperature was close to freezing point.

Conclusions

Taphonomy has a lot to offer forensic science and current research is starting to fill in the gaps in knowledge that inevitably exists in developing areas of science such as this. As a multidisciplinary science it requires contributions from anthropologists, entomologists, soil scientists, microbiologists, biochemists and chemists to work together in the exciting and expanding frontier of forensics. Currently, too little is known in forensic taphonomy from experimental research, and the science is, to date, understandably dependent on the experience of practitioners and the logical inferences and estimates from carefully examined case studies. The time has now come for forensic taphonomy, and an increasing number of studies are now based on carefully designed experimental protocols that should provide the forensic practitioner with a more robust science on which to base his or her work.

References

Bereuter, T.L., Lorbeer, E., Reiter, C., Saidler, H., & Unterdorfer, H. (1996). Post-mortem alterations of human lipids — Part I: Evaluation of adipocere formation and mummification by desiccation. In K. Spindler (Ed.), *Human mummies: A global survey of their status and the techniques of conservation* (pp. 265–273). New York: Wien.

Brady, N.C. (1990). *The nature and properties of soils* (10th ed.). New York: Macmillan Publishing Company.

Cadisch, G., & Giller, K.E. (Eds.). (1997). *Driven by nature: Plant litter quality and decomposition.* Wallingford: CAB International.

Carter, D.O., & Tibbett, M. (2006). Microbial decomposition of skeletal muscle tissue (*Ovis aries*) in a sandy loam soil at different temperatures. *Soil Biology and Biochemistry, 38,* 1139–1145.

Carter, D.O., & Tibbett, M. (2008). Cadaver decomposition and soil processes. In M. Tibbett & D.O. Carter (Eds.), *Soil analysis in forensic taphonomy: Chemical and biological effects of buried human remains* (pp. 29–52). Boca Raton, FL: CRC Press.

Carter, D., Yellowlees, D., & Tibbett, M. (2006). Cadaver decomposition and belowground ecology. *Naturwissenschaften, 94,* 12–24.

Dawson, L.A., Campbell, C.D., Hillier, S., & Brewer, M.J. (2008). Methods of characterising and fingerprinting soils for forensic application. In M. Tibbett & D.O. Carter (Eds.), *Soil analysis in forensic taphonomy: Chemical and biological effects of buried human remains.* (pp. 76–312). Boca Raton, FL: CRC Press.

Dent, B.B., Forbes, S.L., & Stuart, B.H. (2004). Review of human decomposition process in soil. *Environmental Geology 45,* 576–585.

Dix, J, & Graham, M. (2000). *Time of death, decomposition and identification: An atlas.* Boca Raton, FL: CRC Press.

Fitzpatrick, R.W. (2008). Nature, distribution and origin of soil materials in the forensic comparison of soils. In M. Tibbett & D.O. Carter (Eds.), *Soil analysis in forensic taphonomy: Chemical and biological effects of buried human remains.* (pp. 1–28). Boca Raton, FL: CRC Press.

Forbes, S.L. (2008a). Decomposition chemistry in a burial environment. In M. Tibbett & D.O. Carter (Eds.), *Soil analysis in forensic taphonomy: Chemical and biological effects of buried human remains.* (pp. 199–220). Boca Raton, FL: CRC Press.

Forbes, S.L. (2008b). Potential determinants of post-mortem and postburial interval. In M. Tibbett & D.O. Carter (Eds.), *Soil analysis in forensic taphonomy: Chemical and biological effects of buried human remains.* (pp. 221–242). Boca Raton, FL: CRC Press.

Galloway, A. (1997). The process of decomposition: a model from the Arizona-Sonoran desert. In W.D. Haglund & M.H. Sorg (Eds.). *Forensic taphonomy: The post-mortem fate of human remains.* (pp. 139–150). Boca Raton, FL, USA: CRC Press.

Galloway, A., Birkby, W.H., Jones, A.M., Henry, T.E., & Parks, B.O. (1989). Decay rates of human remains in an arid environment. *Journal of Forensic Sciences, 34,* 607–616.

Geberth, V.J. (1996). *Practical homicide investigation: Tactics, procedures, and forensic techniques.* Boca Raton, FL: CRC Press.

Hopkins, D.W., Wiltshire, P.E.J., & Turner, B.D. (2000). Microbial characteristics of soils from graves: An investigation at the interface of soil microbiology and forensic science. *Applied Soil Ecology, 14,* 283–288.

Hunter, J. (1994). Forensic archaeology in Britain. *Antiquity, 68,* 758–769.

Janaway, R.C. (2008). The decomposition of materials associated with buried cadavers. In M. Tibbett & D.O. Carter (Eds.), *Soil analysis in forensic taphonomy: Chemical and biological effects of buried human remains.* (pp. 149–198). Boca Raton, FL: CRC Press.

Mann, R.W., Bass, W.M., & Meadows, L. (1990). Time since death and decomposition of the human body: Variables and observations in cause and experimental field studies. *Journal of Forensic Science, 35,* 103–111.

Mant, A.K. (1950). *A study in exhumation — data.* Unpublished MD dissertation, University of London, London, UK.

Mant, A.K. (1953). Recent work on post-mortem changes and timing death. In K. Simpson (Ed.), *Modern trends in forensic medicine* (pp. 147–162). London: Butterworth and Co.

Mant, A.K. (1987). Knowledge acquired from post-war exhumations. In A. Boddington, A.N. Garland & R.C. Janaway, (Eds). *Death, decay and reconstruction: Approaches to archaeology and forensic science* (pp. 65–78). Manchester: Manchester University Press.

Megyesi, M.S., Nawrocki, S.P., & Haskell, N.H. (2005). Using accumulated degree-days to estimate the post-mortem interval from decomposed human remains. *Journal of Forensic Science, 50,* 618–626.

Micozzi, M.S. (1986). Experimental study of post-mortem change under field conditions: Effects of freezing, thawing, and mechanical injury. *Journal of Forensic Sciences, 31,* 53–961.

Payne, J.A., & King, E.W. (1968). Coleoptera associated with pig carrion. *Entomologist's Monthly Magazine, 105,* 224–232.

Payne, J.A., King, E.W., Beinhart. G. (1968). Arthropod succession and decomposition of buried pigs. *Nature, 219,* 1180–1181.

Rodriguez, W.C., & Bass, W.M. (1983). Insect activity and its relationship to decay rates of human cadavers in East Tennessee. *Journal of Forensic Science, 28,* 423–432.

Rodriguez, W.C., & Bass, W.M. (1985). Decomposition of buried bodies and methods that may aid in their location. *Journal of Forensic Science 30,* 836–852.

Tibbett, M., Carter, D.O., Haslam, T., Major, R., & Haslam, R. (2004). A laboratory incubation method for determining the rate of microbiological degradation of skeletal muscle tissue in soil. *Journal of Forensic Science, 49,* 560–565.

Turner, B. & Wiltshire, P. (1999). Experimental validation of forensic evidence: A study of the decomposition of buried pigs in a heavy clay soil. *Forensic Science International, 101,* 113–122.

Vass, A.A., Bass, W.M., Wolt, J.D., Foss, J.E., & Ammons, J.T. (1992). Time since death determinations of human cadavers using soil solution. *Journal of Forensic Science, 37,* 1236–1253.

Vass, A, Barshick, S.A., Sega, G., Caton, J., Skeen, J.T., Love, J.C. et al. (2002). Decomposition chemistry of human remains: A new methodology for determining the post-mortem interval. *Journal of Forensic Science, 47,* 542–553.

Identification of Australian Aboriginal Mortuary Remains

Marc F. Oxenham

Tom Knight

Michael Westaway

Given that human occupation of Australia likely extends at least 50,000 years into the past (Bowler, Johnson, Olley, Prescott, Roberts et al., 2003) and perhaps as far as 60,000 years (Hiscock, 2008) into the past, the remains of countless individuals are currently scattered across and beneath the Australian landscape. How many of these sets of remains belong to recent victims or homicide or misadventure is difficult to determine, but probably vanishingly small. Australia has a comparatively low rate of murder that peaked at 354 recorded homicides in 2001/4 (Mouzos, 2005). The rate expressed as homicides per 100,000 persons fluctuated between 1.5 and 2.0 from 1990 to 2004 (Mouzos, 2005). In order to gain some comparative perspective there is data recently published by the World Health Organization on youth homicide (persons aged between 10 and 29 years) rates globally. Australia is positioned at 1.6 per 100,000 in comparison to some countries with very low rates: Japan 0.4; France 0.6, Germany 0.8 (Krug, Dahlberg, Mercy, Zwi, & Lozano, 2002). The highest rate for a developed country is the United States at 11.0, while some South American countries have extremely high rates of homicide: Colombia 84.4; El Salvador 50.0; Venezuela 25.0 (Krug et al., 2002). While the homicide rate may be correlated with the probability of clandestine body disposal there is no published data for such behaviour in Australia. Our only clue to the potential frequency with which the bodies of homicide victims may have been secretly disposed of is in the case of contract killings. Given that this category of homicide (only accounting for 2% of all homicides between 1989 and 2002 in Australia) suggests a clear degree of planning, it is worth pointing out that the victim was left at the scene of the crime in the majority of cases (Mouzos & Venditto, 2003: 48). The only other source of data that may shed light on the probability of finding recent human remains in remote or hidden circumstances is the Missing Persons Rate. The Australian Federal Police's web site on missing persons states that some 30,000 people are reported missing each year in Australia and 99.5% are subsequently found. One is left guessing the fate of the 0.5% (some 150 people per year) who are not found. Presumably some of these people are located years later, others eventually contribute to the homicide rate, while others will be added to the death rate through misadventure or natural causes.

The relatively small homicide rate, rarity of clandestine body disposal and low number of unfound missing persons in Australia all indicate a low probability of casual or unintentional discovery of the remains of recent victims of crime or misadventure. In the vast majority of cases where human remains are discovered they will probably derive from historic or pre-European contact contexts (see also Donlon, Chapter 7). Part II, Division 3 (discovery and disposal of Aboriginal remains) of the *Aboriginal and Torres Strait Islander Heritage Protection Act 1984*, is clear as to the requirements of anyone on discovering Aboriginal remains. Section 20, subsection 1 of this Act states:

> A person who, except in Victoria,[1] discovers anything that
> he or she has reasonable grounds to suspect to be
> Aboriginal remains shall report his or her discovery to the
> Minister, giving particulars of the remains and their location.

The obvious problem here is in the identification of remains as Aboriginal; a task that most people without appropriate training or experience would find extremely difficult in many instances. Anecdotal evidence suggests that the public and government agencies, including law enforcement,[2] have frequently disturbed and sometimes collected what subsequently turned out to be Aboriginal remains, presumably on the basis that they may have been dealing with a recent homicide or missing person. The general public, law enforcement and other government agencies have an ethical as well as legal obligation to ensure that efforts are made to determine whether or not unintentionally discovered human remains are Aboriginal and of such antiquity as to be no longer of interest in the pursuance of criminal investigations. In the case of European remains, various State heritage acts may also be relevant. For example, European remains 50 years or older in New South Wales are considered relics under the *New South Wales Heritage Act 1977* and cannot be disturbed without appropriate permits.

   The main purpose of this chapter is to provide a description of the more common forms of mortuary behaviour in precontact and early contact Aboriginal Australia. The focus will be both on the types of funerary treatments that leave a clear archaeological or currently visible signature and the sorts of sites, landscape forms and features favoured by Aboriginal people in disposal of their dead. It is our hope that a greater familiarity with the variability and distinctiveness of past Aboriginal mortuary customs will reduce the occurrence of unnecessary interference with Aboriginal remains. Such a result would not only benefit the efforts of heritage management organisations and community relations but would also, undoubtedly, alleviate law enforcement agencies of the need to engage in some unnecessary investigations at least.

   While it is useful to discuss mortuary variability in Australia by state, the states are delimited by recent political boundaries with no correlations with past Aboriginal mortuary behaviour. Some forms of mortuary behaviour appear to be geographically restricted, such as the presence of large cemeteries in the Murray River region, platform tree burials in the northern half of Australia, and elaborately carved burial trees in New South Wales. Other forms of body disposal occur throughout the continent: ground burial and the stashing of remains in rock crevices, for example. Our chosen format is to discuss mortuary variability by generalised type rather than by region. This is considered to be appropriate because the best rule of thumb is to assume nothing and to expect anything when in the field regarding the identification of Aboriginal mortuary remains. It is in this vein that we have decided not to provide maps summarising mortuary behaviour across the continent (e.g., such maps can be found in Davidson, 1949a; Peterson, McConvell, McDonald, Morphy, & Arthur, 2005; and Thomas, 1908).

Variability in Aboriginal Mortuary Practices

The physical disposal of the deceased is only one part of the funerary or mortuary process. However, given the aims of this chapter, physical disposal of the corpse is the prime focus of this discussion. Aboriginal peoples have engaged in a wide range of body disposal procedures that can be generalised into several categories: burial, cremation, exposure to the elements, mummification, and anthropophagy (consumption of the deceased). Remains that have been buried or mummified are more likely to survive the ravages of time. Nonetheless, some forms of disposal, such as exposure in tree platforms, can still be observed, and the oldest recorded example of cremation in the world is found at Willandra Lakes (Bowler, Jones, Allen, & Thorne, 1970). Cremation appears to have been restricted to the eastern third of Australia, including Tasmania, and does not seem to have occurred in Western Australia (Hiatt, 1969). In addition to these broad categories of mortuary behaviour, body disposal may occur as a single one-off or primary event or over an extended period of time (sometimes measured in years), as in the case of secondary burial behaviours. In the remainder of this chapter a range of mortuary practices and corpse treatments are examined with reference to the ethnographic, ethnohistoric and archaeological literature. This review is far from exhaustive as our aim is only to provide the reader with a broader appreciation of the types of past Aboriginal mortuary behaviour; the remains of which may still be encountered in construction sites, National Parks, farmer's paddocks, and so forth.

Burial

Despite burial having been a very common form of interment in Australia, it is uncommon to find large aggregations of Aboriginal burials, as the use of cemeteries was not a common feature of past mortuary behaviour. For instance, while burial was an extremely common form of body disposal in Western Australia, Davidson (1949a) suggests that isolated burial was the norm, rather than the use of collective burial areas or cemeteries. Pardoe (1988) has suggested that true cemeteries are only seen in the Murray River region of Victoria and South Australia, although he sees the Broadbeach site in Queensland (see Haglund, 1976) as an exception to this rule. Relatively high concentrations of burials are seen in other areas, such as Willandra Lakes in New South Wales, but do not meet the strict requirements of identification as cemeteries in Pardoe's system. Clearly it would be unwise to treat concentrations of burials in other parts of Australia as non-Aboriginal based on our current understanding of past mortuary behaviour. Further, historical accounts of massacres in the recent past (e.g., Clark, 1995) would suggest that the remains of such events may not be entirely uncommon.

By far the most commonly documented traditional Aboriginal burial practice in New South Wales was interment in the earthen ground, specifically in a dug grave. In A.W. Howitt's (1904: 461–467) anthropological work *The Native Tribes of South-East Australia*, 10 out of 12 descriptions of Aboriginal funerary practices in New

South Wales involve the placement of the fully articulated dead body in a humanly constructed pit or 'grave'. Both men and women could be buried in this manner, the elaborateness of the burial seemingly reflecting the social status of the individual involved. An important consideration in the process of Aboriginal ground burial identification and recording is that the often highly dispersed, fragmentary remains evident on the surface today may be equally likely to represent a shallow, simple burial or a very carefully constructed 'tomb'.

Although placement of human remains in natural rocky cavities such as caves and clefts may also be technically considered 'ground burial', important and substantial differences in both mortuary practice and the resultant archaeology are apparent. As such, the essential defining characteristics of ground burial as understood here must be noted:

(a) ground burial was typically conducted in open air locations

(b) an artificial pit or grave was excavated in a naturally loose or soft substrate such as earth, gravel or cultural deposits such as ash and/or shell midden

(c) the body was placed in the pit and the pit was backfilled or the opening covered over.

Ground burials were dug across a range of landscape settings: on alluvial flats, sand dunes, ridge crests, hills and mountaintops. The nature of the associated deposit depended on local environmental and cultural factors. Aboriginal burials are known to occur in natural sediment (e.g., sand bodies) and humanly derived deposits (e.g., oven mounds and middens but not generally in the remains of fires) on the coastal zone or along inland rivers such as the Murrumbidgee (Littleton, 2000; Littleton, personal communication). Depending on the location, the excavated grave could take the form of a vertical pit or shaft, or a horizontal tunnel. An example of the construction and use of the latter was observed by W.D. Wright (1923: 57) during the burial of the Ngunnawal chief Hong Yong at Cuppacumbalong (Tharwa) in what is now the southern Australian Capital Territory:

> After his death at Cuppercumbalong, the men of the tribe got together, tied him up in a complete ball, then cut him open between hip and rib, and through the orifice withdrew the old chap's kidney fat, distributing it in small pieces to every gin in the camp, who stowed the treasure away in the net bags they always carried around their shoulders. His grave was on top of a rocky hill ... and about five or six feet in depth. A tunnel about six feet in length was excavated and the body inserted, with his spears (broken in half), his shield, nulla nulla, boomerang, tomahawk, opossum rug, and other effects. Then the hole was filled in with stones and earth.

Wright's brief description provides us with some important details that are relevant to many other accounts of Aboriginal ground burials from across the state. First, the practice most frequently involved the interment of a newly dead and fully articulated body in a flexed or 'crouched' posture, often tightly bound. The body would subsequently be placed in the grave in an upright 'sitting' position, or laid on its side. Second, the depth of the excavated pit seldom exceeded two metres, and appears to have usually been between four and five feet on the imperial scale. Third, depending on status, various grave goods were sometimes interred with the body. Fourth, heavy objects such as stones could be purposely incorporated into the backfill. As would be expected, there were variations on each of these themes as well as some additional practices and examples of these will be provided below.

Binding of the body into a flexed or crouching position was a widespread Aboriginal practice in the historical period, although the archaeological record indicates that extended position ground burial was also practised in both recent and ancient times at places such as Lake Victoria on the Murray River (Blackwood and Simpson, 1973). Where binding was carried out, careful attention appears to have been paid to the firm fixation of the body into position. The naked or near naked body could be bound solely with fibre cord or several layers of wrapping applied. In this manner the Kamilaroi or Gamilaraay people of the New South Wale's north-west are known to have wrapped their dead into 'mummy-like' bundles.

> While the body was still warm, they brought nets and opossum rugs as wrappers for the corpse, spread them on the ground, and doubled the body into the form of a bale, with the knees and chin touching each other. Then they wrapped the bale in the nets and rugs and tied it tightly. A shallow hole was dug with yam-sticks, in which the body was placed, and being filled in with soil, was covered with logs and deadwood to keep the dingoes out. (Howitt, 1904: 466)

Similar heavy wrapping of the body is known to have been practised in other parts of the state. In 1817 the explorer John Oxley excavated a Wiradjuri burial on the bank of the Lachlan River between Lake Cargelligo and Condobolin. After digging to a depth of 120 cm, Oxley uncovered the body of a 'tall powerful man' set in a flexed position with the arms between the thighs, very carefully wrapped in a number of possum skins and a single large net (Oxley, 1820: 140–141). During the burial process this body had been covered with multiple layers of dried grass and leaves overlain in turn by three to four layers of wood and several feet of soil (Oxley, 1820: 139–140). In Western Australia logs or sticks were sometimes placed over the grave and, in some regions, elaborate platforms were constructed from cross supporting sticks on which stones were placed (Davidson, 1949a). Further, the custom of binding the corpse occurred in Western Australia, and in some cases the limbs of the deceased would be broken (Davidson, 1949a). The discovery of such remains might at first glance appear to be consistent with foul play/homicide.

An alternative wrapping material to animal skin was tree bark. Another description from Howitt (1904: 464–465) indicates the use of this substance at Dungog in the Hunter Valley:

> The body was doubled up, heels to hips and face to knees, and the arms folded. It was then wrapped up in sheets of Ti-tree bark secured by cords of string-bark fibre. A hole was dug in easy soil and in a well-shaded locality, about two feet deep and circular. The body was dropped in sideways, and after putting a stone hatchet and a club beside the body, the grave was filled in, and the ceremonies ended.

Through the course of the 19th century, traditional wrappings were supplemented or replaced with European textiles. In this sense, the distribution of blankets to Aboriginal people at missions, stations and through government outlets appears to have provided an alternative to animal skin cloaks. Helms

(1895: 404–406) noted the use of a European blanket wrapping in the case of a pit burial unearthed near Jindabyne:

> The knees had been drawn up to the abdomen and lashed with bast (bark fibre), the elbows had been laid close to the sides, and the hands were placed flat in front of the face … It was evident that the body had been lashed together into the smallest possible compass by bast being coiled around it in all directions. After being tied up it had then been wrapped in a blue blanket, perished fragments of which still remained and then in thick fibrous bark that was well lashed round it.

A similar contemporary account comes from the lower reaches of the Wollondilly River in the Southern Highlands:

> [we] found the skeleton well wrapt [wrapped] in what had once been an old coat, a blanket, and an opossum rug. The skeleton was doubled up in the usual manner, the arms drawn up to the breast, and the legs against the abdomen, placed on the right side, and facing the south east. (Etheridge, 1893a: 595).

In both these instances the bodies had been buried at elevated landscape positions in pits over six feet deep dug into solid ground. In addition to earth the backfill included carefully placed layers of grass, boulders, rocks, and pieces of timber. The robustness of the backfill in these cases stands in stark contrast to the Aboriginal ground burial practices observed in the mountains near Murwullimbah on the far north coast:

'They made a hole and put the corpse in it in a sitting posture and covered it with a sheet of bark never filling any earth at all.' (Yardley, 1899 in Turnbull, 1991: 111–112).

Mummification

The remains of another mortuary treatment likely to be encountered in modern times, and reported on by Hamlyn-Harris (1912) for the Torres Straight Islands, is that of deliberate mummification. Hamlyn-Harris notes that after initial mourning the body is placed on a bamboo platform over 2 m high, under which a fire is lit for the benefit of the deceased. The body is allowed to decompose for 4 to 5 days and is then placed in a canoe with a hole in the bottom and taken to the sea. The skin is removed and an incision made to remove the intestines and testicles (if male), the eyes are punctured to release fluids and internal organs are discarded in the sea. The skin of the palms of the hands and feet, including fingernails and toenails, are removed, dried and worn around the neck of the widow. The corpse is washed in the sea and moved to land, where an incision is made in the base of the skull and the brain removed. Pieces of dried sago palm were then placed inside the body cavity to prevent collapse and shrinking during the drying process. The incision was then sewn up and new incisions are made between fingers and toes and at the knees for drainage. The body is then attached to a bamboo frame and hung 2 m to 3 m high to dry. Before completely dry it would be decorated with ochre and coconut oil, and shells would be placed in the eyes and so forth. Drying once complete, the body would be taken down and displayed until it began to disintegrate. The head would be retained by the widow while the corpse is placed in a garden where it eventually disintegrates.

The use of drying frames is also reported for other parts of Queensland. Semon (1899: 222–223) notes that:

> In Central Queensland the corpses are first dried whole
> in hollow trees, and the bones buried later on in the
> ground or within these trunks. Some tribes erect
> wooden scaffolds to prevent dingos and other animals
> from disturbing their drying corpses. Sometimes the
> dead are mummified by smoke, and carried about for
> some time by the wandering tribe before they are
> buried. When this takes place, they generally encase the
> bodies or bones in bark.

Semon's description is particularly interesting in highlighting the main components of a common theme in Aboriginal secondary burial behaviour: initial treatment of the corpse followed by a form of curation and transport of the remains around the landscape and subsequent final storage of the remains. This process of drying the corpse followed by a lengthy period of curation/transportation of the remains is also noted by Lethbridge (e.g., see quotation in Moorwood, 1982) and would seem to be a fairly common form of mortuary practice in the ethnohistoric period of Queensland at least.

Mounds and Other Grave Markers

An interesting feature of Aboriginal ground burials in many parts of New South Wales was the construction of a mound of raised earth over the top of the burial pit. A.C.R. Bowler (1902: 67) noted that the western Wiradjuri people constructed mounds over the graves of both men and women:

> When a male or female dies they first tie the body up in a
> sitting position, with the head resting on the top of the
> knees. They then proceed to the nearest sand hill, and with
> sharp pointed sticks, called co-nies, dig a round hole from
> three to four feet deep, in which they place the body, in a
> sitting position, they then fill in the hole with earth and
> leaves, making a mound on the top like a sugar-loaf.

Most records indicate the mounds as neat and rounded in form, approximately 2 m to 3 m in diameter and 1 to 1½ m in height (e.g., Etheridge, 1893a; Govett, 1836; Helms, 1895; Meredith, 1989: 45–46; Oxley, 1820: 138–141). However, dimensions and precise form could vary widely and there are accounts of some very large burial mounds. For example, Atkinson (1853 in Clarke, 1990: 82–84) described an Aboriginal 'tumulus' near Moss Vale as an earthen oblong mound resembling 'a large hillock some 100 feet long, and 50 in height'.

Mounds are also a relatively common form of burial marker in Western Australia. Davidson (1949a) suggests that mounding in Western Australia was commonly associated with funerary behaviour that required the grave to be left open for a period of time. A formalisation of this behaviour led to the development of mounding rules. For example:

> [i]n the Laverton area. The Warburton Range and
> eastward, and among the Andigarina, these mounds are
> conical in shape and are regarded as representing the
> Moon-man, the first human being killed by the Wati

> Kuthara, the two ancestral culture heroes so important
> in the mythology of South Australia and parts of
> western Australia.

> Special mounds of crescent or semi-circular shape, which
> partially enclose the head of the grave, are raised in such
> widely separated areas as Esperance and Walebing, and
> among the Wirangu Wailpi of South Australia.
> (Davidson, 1949a: 85)

Apart from more obvious forms of grave makers, such a mounds and carved trees, a range of more portable objects have been placed on or by graves during the funerary process. Mourning caps, constructed from pipe clay or gypsum, are known for much of the southern half of the continent. While they do not seem to have been placed on graves in Western Australia, Davidson (1949b: 65) notes that complete caps were placed on graves 'along the Murray and Darling Rivers, in northeastern South Australia and adjacent areas, and presumably along the tributaries of the Darling'. Shaved sticks are also known to have been used as grave markers in Western Australia.

> At Kellerberrin they [shaved-sticks] are arranged in three
> rows of fences, six inches high, to contain the crescent of
> boughs and leaves. Sticks with red horizontal marks also
> ornamented the edge of the grave at Geraldton.
> (Davidson, 1949a: 85)

While grave goods are treated as a separate category (see below) it is worth noting here that the types of objects placed inside graves, and often referred to as grave goods or grave furniture, could also be placed on top of a filled grave and act, perhaps unintentionally, as a form of grave marker.

Carved Trees

An additional burial practice peculiar to certain parts of New South Wales was the carving of tree trunks adjacent to burial mounds. Such burial trees or 'taphoglyphs' appear to have been created exclusively for the graves of 'chiefs', celebrated warriors or other men of importance (Black, 1941: 18).

> In the grave the corpse was placed in a 'squatting'
> position. The head bent over the knees and covered with
> bark, over which was raised a large mound of soil, and if
> a man of influence from one to four trees around the
> grave were elaborately carved (the bark first being
> removed and placed in the grave). To a women's (sic)
> burial and grave less attention was given, and trees were
> never carved. (Richards, 1902: 166)

> The blaze on the tree was also carved in tribal markings,
> to show the man's status in the case of the Eulomogo
> ('clever man'), and carved trees also marked the grave of
> a Eula (head man), but the ordinary man or co-ba had
> no tree marked that I know of. (Garnsey, 1946: 7)

The designs were carved into the tree trunk on a surface from which a slab of bark had been carefully removed. The result was a blaze effectively framing the carved design or 'glyph'. Glyph designs were generally scroll and straight line styles, with occasional representations of humans or animals (McCarthy, 1940: 165). An important burial could be marked by up to five carved trees, the trees selected usually positioned at cardinal points in relation to the grave.

Research on the distribution of carved burial trees indicates they were most common in the New South Wales central-west and certain parts of the south-west slopes and southern highlands (Black, 1941; Etheridge, 1918). Extant examples of such burials include the Wiradjuri chief Windradyne near Sofala and Yuranigh near Molong. A less known observation is that a form of tree carving occurred in Western Australia.

> In the Southwest [of Western Australia] trees near the grave are sometimes carved. Notches and 'uncouth' figures, daubed red, are mentioned for the Harvey River area. Circles and other carved ornamentations are reported for Perth, circles for the 'Southwest'. Notches are cut on two trees for each grave, an even number of notches for a man, an uneven for a woman, by the tribes from Esperance. (Davidson, 1949a: 85)

Tree Burials

Two forms of tree burial are described here: placement of the corpse on a platform within a tree; stowage of remains within a hollow of the tree itself. Generally storage of remains within a hollow tree forms the terminal phase of a secondary burial process, although as Semon's (1899) account of mummification in Queensland suggests (see previous quote in mummification section), the initial body preparation stage can begin and end in a hollow tree. Muirhead (1887: 28–29) provides a graphic account of the procedures leading up to a hollow tree internment:

> [T]he corpse would be temporarily deposited in a grave, covered only with bark, and be there allowed to remain for two months. A half-circle would then be dug round one side of the grave, the body be chopped up, put into fresh bark in as small a space as could be conveniently managed, and be given to the mother or sister of the deceased to carry to all meetings of the tribe, or until the death were avenged. Remains are sometimes carried in this way for two years. When tired of carrying them about, they are dropped down the pipe of a hollow tree and left there, and a ring of bark is stripped off that and the neighbouring trees to mark the spot.

Tree platform exposure has also been reported for Western Australia although the custom may be a more recent import from the Northern Territory (Davidson, 1949a).

Historical accounts from New South Wales suggest the use of hollow trees as receptacles for the dead either in accordance with the social status of the deceased individual or in locations where the ground was simply too hard to undertake ground burial. Parker (1905: 92) wrote that along the upper Barwon River hollow trees were generally used as burial places for certain body parts such as skin and internal organs, or the complete corpses of lower ranking members of Aboriginal society:

> Even in our district the dead were sometimes placed in hollow trees. I know of skeletons in trees on the edge of the ridge on which the home station was built. These are said to be for the most part the bodies of worthless women or babies.

Alternately, in the southern parts of the state it would appear that large hollow trees were sometimes used as alternative primary burial sites for adult men and women. In the Monaro, certain trees with elevated accessible voids were described as Aboriginal 'sepulchres' containing bodies bound in the same fashion as those in ground burials (Flood, 1980: 120; Helms, 1895: 399). Similar practices were undertaken in the Boorowa district where a number of complete skeletons were discovered in hollow trees in the late 1800s and early 1900s (Lloyd, 1990: 5).

Cave/Crevice Interments

For want of a better term, cave or crevice interments are somewhat analogous to hollow tree burials in that they represent remains stowed (not buried) in a small, perhaps secrete or less than obvious, place as the terminal phase of an often extended mortuary process. The best descriptions of this form of mortuary behaviour are described for central Queensland and are worth quoting in detail.

> The desiccated corpse, sometimes only a bundle of defleshed bones, was then placed inside tightly rolled bark cylinders up to 2500 mm [long]. Cylinders were elaborately bound with hair, fur, and fibre string, and sometimes finely-woven bands. Some were painted with alternate bands of ochre in varying combinations of red, orange, yellow and white. One example even features a white hand stensil [stencil] on the bark.
>
> This complex burial preparation appears to have been reserved for males between 18 and 40 as part of inquest rites to determine those responsible for the individual's death, and for children under about eight years. Adolescents, females, and the elderly were not treated in this manner ...
>
> Burial sites are found at ground level or in inaccessible locations as high as 30 m up vertical cliffs. Some have burial art painted and stencilled around entrances. Only 32 examples of burial art have been recorded, some at sites containing multiple burials. Half these sites contained adult burials, two had adult and child remains, four had only child burials, and the remainder had been pillaged before recording. (Walsh, 1988: 128)

Clearly, the presence of bark cylinders in caves and crevices should be enough to alert most people to the presence of an Aboriginal interment that should not be disturbed, let alone removed, in any form whatsoever.

Despite the fact that the process of placing the dead in caves and crevices is rarely described in accounts from New South Wales, there are numerous records of such places in the landscape being known Aboriginal burial sites and/or locations where skeletons have been found. Bodies are known to have been placed in almost inaccessible voids high on cliff faces, small rock shelters in the hills, and in large caverns. Although such burial was by no means restricted to karst terrain where weathering of local limestone has resulted in extensive and often spectacular cavernous formations, these geological zones appear to have been associated with considerable mortuary activity. Examples include the cave systems at Bungonia, Yarrangobilly and Rosebrook (Etheridge, 1893b; Flood, 1980: 120; Leigh, 1893: 79; Wilson, 1968:

110;). At London Bridge, south of Queanbeyan, Brennan (1907: 208) found numerous Aboriginal remains in a limestone cave:

> In January, 1874, I discovered on the London Bridge Estate, the property of Mr John McNamara, a veritable catacomb on a small scale. It was a limestone cave, wherein were found many hundreds of human bones and skulls, centuries old. I had several bags of them conveyed to Queanbeyan, where they were carefully inspected by three surgeons, including Coroner Morton, who pronounced them to be the skeletons of the Aborigines of former times.

In the mountainous country to the west of this location, multiple Aboriginal burials have also been found in the limestone terrain on the upper Goodradigbee River. Aboriginal human remains in this area include entire extended individuals placed on natural rock platforms in comparatively spacious caverns and secondary burials where disarticulated bones loose or wrapped in parcels were positioned in small grottos and crevices (Bluett, 1954: 13; Cooke, 1988).

Grave Goods

A number of historical accounts describe the purposeful inclusion of certain objects or grave goods with the body. The presence of such items associated with human remains is often the best way to identify the remains as Aboriginal. Most descriptions tell us these items were the personal property of the deceased, although other 'offerings' brought by participants in the funeral may also have been included. Grave goods included spears, spear throwers, clubs, stone axes, boomerangs, stone flakes, bone points, skin cloaks, pendants, necklaces, headbands and items of ceremonial clothing (Coe, 1986; Fraser, 1883: 229; Howitt, 1904: 461–466; Witter, Fullagar, & Pardoe, 1993; Wright, 1923); in short, status items or implements important to the deceased. Whatever the rationale behind this ritual activity, some groups were meticulous in ensuring the dead were accompanied by all of their worldly possessions.

> The Wolgal were very particular in burying everything belonging to a dead man with him; spears and nets were included; even in one case a canoe was cut into pieces so that it could be put in the grave. (HoWitt, 1904: 461–462)

Depending on local conditions, certain artefacts included as grave goods may be very well preserved and survive centuries or even thousands of years of burial at least as well as human bone. A ground burial unearthed by flood erosion on the Monaro during the 1990s was found to contain stone tools, bone points, macropod mandibles and 327 kangaroo and wallaby teeth (Cohen, 1993; Feary, 1996). The macropod teeth were finely drilled and constituted the remains of a large necklace. This burial contained two skeletons, a middle aged female and a young adult male, and was subsequently dated to 7000 years ago (Feary, 1996).

It should be noted that some burials dating to the later part of the nineteenth century contained grave goods of European origin (see also Donlon, Chapter 7). In addition to the presence of blankets and clothing already mentioned, certain utilitarian objects of glass, metal and ceramic were viewed as suitable for inclusion with the dead. In one case Etheridge (1893a) noted the presence of an iron spear head, an old comb, a thimble, two iron spoons, a bullet mould, a quart pot, a clay tobacco pipe, the top of a metal powder case with shot, some shirt buttons, and a bottle of castor oil that had been placed directly under the head of the skeleton. Similar items, including a pair of scissors, a knife and fork and an old umbrella, were found in association with an Aboriginal burial discovered at Boorowa in the early twentieth century (Lloyd, 1990: 5). It needs to be stressed that the presence of European goods in a grave cannot be used as an excuse to disturb the remains, even if you consider the remains to be European. As mentioned in the introduction, various states have their own heritage legislation protecting human remains 50-plus years old.

Grave goods are also associated with forms of interment that are more readily identifiable as Aboriginal: the bark cylinders referred to in the previous section on cave/crevice burials. Walsh (1987) has recorded a wide range of objects often found in the bark cylinders (or cylinder coffins) of central Queensland, including European artefacts such as a steel axe and felt hat in one cylinder belonging to a child. More commonly, the cylinders can contain various animals (bones, feathers, quills or mummified remains), grass, nuts, shell pendants, dilly bags, wooden shields and even small boomerangs (Walsh, 1987).

Extended or Secondary Mortuary Practices

It is worth treating mortuary practices that involve multiple and an often complex series of body treatments as well as extended periods of curation as a separate category. In many cases of secondary interment, the corpse, or what is left of it, receives some form of final treatment: cremation, pulverisation, ground burial, stowage in a hollow tree of rock crevice, for example. In many cases there may be very little left of the original corpse at the time of final interment or treatment. In other instances portions of the corpse may be curated or transformed into sacred objects that may remain intact for considerable periods of time. Hiatt (1969) has suggested that (with some exceptions) extended funerary rituals are generally confined to the northern half of the continent while primary forms are found mostly in the southern half. While the reasons for such extended funerary rituals are complex, an important component often involves a search for the murderer of the deceased. It was a widely held belief among many Aboriginal groups that sorcery was the cause of most deaths. One way to locate the sorcerer was to transport the remains of the deceased around the landscape until a sign was received indicating the place of the initial sorcery and/or the identity of the actual sorcerer. Several good accounts of extended or secondary burial rituals recounted by Walter Roth (1907), a former Magistrate, Chief Protector of Aborigines (for Queensland) and a member of the Anthropological Institute, London, are presented for Queensland. Peterson's (1976) account of extended mortuary customs in northeast Arnhem Land, based on Donald Thomson's field notes, forms the other case study.

In the Pennefather River region, western Cape York Peninsula, Roth (1907) noted that burial ceremonies varied by age and sex of the deceased, with old men and old and young women being buried within a day or two of death near the camp, while children were disposed of immediately. Children were sometimes wrapped in bark and carried until they desiccated, after which they were placed (not buried) in the roots of a tree or within a cave. With the death of a young man the corpse is bound in a sheet of bark cloth and slung to a pole supported by two forked sticks; or alternatively, the body may be slung naked except for a dilly bag over the head. The strung corpse is mourned until such time as it has become dried and is eventually cremated, with the exception of the head, soles of the feet, and fleshy portions of the fronts of the thighs. The head was carried about in a piece of bark or dilly bag by the mother, while the fibulae (a leg bone) are wrapped in bark and decorated with emu feathers and subsequently worn by a close relative.

At Princess Charlotte Bay Roth (1907) noted that while the dying individual is removed from the camp of the living, the corpse is brought back to the camp on death and buried within the camp area. After a certain period, sometimes only several days, the body is exhumed, laced into a sheet of bark and transported from camp to camp (sometimes for months) until a close relative determines who the murderer was.

At Cape Bedford a grave was dug in the centre of the camp and sticks placed within the grave followed by grass and bark to create a platform. The corpse was then placed within the grave and covered in bark and soil. Mourners covered their heads with dilly bags while the deceased's wife would accept a rather severe beating from the men. Following a period of time, during which the corpse is well decomposed, it is wrapped in bark and then carried around on the head of the brother until the place where the deceased was doomed (and the murderer identified) is located. The corpse is eventually buried or placed in a cave (Roth, 1907).

Roth's (1907) account of mortuary practices at the Bloomfield River is interesting in pointing out differential treatment for prominent males and low status males and all females. Low status males and all females were initially wrapped in bark and later unwrapped for viewing. At that time mourners may cover their own body with the liquid exudate of the corpse. The body is later buried in a flexed position within the bark wrapping. For high status males the body is buried beneath a purpose-built hut and later exhumed for viewing. A rather elaborate 'postmortem' is then performed to discovery the source of sorcery. From Roth's description of this treatment of the body it would seem likely that damage to the skeleton could be erroneously interpreted, from a forensic standpoint, in terms of homicide or clandestine body disposal. After the postmortem examination much of the upper portion of the body is sewn into bark sheet and then carried around until the murderer has been located and the remains can be buried. The lower half of the body is generally cremated or reinterred.

The following account is based on Peterson's (1976) work on Donald Thompson's work in Arnhem Land, Northern Territory, in the 1930s. The body was first prepared by way of removing head and facial hair, often by using beeswax, which was then kept for further treatment and ceremonies. Most corpses were painted with the clan design after which it could not be seen by women or children and was usually covered in bark, leaving the face free. Soon after painting, 'burial' occurs either in the ground or in a tree. Interestingly, there is reference to the possibility of burial in a collective burial ground, although no data is given on the size (number of burials) or if the burial ground only houses the corpse temporarily. If buried, the head is positioned either facing the clan well or east. Burial with heavy stones and logs generally indicates the bones are to be left, as no appropriate living member is around to exhume and carry the bones.

Generally, exhumation is expected and the body is first covered in a bark sheet with poles and stones placed on the soil to prevent scavenging by dogs, dingoes, lizards and so on. If the deceased is a child, the grave will be in the camp of the parents whereas an adult will be buried outside the camp or in it if the camp is to be immediately abandoned. In some cases there are collective burial grounds. An alternative to burial, depending on the age of the deceased, is the placement of the corpse on a tree platform. Children and the old were usually buried in the ground, while active adults were placed in trees where the flesh rapidly dries and the bones become cleaner. Another reported mode of disposal involved eating the deceased, although there is little verification of this custom for the region.

A month or two after the primary disposal, the body is exhumed or recovered, with subsequent treatment of the flesh varying depending on area and burial type. In some cases the flesh from a grave burial may be returned to the ground while flesh from a platform burial is placed in paperbark in a tree to be destroyed naturally. In other instances, the flesh may be placed in a special hollow log. As for the bones, they are washed and wrapped in paperbark and transported by close relatives as they move around the countryside. Eventually, perhaps after several weeks, the final burial takes place. A coffin is made from a special hollow log that can range in size from 1.25 to 4.50 m long. Finally, the bones are smashed and inserted into the log coffin that is then erected vertically and left to the vagaries of the elements.

Conclusions

> The tombs are enclosed by brush fencing, the form of the enclosure being of a diamond-shape; the tomb in every instance is exactly in the centre; all the grass inside of the fence is neatly shaved off, and the ground swept quite clean. It is kept in this tidy condition for two or three years; after the lapse of that time, however, the whole arrangement is left to dwindle to decay, and after a few more years the very site of it is forgotten
> (Beveridge, 1883: 29–30)

Much of the artificial structure associated with Aboriginal burials did not last beyond a limited space of time, nor was it intended to. Carved trees, wooden platforms, bark coffins, and even structures of packed earth stand little chance of surviving many decades, centuries or even thousands of years of exposure to the elements and human agency. Unfortunately in Australia the latter included a period of purposeful location and desecration of burial sites during the 19th century aimed at the retrieval of Aboriginal bones destined for museums and private collections (Turnbull, 1991). As a result, what remains today of often sophisticated and prolonged funerary rites and physical processes of interment are either surface scatters of human bone, or subsurface skeletal material possibly associated with cultural deposits such as artefacts (grave goods), and/or evidence of grave structure (e.g., backfill and pit outline). The state of preservation of these remains and their exact manifestation is in turn highly influenced by the nature of local geomorphology, an assessment of which is beyond the scope of this work. Likewise, this study is not presented as a 'how to' guide on the details of field recognition of burial sites or practicalities of their management as excellent publications to that end already exist (e.g., Hope & Littleton, 1995a, 1995b).

The aim of this chapter has been to provide examples of the range of mortuary practices known to have been carried out in Aboriginal Australia, and in turn to illustrate some key attributes of burials that may assist as an adjunct in their identification. In step with this objective the following key points are of relevance: (a) Aboriginal burials are not restricted to any particular part of the landscape. Historical references and archaeological finds indicate that a broad range of topographic zones and natural features were associated with mortuary activity. In this regard it is also important to consider that the current landscape form may not be a reliable indicator of an area's 'precontact' morphology. Landscaping, mining, agriculture and accelerated erosion or deposition processes may both truncate and cap prehistoric cultural deposits including burial sites. (b) Burials may manifest themselves in a range of subtle ways (e.g., highly fragmented bone scatters, smears in the soil, single skeletal components) that provide only the slightest indication of what may be associated in adjoining subsurface or otherwise obscured contexts. Comprehensive and expert investigation of seemingly minor finds is the best way to avoid inadvertent loss of or further damage to significant and culturally sensitive sites. (c) The manner in which skeletal material presents itself may provide clues indicating Aboriginal origin. Aboriginal burial activity was governed by purposeful, reasoned behaviour. Primary evidence of this includes the orientation and layout of the body. (d) Aboriginal burials may include a range of grave goods, including 'traditional' Aboriginal artefacts of bone, stone, wood and fibre, and/or post-contact items. Depending on their level of preservation, such items can play a major role in the determination of the cultural origin of human skeletal material. (e) Aboriginal burials are protected by law throughout Australia and are of great importance to Aboriginal people. If a burial is discovered, timely and appropriate action must be undertaken to ensure that a proper conservation and management plan can be implemented.

Endnotes

1   The variation in requirements governing Victoria are outlined in section 21Q of the Act.
2   Published accounts involving the police include the Broadbeach Burial Ground on the Gold Coast (Haglund, 1976) and the Angophora Reserve rock shelter in New South Wales (MacDonald, 1992).

References

Aboriginal and Torres Strait Islander Heritage Protection Act 1984. Retrieved May 1, 2007, from http://www.austlii.edu.au/au/legis/cth/consol_act/aatsihpa1984549/

Australian Federal Police. (2005). *Missing persons.* Retrieved May 1, 2007, from http://www.afp.gov.au/national/missing.

Beveridge, P. (1883). Of the Aborigines inhabiting the great lacustrine and riverine depression of the Lower Murray, Lower Murrumbidgee, Lower Lachlan and Lower Darling. *Journal and Proceedings of the Royal Society of New South Wales, 17,* 19–74.

Black, L. (1941). *Burial trees: Being the first of a series on the Aboriginal customs of the Darling Valley and central New South Wales.* Melbourne, Australia: Robertson & Mullens.

Blackwood, R., & Simpson, K.N.G. (1973). Attitudes of Aboriginal skeletons excavated in the Murray Valley region between Mildura and Renmark, Australia. *Memoirs of the National Museum of Victoria, 34,* 99–150.

Bluett, W.P. (1954). *The Aborigines of the Canberra district at the arrival of the white man*. Canberra, Australia: Canberra Historical Society.

Bowler, A.C.R. (1902). Burial rites. *Science of Man*, 5, 67.

Bowler, J.M., Johnson. H., Olley, J.M., Prescott, J.R., Roberts, R.G., Shawcross, W. et al. (2003). New ages for human occupation and climatic change at Lake Mungo, Australia. *Nature*, *421*, 837–840.

Bowler, J.M., Jones, R., Allen, H., & Thorne, A.G. (1970). Pleistocene human remains from Australia: A living site and human cremation from Lake Mungo, western New South Wales. *World Archaeology*, 2, 39–60.

Brennan, M. (1907). *Reminiscences of the gold fields and elsewhere in New South Wales, covering a period of forty-eight years' service as an Officer of Police*. Sydney, Australia: William Brooks.

Clark, I. (1995). *Scars in the landscape: A register of massacre sites in western Victoria, 1803–1859*. Canberra, Australia: Australian Institute of Aboriginal and Torres Strait Islander Studies.

Clarke, P. (1990). *Pioneer writer: The life of Louisa Atkinson, novelist, journalist, naturalist*. Sydney, Australia: Allen & Unwin.

Coe, M. (1986). *Windradyne: A Wiradjuri Koorie*. Sydney, Australia: Blackbooks.

Cohen, S. (1993). Burial site bones baffle the boffins. *GEO Australia 15*, 52–61.

Cooke, H. (1988). An investigation into the prehistory of Blue Waterholes and Cooleman Plain, New South Wales. Unpublished BA Hons dissertation, Australian National University, Canberra, Australia.

Davidson, D.S. (1949a). Disposal of the dead in Western Australia. *Proceedings of the American Philosophical Society, 93*, 71–97.

Davidson, D.S. (1949b). Mourning-caps of the Australian Aborigines. *Proceedings of the American Philosophical Society, 93*, 57–70.

Etheridge, R. (1893a). Ethnological observations in Australia. *Nature, 47*, 594–596.

Etheridge, R. (1893b). Aboriginal skull from a cave at Bungonia. *Records of the Geological Survey of New South Wales*, 3, 128–132.

Etheridge, R. (1918). The dendroglyphs, or 'carved trees' of New South Wales. *Memoirs of the Geological Survey of the New South Wales* (Ethnological series No. 3). Sydney, Australia: Department of Mines, Geological Survey of New South Wales.

Feary, S. (1996). An Aboriginal burial with grave goods near Cooma, New South Wales. *Australian Archaeology*, *43*, 40–42.

Flood, J.M. (1980). *The moth hunters: Aboriginal prehistory of the Australian alps*. Canberra, Australia: Australian Institute of Aboriginal Studies.

Fraser, J. (1883). The Aborigines of New South Wales. *Royal Society of New South Wales Proceedings 16*, 193–233.

Garnsey, E.J. (1946). *A treatise on Aborigines of Dubbo and district, their camplife, habits and customs*. Unpublished manuscript (AIATSIS PMS 3467).

Govett, W.R. (1836). *Sketches of New South Wales, written and illustrated for The Saturday Magazine in 1836–37, together with an essay on the Saturday Magazine by Gaston Renard and an account of his life by Annette Potts*. Melbourne, Australia: Gaston Renard.

Haglund, L. (1976). *The Broadbeach Aboriginal burial ground: An archaeological analysis* .Brisbane, Australia: University of Queensland Press.

Hamlyn-Harris, R. (1912). Papuan mummification as practised in the Torres Strait Islands, and exemplified by specimens in the Queensland Museum collections. *Memoirs of the Queensland Museum, 1*, 1–6.

Helms, R. (1895). Anthropological notes. *Proceedings of the Linnaean Society of New South Wales, Ser. 2, 20*, 387–407.

Heritage Act 1977 (NSW). Retrieved May 1, 2007, from http://www.austlii.edu.au/au/legis/nsw/consol_act/ha197786/

Hiatt, B. (1969). Cremation in Aboriginal Australia. *Mankind*, *7*, 104–119.

Hiscock, P. (2008). *Archaeology of ancient Australia*. London and New York: Routledge.

Hope, J., & Littleton, J. (1995a). *1 Finding out about Aboriginal burials.* Murray Darling Basin Aboriginal Heritage Handbooks. Sydney, Australia: Mungo Publications.

Hope, J., & Littleton J. (1995b). *2 Protecting Aboriginal burial sites.* Murray Darling Basin Aboriginal Heritage Handbooks. Sydney, Australia: Mungo Publications.

Howitt, A.W. (1904). *The native tribes of south-east Australia.* Canberra, Australia: Australian Institute of Aboriginal and Torres Strait Islander Studies.

Krug, E.G., Dahlberg, L.L., Mercy, J.A., Zwi, A.B., & Lozano, R. (2002). *World report on violence and health.* Geneva: World Health Organization.

Leigh, W.S. (1893). Notes on the Rosebrook Caves, near Cooma. *Records of the Geological Survey of New South Wales, 3,* 77–79.

Littleton, J. (2000). Taphonomic effects of erosion on deliberately buried bodies. *Journal of Archaeological Science, 27,* 5–18.

Lloyd, H.V. (1990). *Boorowa: Over 160 years of white settlement.* Panania, Australia: Toveloam Press.

McCarthy, F.D. (1940). The carved trees of New South Wales. *Australian Museum Magazine, 7,* 161–166.

McDonald, J. (1992). *The archaeology of the Angophora Reserve rock shelter: (Or helping the police with their enquiries)* (Environmental Heritage Monograph Series No. 1.) Sydney, Australia: NSW National Parks and Wildlife Service.

Meredith, J. (1989). *The last Kooradgie: Moyengully, chief man of the Gundungarra people.* Kenthurst: Kangaroo Press.

Moore, D. (1980). The Aboriginal tribes of New South Wales. In C. Haigh & W. Goldstein (Eds.), *The Aborigines of New South Wales* (pp. 11–13). Sydney, Australia: NSW National Parks & Wildlife Service.

Mouzos, J. (2005). *Homicide in Australia: 2003–2004.* National Homicide Monitoring Program (NHMP) Annual Report (Australian Institute of Criminology Research and Public Policy Series No. 66). Canberra, Australia: Australian Institute of Criminology.

Mouzos, J., & Venditto, J. (2003). Contract killings in Australia (Australian Institute of Criminology Research and Public Policy Series No. 53). Canberra, Australia: Australian Institute of Criminology.

Morwood, M.J. (1982.) *The ethnography of Aboriginal groups in the Central Queensland Highlands. Cultural heritage management* (Monograph series No. 1.) Brisbane, Australia: Department of Aboriginal and Islanders Advancement, Archaeology Branch.

Murihead, J. (1887). Belyando River. In E.M. Curr (Ed), *The Australian race.* (Vol. 3, pp. 26–35). Melbourne, Australia: John Ferres, Government Printer.

Oxenham, M.F., & Matsumara, H. (2008). Oral and physiological palaeohealth in cold adapted peoples: Northeast Asia, Hokkaido. *American Journal of Physical Anthropology, 135,* 64–74.

Oxley, J. (1820). *Journals of two expeditions into the interior of New South Wales, undertaken by order of the British Government in the years 1817–18.* London: Murray.

Pardoe, C. (1988). The cemetery as symbol. The distribution of prehistoric Aboriginal burial grounds in southeastern Australia. *Archaeology in Oceania, 23,* 1–16.

Parker, K.L. (1905). *The Euahlayi Tribe: a study of Aboriginal life in Australia.* London: Constable.

Peterson, N. (1976). Mortuary customs of northeast Arnhem Land: an account compiled from Donald Thomson's fieldnotes. *Memoirs of the National Museum Victoria 37,* 97–108.

Peterson, N., McConvell, P., McDonald, H., Morphy, F., & Arthur, B. (2005). Social and cultural life. In B. Arthur & F. Morphy (Eds). *Macquarie atlas of indigenous Australia: Culture and society through space and time* (pp. 88–107). Sydney, Australia: The Macquarie Library Pty Ltd.

Richards, C. (1902). 'Wirra-Dthoor-ree Wir-rai' Yar-rai Wir-rach' Ar-ree'. Wir-ra' Jer-ree'. *Science of Man, 5,* 166.

Roberts, R.G., Jones, R., & Smith, M.A. (1990). Thermoluminescence dating of a 50,000 year-old human occupation site in northern Australia. *Nature, 345,* 153–156.

Roberts, R.G., Jones, R., Spooner, N.A., Head, M.J., Murray, A.S., & Smith, M.A. (1994). The human colonisation of Australia: Optical dates of 53,000 and 60,000 years bracket human arrival at Deaf Adder Gorge, Northern Territory. *Quaternary Science Reviews, 13,* 575–583.

Roth, W.E. (1907). Burial ceremonies and disposal of the dead. *Records of the Australian Museum*, 6, 365–403.

Semon, R. (1899). *In the Australian bush and on the coast of the coral sea*. London: Macmillan.

Thomas, N.W. (1908.) The disposal of the dead in Australia. *Folklore, 19*(4), 388–408.

Turnbull, P. (1991). 'Ramsay's Regime': The Australian Museum and the procurement of Aboriginal bodies, c. 1874–1900. *Aboriginal History, 15*, 108–121.

Walsh, G.L. (1987). The Chesterton Range: Its sites and management. Unpublished report (draft). Brisbane, Australia: Queensland National Parks and Wildlife Service.

Walsh, G.L. (1988). *Australia's greatest rock art*. Bathurst, Australia: EJ Brill/Robert Brown & Associates.

Wilson, G. (1968). *Murray of Yarralumla*. Melbourne, Australia: Oxford University Press.

Witter, D., Fullagar, R., & Pardoe, C. (1993). The Terramungamine incident: A double burial with grave goods near Dubbo, New South Wales. *Records of the Australian Museum, Suppl. 17*, 77–89.

Wright, W.D. (1923). *Canberra John*. Sydney, Australia: Andrew & Co.

The Role of the Biological Anthropologist in Mass Grave Investigations

Tim Anson

Michael Trimble

Recent (in the last 5 to 10 years) events in world history associated with violence have seen loss of life and property on massive scales. Such events are not particularly new or uncommon in world history. However, postevent examination and treatment of victims in the modern era is new and is reflective of a global society intent on documenting and exposing details of mass killing events. Civil strife in the Balkans, continued unrest in parts of Africa, open warfare in the Gulf region, abusive dictatorships and natural disasters like the Indonesian tsunami and Pakistan earthquake have resulted in widespread death and destruction. In the last 20 to 30 years, other conflicts such as those seen in Central and South America have left a legacy of broken families and devastated communities. Principal among the reasons for the great loss of life from human-made disasters is the elimination of political opposition and the genocidal product of ethnic cleansing. A common characteristic shared by these examples has been the creation of mass graves.

The definition of exactly what constitutes a mass grave will not be addressed here. The reader is directed to Haglund (2002) for an extensive and erudite summation of previous attempts at defining a mass grave. Similarly, the reasons for excavating mass graves will not be discussed at any length (see Hanson, Chapter 2, for an archaeological perspective on mass graves). Rather, the baseline methods and practical approaches of conducting a mass grave investigation are the focus of this discussion with particular reference to the multivariate team required and the biological anthropologist's role within that team.

The authors draw on their experience working as part of an investigative team (Mass Graves Investigative Team or MGIT) working in Iraq during 2004–2006. The methods and procedures outlined here have been developed over the last 2 to 3 decades by personnel in the United States Army, and the Army Corps of Engineers (USACE). During the writing of this work, the authors were not at liberty to provide details of locations investigated; names of the investigating bodies; or specific reasons for conducting the investigations. The principal reason for this is the ongoing and current prosecutorial nature of the investigation and aim of building an evidential case for a war crime tribunal in Iraq.

The Team: An Overview

The term 'forensic team' as it is applied here refers to the entire forensic group, which consists of two main subgroups. The two chief aspects of mass grave investigation require the use of: a field team; and a laboratory team. The field team has a three-tiered structure. This structure consists of a Program and Field Director (two tiers) and then the core of the unit that is composed of subject matter experts in (a) archaeology, (b) evidence management, (c) unexploded ordinance/safety, (d) osteology, photography, (e) GIS mapping and survey/geomorphology, and (f) heavy equipment operations (see Figure 5.1). The laboratory team should include specialists in (a) biological anthropology/forensic analysis, (b) osteological technicians, (c) IT/database applications, (d) intake/archives, (e) cultural objects analysis, (f) digital imaging, (g) radiography, (h) evidence management and (i) administration (Figure 5.2).

The logistical reality of mass grave investigation is often a scenario of information recovery in inhospitable circumstances under difficult conditions. Those responsible for mass grave creation are compelled to hide their crimes. As a consequence, mass graves are often located in remote and inaccessible areas. Furthermore, harsh climatic conditions can make the recovery teams' work even more difficult. Although this may be a familiar story for archaeologists one must consider the added security risks associated with working in recent or current war zones or otherwise anarchic locations. Once material has been recovered the project director is faced with issues of transportation, chain of custody, personnel requirements/safety and postexcavation processing. In the past, the best option was to have postexcavation processing facilities located at or near the location of the mass grave. However, safety in a combat environment, the need for specialised equipment and facilities plus proximity to an established settlement affording ready access to a variety of required supplies may preclude location of the laboratory in the field.

Logistical operations of a large-scale mass grave investigation are a considerable issue for the project director. Issues of equipment, personnel, security, living quarters

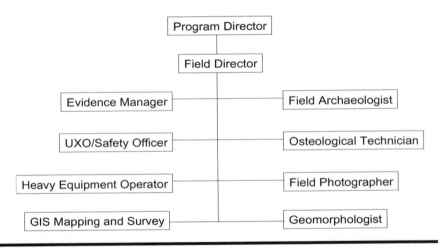

Figure 5.1
Structure and departments of the archaeological field team, Mass Graves Investigation Team 2004–2007.

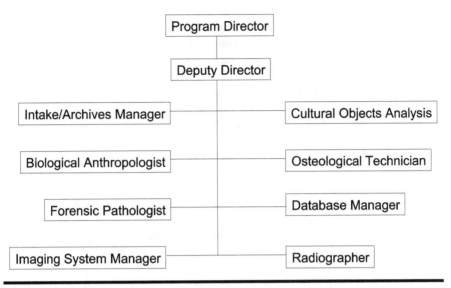

```
                    ┌──────────────────┐
                    │ Program Director │
                    └────────┬─────────┘
                    ┌────────┴─────────┐
                    │ Deputy Director  │
                    └────────┬─────────┘
┌────────────────────────┐   │   ┌─────────────────────────┐
│ Intake/Archives Manager │───┼───│ Cultural Objects Analysis │
└────────────────────────┘   │   └─────────────────────────┘
┌────────────────────────┐   │   ┌─────────────────────────┐
│ Biological Anthropologist │──┼───│ Osteological Technician  │
└────────────────────────┘   │   └─────────────────────────┘
┌────────────────────────┐   │   ┌─────────────────────────┐
│ Forensic Pathologist    │───┼───│ Database Manager         │
└────────────────────────┘   │   └─────────────────────────┘
┌────────────────────────┐   │   ┌─────────────────────────┐
│ Imaging System Manager  │───┴───│ Radiographer            │
└────────────────────────┘       └─────────────────────────┘
```

Figure 5.2

Structure and departments of the Forensic Analysis Facility, Mass Graves Investigation Team 2004–2007.

information transfer, water, meals and sanitation issues, plus many more too numerous to mention, should be handled by an individual dedicated to logistical management. Such an individual should also be proficient in handling logistical problems as they arise and be able to assist the director with day-to-day operations of all field team activities. This latter criterion could incorporate many activities from ensuring the readiness of life support areas (i.e., accommodation facilities), through to liaison with military personnel regarding transportation and security.

Haglund (2002) identifies the need for archaeologists during the excavation and recovery processes. This requirement is supported here; however, ultimately it is up to the judicial system/courts to decide how evidence can be collected and what evidence can be used by prosecutors. In addition to archaeological specialists, the field team should also include individuals capable of fulfilling various other specialised tasks.

A person skilled in the operation and maintenance of heavy equipment/machinery is vital to the excavation of large trenches needed to expose mass graves. Mass grave investigation in the context of this discussion requires the use of an excavator and, more importantly, a skilled operator. An excavator, as opposed to a backhoe, allows the operator to work in 360° space. It is also important that the machine be adequately large enough to handle large scale excavation. Work in the Iraq context required the use of a 50,000 to 80,000 lbs (22.7 to 36.3 metric tons) track excavator. In the hands of a skilled operator excellent forensic detail is recoverable with little or no damage to cultural features, forensic evidence and human remains. Excavation method principally involves use of machinery to remove overburden, a process that is closely monitored by the program and/or field director. At the first sign of cultural material, hand excavation by archaeologists commences. This process is repeated across the trench until the entire grave is exposed.

The next key subject-matter specialist required is a geographical information systems (GIS) survey manager. Through this individual a great deal of valuable forensic information can be retrieved through the use of electronic survey and GIS applications. For example, site formation processes; graphic representation (e.g., 3-D) of evidence both for written reports and court room proceedings; and standard archaeological site recording can all be achieved through computerised manipulation of survey data.

When excavators of mass graves are seeking to build a legal case, a principal concern is maintenance of evidence integrity. As a consequence, there is the need for the inclusion of a team member (evidence manager) dedicated to issues of evidence and law. The specialist in this role is mainly concerned with the maintenance of chain of custody and the safe transfer of evidence from the field to the laboratory. Chief among the tasks of this role are ensuring that the protocols of evidence sealing are followed, that chain of custody paperwork is completed, and that evidence is always secure or in the custody of a legitimate team member.

The evidence manager ensures that all field protocols are followed and that at the time of recovery both clothing and skeletal material are left intact and recovered together. The main advantages of this approach are that commingling of skeletal material is minimised; and the association between the individual set of skeletal remains and associated cultural objects (including clothing) is maintained.

On arrival at the laboratory facility (Figure 5.3), skeletal material is separated from its associated cultural objects in a controlled and secure environment. Maintenance of the relationship between the two sets of evidence is achieved through the assignment of a shared alphanumeric sequence. This sequence contains information identifying the site, evidentiary order, category and number of objects recovered within that category. At this stage in the process, cultural objects are processed in a laboratory separate to that used for processing skeletal material.

The Role of the Biological Anthropologist

As mentioned above, no specific details of the authors' experience in Iraq can be relayed here, but it is possible to discuss the operations and procedures used to process evidence, and to interpret and present the findings. Procedures related to the analysis of human remains outlined here were employed during laboratory analysis of Iraqi mass graves inspected during 2004–2006. Information and evidence recovered during this period were to be directly used in the prosecution of Saddam Hussein[1] and other regime members suspected of allowing the mass murder of Iraqi civilians.

The laboratory-based operations of the biological anthropologist focus mainly on the creation of a biological profile. That is, diagnostic characteristics of the human skeleton are assessed to form a profile of the individuals' age, sex, stature and health history. By the very nature of mass grave scenarios, it is likely that the analyst will be confronted with skeletal injuries caused at the individuals' time of death. It is therefore necessary for the biological anthropologist to be familiar with the various signs/characteristics of the different injury force types that can manifest in bone. Furthermore, interpretation of bone injury characteristics aid in the identification of event timing. In the context of a legal exercise, it is important to know when the injury was caused. Did the injury occur during the life of the individual at or around the time of death, or as a result of natural deterioration in the postmortem environment?

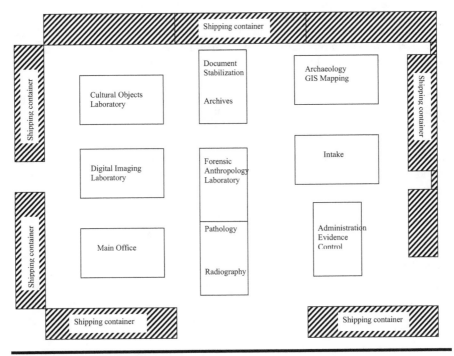

Figure 5.3

Physical layout of the Forensic Anthropology Facility compound, Mass Graves Investigation Team 2004–2007.

In addition to the standardised approach of biological anthropological analysis, the Iraq experience was coupled with a strong forensic theme. As a consequence, a great deal of emphasis was placed on chain of custody and the importance of maintaining viable evidence. This was achieved through the maintenance of tracking forms, an internal document formalising the custody of evidence and detailing individual responsibility throughout the processing and analysis procedures.

Forensic procedures used for the analysis of skeletal remains relied heavily on the standard methods for recovering biological information from the human skeleton. The widely accepted techniques of biological anthropology (see Littleton & Kinaston, Chapter 11, for a detailed discussion of such techniques) were used to determine age-at-death, sex, stature, and type and timing of injuries/pathologies. Laboratory analyses typically commenced by laying out the remains in full and correct anatomical position. This was done on stainless-steel gurney tables that allowed movement of cases around the laboratory. During this process, the analyst gained a familiarity with the particular set of remains preparing them for subsequent aspects of the analysis.

Following layout, a thorough inventory of the components was carried out recording presence and absence of elements on standardised inventory forms like those provided by Buikstra and Ubelaker (1997). Once again, this process allows the forensic analyst to familiarise themselves with the case in question. In this way it is possible to preliminarily observe or identify characteristics of age or sex and perhaps the more subtle signs of trauma. It is also during this phase of the investigation that the analyst may decide to reconstruct fragmented bone elements. On a number of occasions crania were found to be in an extensively fragmented state. Commonly, this was seen as a characteristic of the high velocity projectiles used. Therefore, in order to recover information regarding perimortem and projectile trauma it was often necessary to rebuild crania. Through this approach it was possible, in a number of cases, to identify specific details of projectile trauma including entrance and exit points. This information has significant implications with regard to modus operandi and cause/manner of death. Reconstructions of other (i.e., postcranial) bones of the skeleton provided similar results in a number of cases.

Preservation of the Iraq mass grave victims was generally very good, a factor reflective primarily of the base nature of the soil and, second, the relatively short period of time the remains were in the ground. It was suspected that the graves in question were approximately 20 years old and dated to 1987–1988 in association with the so-called *Anfal* campaign. As a consequence, forensic analysis of skeletonised material was relatively straightforward.

Sex Determination

Following completion of the inventory, a sex determination was made. Sex determination was restricted to adult individuals only, a status determined during preliminary inspection. In most cases it was possible to reliably determine the sex of an individual based on morphological features of the skeleton. These observations were reliant on published research using large samples of skeletal material of known age and sex. The sexually dimorphic characteristics of both the pelvis and crania were used where possible. This highlights once again the advantage of reconstructing fragmented skeletal elements. Vertical head diameter of humeri and femora was also routinely used to determine sex. Observations of sex were recorded on standardised forms created for this project.

Age Determination

Subadults

As with sex, age determination of the Iraq mass grave victims followed standardised methods reported in widely published literature. Principal among the reference guides used were Buikstra and Ubelaker (1994), and Scheuer and Black (2000). Due to the clear morphological differences between adults and subadults, a variety of methods were used to determine age-at-death. Generally speaking, it was possible to accurately determine age-at-death based on developmental characteristics of the skeleton. The age of subadult individuals was estimated using any or all of the following methods: dental development, dental eruption, limb bone lengths, epiphyseal appearance and union.

Adults

A variety of published methods (Buikstra & Ubelaker, 1997; Byers, 2005; White & Folkens, 2000) for the determination of age-at-death of adult skeletal material were applied during the course of Iraq mass grave analysis. The principal methods used included: pubic symphysis morphology, sternal rib end morphology, auricular surface morphology, ectocranial suture closure, tooth root opacity (Lamendin, Baccino, Hunbert, Tavernier, & Nossintchouk, 1992).

Interpretation

At the completion of case analyses, all recovered data was loaded into a Microsoft Access database. This allowed condensation of fields of data providing clearer details of trends across the entire group of mass grave victims. For example, in addition to demographic information of age and sex ratios, one is able to identify the most common forms of injuries, the most commonly affected skeletal elements, and the main cause of perimortem injury. Such information can then be used by others to interpret or infer details related to the creation of a given mass grave.

This can be illustrated through the findings of one complex of mass graves worked on by the authors. In this case, a site located in northern Iraq was found to have two mass graves within close proximity of each other (approximately 50 m apart). Despite their close proximity the graves exhibited significantly different victim profiles. One grave contained 123 individuals, all of whom were adult women or children. In fact the vast majority of individuals were aged 12 years or less at the time of death. In contrast, the second grave contained 64 individuals all of whom were adult males.

Characteristic trauma patterns exhibited by the two groups showed two interesting and very distinct mass murder events. Virtually all of the women and children in the one grave had been executed with a single gunshot injury to the back or side of the head. In contrast, nearly all of the male victims in the other grave exhibited multiple gunshot injuries in a wide variety of cranial and post cranial locations. Such distinct profiles prompt a number of questions regarding actions of the perpetrators. For example, a single bullet to the head versus multiple projectile injuries to the head and body could indicate the use of different weapons to inflict such injuries. Were the women and children executed using hand guns, while the men were sprayed with automatic gunfire? Naturally, ballistic investigation would shed further light on this question.

Similarly, a breakdown of the most commonly injured bone in the skull, combined with details of projectile trajectory, can allow inference regarding position and intent. Among the women and children the most commonly injured cranial bone was occipital with a posterior to anterior trajectory. It would be difficult not to interpret this as deliberate individual execution from a relatively close range.

Furthermore, do the different execution styles indicate a variance in the groups carrying out the murders? Can it be implied, for example, that special or secret service personnel were more likely to use a single bullet to the head, whereas multiple injuries were caused by regular army personnel (or, automatic weapons were the pre-ferred choice of regular army personnel)? And, what does the difference between execution styles say regarding the motives of the perpetrators? Can the multiple injuries inflicted on the men be interpreted as a more spiteful approach to the given task? Were the perpetrators intent on terrorising their male victims before finally killing them, whereas a more methodical and less vindictive method was used to eliminate the women and children? It is also possible to suggest that the two distinct methods could represent a variance in the timing of the two events.

Another interesting inference to come from the condensed data of the men's trench included the observation of a high frequency of projectile injuries to the posterior knee. This was thought by analysts to represent a deliberate tactic by perpetrators to disable the victims before inflicting the final volley of machinegun fire. It is necessary to emphasise, however, that it is not the role of the biological anthropologist to provide or make such inferences or ask such questions. Furthermore, it is not up to the biological anthropologist to make claims or statements as to the ultimate fate of mass grave victims and the cause of death of individuals. That is, the biological anthropologist may present the findings of their observations for age, sex and trauma, but may not make comment on cause of death or the intent/actions of perpetrators. These are the duties of other specialists. A qualified forensic pathologist is able to legally 'sign off' on cause of death and is an integral part of the mass grave investigation. Speculation regarding the findings of forensic analysis of skeletal material is a matter for lawyers and in association with other evidence and research, aids in their reconstruction of mass murder events.

In order to strengthen the findings of forensic skeletal analysis, a peer review system is recommended. With the inclusion of a system for formal review of the findings of forensic analysis an added degree of robustness is added to the body of work. This in turn creates a greater level of information reliability that is more likely to stand up to external testing and cross examination. In the Iraq instance, two peer reviews of each case were required. The principal aims of the review were to identify any conspicuous errors made by the analyst. However, in the situation where each page is considered to be a legal document, peer reviewers additionally checked for signatures, correct dates and any other errors that may detract from the documents validity. Peer reviews were generally conducted immediately after completion of the analysis in an attempt to reduce over handling of skeletal material.

Conclusions

The role of biological and cultural anthropologists in mass grave examination is to analyse human skeletal remains and associated grave goods/evidence, in the context of a forensic investigation. The application of traditional methods remains the same; however, established procedures and protocols must be maintained in order to preserve crime scene and evidence integrity. In the end, strict adherence to legally acceptable procedures and sound scientific analysis, enable subject matter experts to document in an impartial and responsible way evidence associated with mass murders and genocide.

Endnote

1   On the 30th December 2006 at around 6.00 a.m., Saddam Hussein was executed, by hanging, in Baghdad, Iraq.

References

Buikstra, J.E., & Ubelaker, D.H. (Eds.). (1997). *Standard for data collection from human skeletal remains* (Arkansas Archaeological Survey Research Series No. 44). Fayetteville, AR: Arkansas Archaeological Survey.

Byers, S.N. (2005). *Forensic anthropology laboratory manual*. Boston: Pearson, Allyn and Bacon.

Haglund, W.D. (2002). Recent mass graves, an introduction. In W.D. Haglund & M.H. Sorg (Eds). *Advances in forensic taphonomy* (pp. 243–261). Boca Raton, FL: CRC Press.

Lamendin, H., Baccino, E., Hunbert, J.F., Tavernier, J.C., Nossintchouk, R.M., & Zerilli, A. (1992). A simple technique for age estimation in adult corpses: The two criteria dental method. *Journal of Forensic Science 37*, 1373–1379.

Scheuer, J.L., & Black, S.M. (2000). *Developmental juvenile osteology*. London: Academic Press.

White, T.D., & Folkens, P.A. (2000). *Human osteology*. San Diego: Academic Press.

Human, Sheep or Kangaroo: A Practical Guide to Identifying Human Skeletal Remains in Australia

Marc Oxenham

Richard Barwick

One of the most common questions asked of a forensic anthropologist is: human or not? From experience the answer is generally in the negative, with the remains more often than not belonging to a sheep or kangaroo or similarly sized domestic or indigenous animal (Croker & Donlon, 2006). The main aim of this chapter is to provide a practical illustrated guide to differentiating between human and nonhuman skeletal remains. As most of the difficulty tends to centre on the similarity between human bones and those of similarly sized animals the authors have selected two animals with similarly sized, and arguably similarly shaped, bones to compare and contrast with those of an adult human. Space constraints have necessitated a number of sacrifices, the first being that the comparisons are limited to the main adult bones of a human, kangaroo, and sheep. Subadult (juvenile) bones are not dealt with here, and if you suspect the presence of such bones in an assemblage or at a crime scene you should refer to a specialist osteologist. Subadult bones, whether human or nonhuman, can be easily distinguished by the lack of fusion, or partial, fusion of their epiphyses (the joint surfaces at either end of a long bone for instance). When the epiphysis of a bone has not fused to the main body of the bone the region of nonfusion appears uneven and billowed in appearance. We have excluded detailed illustrations of the skulls of our comparative sample, although the basic morphology of each can be seen in Figures 6.1, 6.2 and 6.3. Finally, only the larger bones have been illustrated and described in this guide due to the difficulties in differentiating between many of the smaller bones; finger, toe and rib bones for instance.

Our presentation method has been to illustrate the basic bony anatomy of a human, sheep or kangaroo by preparing a series of figures (drawn by Richard Barwick) that illustrate the key features of each bone. It is appreciated that many people will not have the time or inclination to learn technical anatomical or positional terms. However, it is necessary to use some, albeit limited, technical terms if only for the sake of brevity of descriptions. All such terms are labelled on the appropriate illustration and mentioned in the accompanying text. It is also a convention in anatomy and osteology texts to use terms that specify the relative orientation of the bone or body part of interest. For our purposes we believe it is sufficient for someone using this guide in the field to orient their unknown bone in a way that approximates the orientation of the illustration of interest. For those readers with familiarity in standard anatomical positioning, the vast majority of illustrations are rendered with an anterior (front), posterior (back) and/or lateral/medial (side) view with the superior (top) portion of the bone to the top of the illustration.

In using this guide there is also the assumption that you are dealing with a single individual and with relatively complete (rather than fragmentary) material. Nonetheless, even when dealing with a large pile of bones it is assumed that only human bones are of interest. The discovery of a single bone that appears to be human should be cause enough to contact the police and have a specialist examine the material. Before attempting to identify your unknown bone(s) it is advised that the first three figures (of a complete articulated human, kangaroo and sheep skeleton) and their accompanying explanatory text are reviewed. Differences in the proportions of limb bones can be important in identifying a skeleton. For instance, kangaroos can have leg bones of a similar size to humans but with relatively small forelimbs (arms). As a final word of caution, illustrations are not reproduced at natural size nor are the bones in each illustration drawn to relative size. The lower case 'reb' in the following illustrations is Richard's signature.

.

Plate 6.1

Articulated human skeleton (*Homo sapiens*). Anatomical position (viewed from the front). Main bones illustrated and described below are labelled. Note that the arm bones (humerus, radius and ulna) are a little shorter than those of the leg. Compare this to the marked difference in the upper and lower limbs of a kangaroo (Plate 6.2). The femur (thigh) is the largest and most robust bone in the human skeleton.

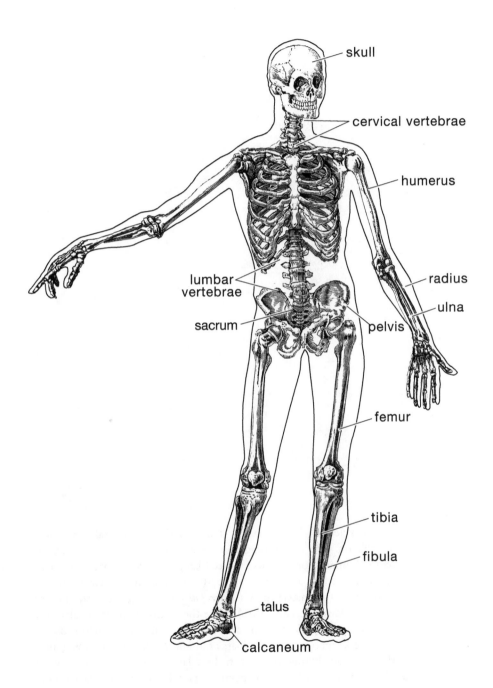

skull

cervical vertebrae

humerus

radius

ulna

lumbar vertebrae

sacrum

pelvis

femur

tibia

fibula

talus

calcaneum

Plate 6.2

Articulated kangaroo skeleton (*Macropus sp.*). This is a side (or lateral) view of a generic kangaroo skeleton. The larger kangaroo species can stand taller and weigh more than an average human. For instance, the red kangaroo (Macropus rufus) can reach a standing height of 1.8 m and weigh up to 90 kg, while the kangaroo used in the following illustrations, the eastern gray (*Macropus giganteus*), is a little shorter but of a similar weight (Dewey & Yue, 2001). Note the relatively much smaller arm bones (although those of a large kangaroo can be as big if not larger than those in an adult human) in the kangaroo (see also Plates 6.6 and 6.7). It is the tibia (shin, see Plate 6.12) that is relatively much longer in these large kangaroos and can even be much longer than a human's tibia. Apart from the fact that kangaroos have caudal (tail) vertebrae, the other chief difference to a human skeleton is in the shape of the kangaroo pelvis (see Plate 6.9).

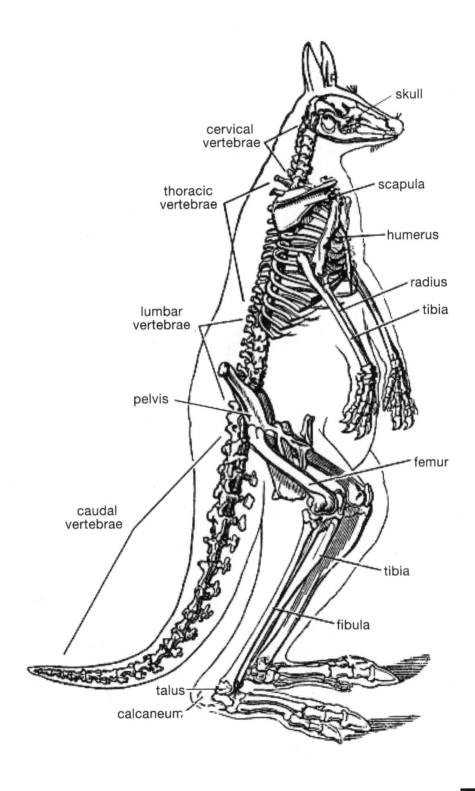

skull

cervical vertebrae

thoracic vertebrae

lumbar vertebrae

pelvis

caudal vertebrae

scapula

humerus

radius

tibia

femur

tibia

fibula

talus

calcaneum

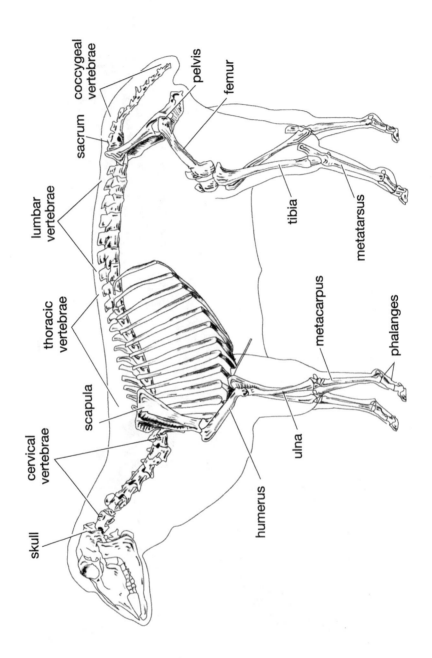

Plate 6.3

Articulated sheep skeleton (*Ovis sp.*). This is a side (or lateral) view of a generic sheep skeleton. The most common species of domestic sheep is *Ovis aries,* of which there are over 200 breeds. Such sheep can grow up to 1.8 m long, 1.27 m high at the shoulder and weigh up to 200 kg (Reavill, 2000). As seen with humans, the fore-limbs are slightly shorter than the hind limbs, but not to the same extent as that seen in kangaroos. Sheep also have caudal (or coccygeal) vertebrae and while their pelvis can be easily confused with that of a kangaroo, it is very different from the pelvis of a human (see Plate 6.9). Sheep, like kangaroos, have specialised and much enlarged metacarpal (hand) and metatarsal (toe) bones that, while they may be confused between these two animals, are very distinct from those seen in humans. It is also worth noting that the skeleton and individual postcranial bones (all bones excluding the skull and jaw) of the cow (apart from its larger size), and also the pig for that matter, are quite similar to those of the sheep.

Plate 6.4

Scapula (shoulder blade). Left side shown: all views from the rear of a human, kangaroo and sheep. The hollowed out region (glenoid fossa, to the top of the illustrations) is for articulation with the humerus (forming the shoulder joint). Opposite the glenoid fossa is the spinal border of the scapula. The human scapula is distinct in having a very elongated shape (the spinal border extends well below the spine), a quite concave inferior (lower) border and a very prominent acromion process that sweeps forward and forms an 'L' shape when looked at from above (the acromion is an extension of the scapula spine). The kangaroo has some superficial similarities to the human scapula including a pronounced acromion, although it does not have the forward projection seen in humans. The scapula of the sheep is very triangular in comparison, roughly divided in half by the spine, has a distinct neck below the glenoid fossa, and has virtually no expression of the acromion (the spine ends abruptly at the neck). Both the sheep and kangaroo scapulae can be placed flat on a table while the human scapula cannot due to the presence of a hook-like process called the coracoid process; a feature absent in both the kangaroo and sheep.

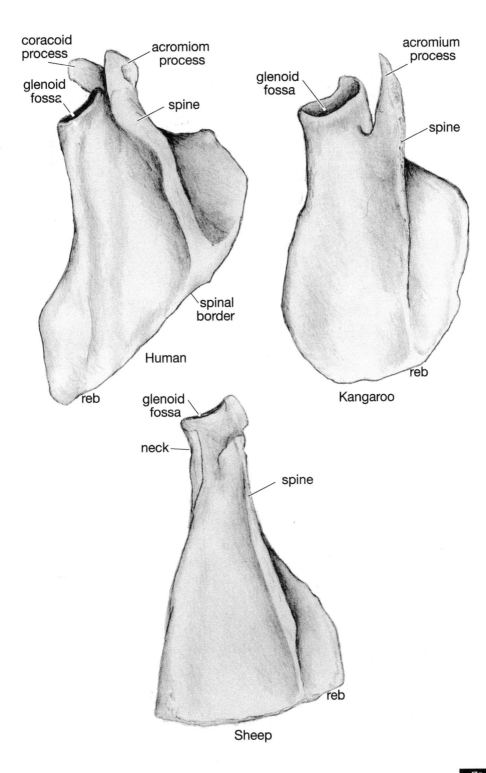

coracoid process

acromiom process

glenoid fossa

spine

spinal border

Human

reb

acromium process

glenoid fossa

spine

reb

Kangaroo

glenoid fossa

neck

spine

reb

Sheep

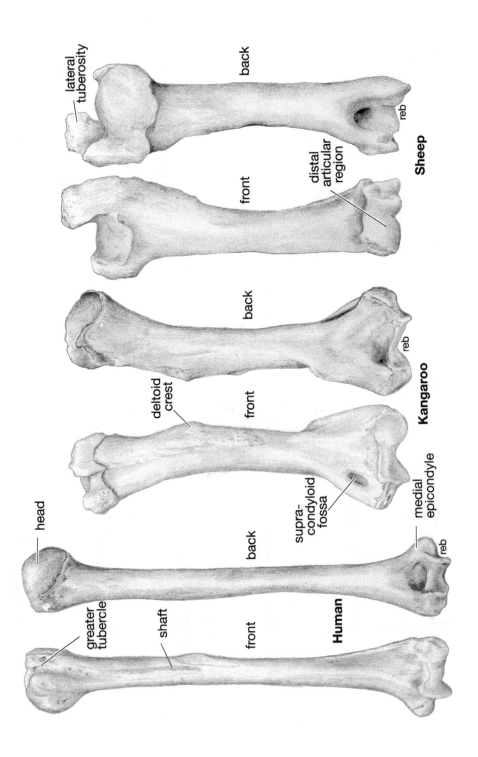

Plate 6.5

Humerus (upper arm). Left side shown: front and rear of a human, kangaroo and sheep. In differentiating between the three the human humerus is much larger than the sheep. The important anatomical features of the human humerus (with counterparts variously expressed and named in the other animals) to note are the head (forms part of the shoulder joint), greater tubercle, medial epicondyle (a side facing projection on the lower portion of the bone) and the lower (distal) articular region. The human humerus is relatively long and thin in comparison to the sheep and kangaroo. In the human and kangaroo humerus there is little difference between the height of the head (for the shoulder joint) and the greater tubercle. In the sheep the (lateral) tuberosity (equivalent to the human greater tubercle) is very pronounced and extends considerably above the head. The lower (distal) articular region of the sheep humerus (elbow) is very narrow from side to side in comparison to both humans and kangaroos. The lower end of the human and kangaroo humerus are both relatively wide and have prominent medial (inner side) prominences (epicondyles). The kangaroo humerus has a very distinctive raised ridge or sharp crest (the deltoid crest) running down the anterior (front) of the shaft. In the human humerus there is a blunt and slightly raised area on the lateral (side) of the shaft that marks the insertion of the deltoid muscle. A subadult kangaroo humerus with unfused epiphyses (upper and lower articular ends) may be confused with a human child's humerus, although the prominent supracondyloid foramen in the kangaroo humerus will help in correct identification.

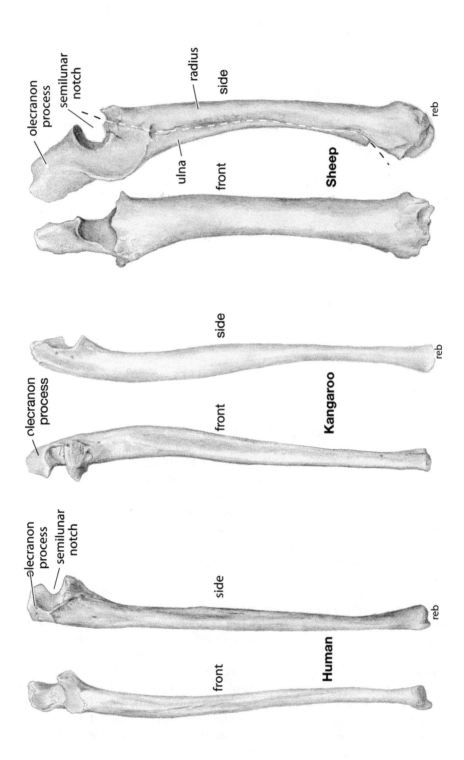

Plate 6.6

Ulna (forearm bone). Left side shown: front and side of a human, kangaroo and sheep. The important feature to note with the human ulna is that it has a low (non-projecting) olecranon process (tuberosity or blunt projection of bone on top of the ulna that you can feel as the hard bony part of your elbow) that does not extend very far above the upper most part of the lunar notch. This is in marked contrast to the prominent olecranon processes of the kangaroo and, particularly, the sheep. The shaft of the human ulna is triangular in cross-section while that of the kangaroo is quite flat from side to side (blade-like). The ulna and radius of the sheep are fused (see labels in the illustration pointing to the ulna and radius portions of this fused bone) and if the ulna is found separated, usually only the top third will be present or easily identifiable. The ulna of the sheep is so compressed from side to side as to appear blade-like.

Plate 6.7

Radius (forearm bone). Left side shown: front and rear of a human and kangaroo. The radius (fused with the ulna) of the sheep is illustrated in Plate 6.6. The kangaroo radius is quite similar to the human form and the two could easily be confused. In differentiating between the two the shaft of the kangaroo radius is more curved, the neck is not as pronounced as in the human and the lower (distal) end of the bone does not flare out as much as in the human radius which has a significant side to side (mediolateral) flare. The sheep radius is relatively flat anteroposteriorly (front to back) and relatively broad mediolaterally (from side to side) for the length of the shaft and appears somewhat squat in comparison to the human radius. The sheep radius does not have the distinctive radial tuberosity (for the biceps muscle) seen in the kangaroo and human radii.

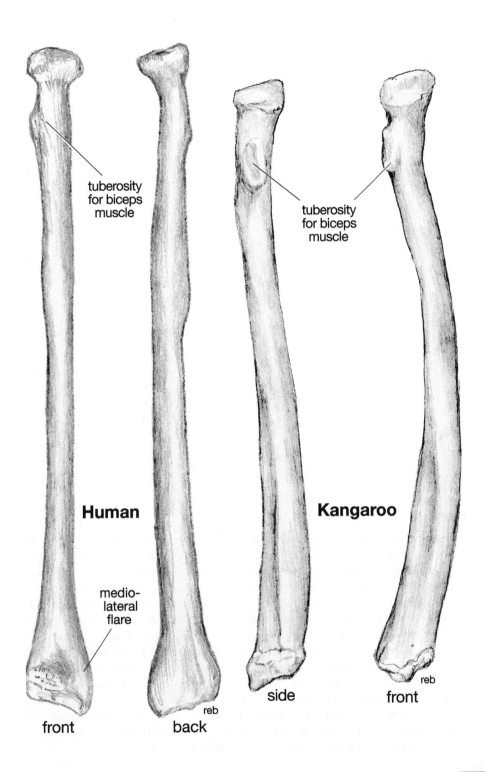

tuberosity
for biceps
muscle

tuberosity
for biceps
muscle

Human

Kangaroo

medio-
lateral
flare

front

back

reb

side

front

reb

Plate 6.8

Vertebrae (back bones). Three types of human vertebrae are illustrated (cervical, thoracic and lumbar) in top (dorsal), side and bottom (ventral) views. For comparison an example of a kangaroo and sheep thoracic vertebra is illustrated in a front to side (anterolateral) view as well as a sheep lumbar vertebra viewed from the front and rear. To anyone with little experience with bones the vertebrae may be quite challenging. However, there are distinctive features of the sheep and kangaroo vertebrae that can be used to differentiate them from human bones. Regardless of which vertebra is examined, human vertebrae tend to have blunter, thicker and shorter projections (the various transverse and spinous processes) and the vertebral body tends to be lower and wider than those seen in sheep and kangaroos. The transverse processes of the kangaroo vertebrae have a distinctive upward hook that looks something like a pair of horns. The thoracic vertebrae of the sheep have very pronounced and extended spinous processes and very short blunt transverse processes. The lumbar vertebra of the sheep has very pronounced, extended and straight transverse process.

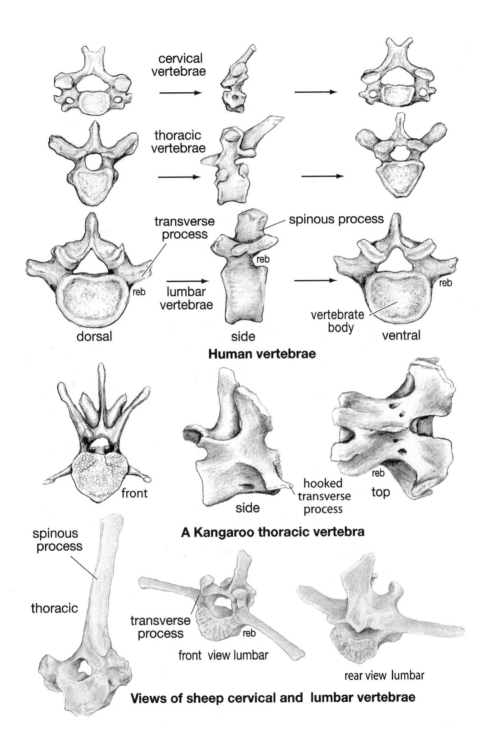

cervical
vertebrae

thoracic
vertebrae

transverse
process

spinous process

reb

lumbar
vertebrae

reb

vertebrate
body

dorsal

side

ventral

Human vertebrae

front

side

hooked
transverse
process

reb

top

A Kangaroo thoracic vertebra

spinous
process

thoracic

transverse
process

reb

front view lumbar

rear view lumbar

Views of sheep cervical and lumbar vertebrae

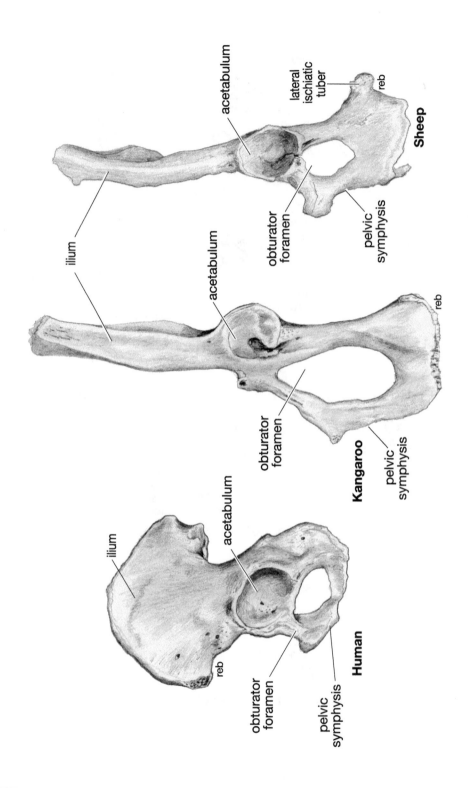

Plate 6.9

Os coxae (pelvis). Lateral or side view of left bone of a human, kangaroo and sheep. The human pelvic bone is very distinctive in comparison with the kangaroo and sheep which are superficially quite similar in appearance to each other. The human pelvis has a very broad fan-like upper (ilium) portion in comparison to the kangaroo which resembles a narrow triangular column-like structure. The iliac portion in the sheep is intermediate between the human and kangaroo in having a distinctive flaring from front to back. The lower, rear portion of the sheep os coxae is distinctive in displaying strong lateral hook-like projections (lateral ischiatic tubers). The lower part of the sheep and kangaroo pelvis extends far below the hip socket (acetabulum) creating a large elongated opening (obturator foramen). In humans the obturator foramen is squashed from top to bottom. The two sides of the pelvis are fused along a very long pubic symphysis in both the kangaroo and sheep. The two sides of the human pelvis also join (in life) by way of cartilage at the sacrum and in the pubic area but will normally be seen as separate bones in dry skeletal remains.

Plate 6.10

The sacrum is situated between the two pelvic bones and a rear view of a human, kangaroo and sheep is shown. The human sacrum is a squat, broad (at the top) triangular bone made up of 4 to 6 (usually 5) fused segments that ends in a small blunt point where the vestigial tail (coccyx) is attached. Along the rear of the human sacrum are a series of short, blunt raised projections and/or a slightly raised ridge of bone called the median crest. In the kangaroo the sacrum is superficially similar to the sheep and the number of fused segments is variable. The spinous processes of the fused segments are very prominent and sharp along the median crest. The sacrum in the sheep is made of 4 segments that can show varying levels of fusion or nonfusion. The sacrum is narrower than in the human and the median spine (on the rear) tends to project much more and is rather sharp.

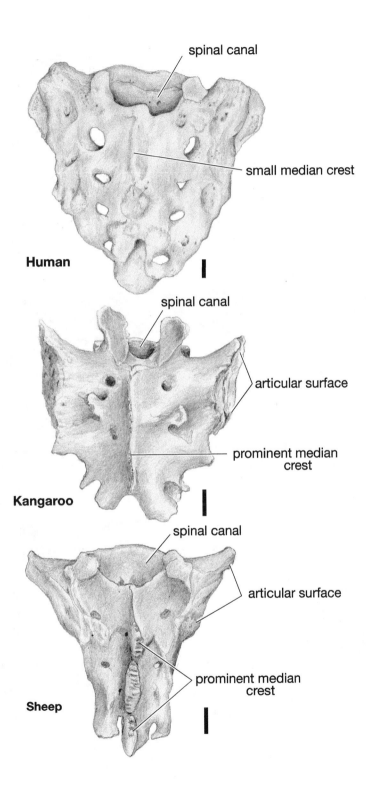

spinal canal

small median crest

Human

spinal canal

articular surface

prominent median crest

Kangaroo

spinal canal

articular surface

prominent median crest

Sheep

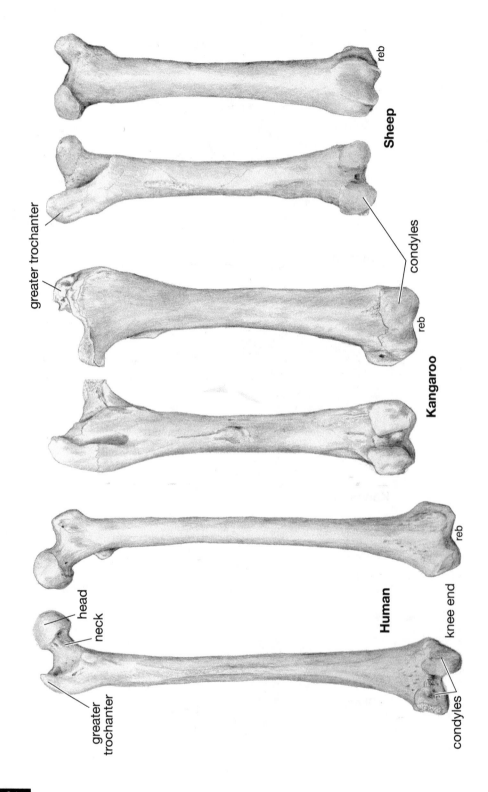

Plate 6.11

Femur (thigh bone). Left side shown: front and rear of a human, kangaroo and sheep. The human femur is a very large bone, much longer than that seen in sheep and kangaroos. The sheep and kangaroo femur are superficially similar and characterised by a femoral head (for the hip articulation) that is markedly lower than the upward projection of the greater trochanter. The human femur is distinctive in having a ball-like femoral head and a very pronounced and relatively narrow neck on which the femoral head is attached. The lower end (distal or knee) of the human femur is again distinctive in flaring out to form relatively large articular condyles. The lower end of the kangaroo and sheep are relatively quite narrow (from side to side).

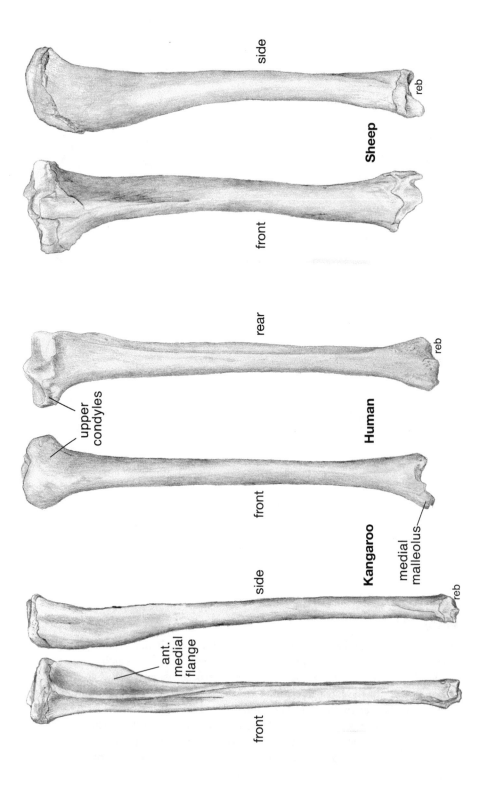

side

reb

Sheep

front

rear

reb

upper
condyles

Human

front

Kangaroo

side

medial
malleolus

reb

ant.
medial
flange

front

reb

86

Plate 6.12

Tibia (shin). Left side shown: front and rear of a human, kangaroo and sheep. The tibia of one of the large kangaroos can be longer than that of a human, but differs in being roughly circular in cross-section for much of its lower half and is wedged-shaped or triangular in the upper half. The kangaroo tibia also displays a very pronounced and extremely mediolaterally (side to side) compressed ridge (labelled as the anterior tibial flange) that projects from the front and top of the shaft. In contrast, the human, and also sheep to a degree, tibia does not appear as narrow and is more triangular in cross-section for most of its length. The upper condyles of the human tibia (part of the knee joint) are relatively much larger and more rounded in outline than those of either the sheep or kangaroo. The distal (lower) end of the human tibia is simpler than that of the sheep, although similar to the kangaroo, in being relatively flat or convex with one prominent downward projection called the medial malleolus (forms the bony bump on the inside of your ankle).

Plate 6.13

Fibula. Left side shown: front and rear of a human and kangaroo. The fibula is a long thin bone that runs parallel to the outside of the tibia and its distal (lower) end forms the outer bony bump of the ankle (lateral malleolus). Only the upper (fused to the tibia and present as a small tuberosity) and lower extremities (unfused) of the fibula are present in the sheep. The fibula of the kangaroo is very long and thin with the upper (bulbous head) and lower (flaring, front to back) extremities superficially similar to a human's. In distinguishing between the two, the shaft of the human fibula is triangular in cross-section for much of its length and is relatively quite broad anteroposteriorly (front to back). The shaft of the kangaroo fibula is relatively much thinner and narrower with the top half of the shaft being somewhat semi-circular in cross-section and the lower half being very thin and blade-like, albeit quite concave on the medial (inner) side.

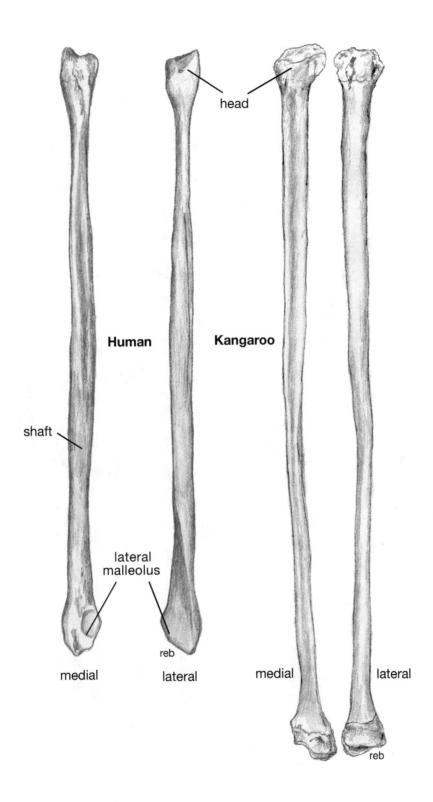

Human **Kangaroo**

head

shaft

lateral
malleolus

reb

medial   lateral   medial   lateral

reb

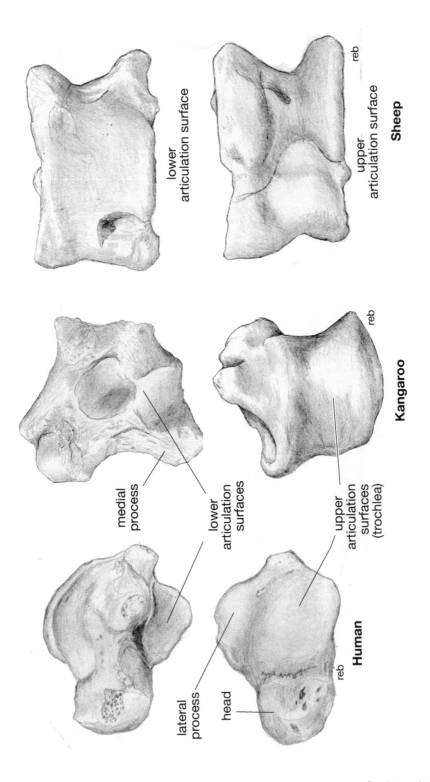

Sheep

lower articulation surface

upper articulation surface

reb

Kangaroo

medial process

lower articulation surfaces

upper articulation surfaces (trochlea)

reb

Human

lateral process

head

reb

Plate 6.14

Talus or astragalus (foot bone). Left side shown: upper and lower aspects of a human, kangaroo and sheep. The human talus (or astragalus) is distinct in having a large prominent trochlea (articular area for the bottom of the tibia) as well as a distinct head at the front of the bone. The kangaroo talus is superficially similar to the human talus, but it has a prominent medial projection (medial process) as opposed to the prominent lateral projection (lateral process) seen in the human. Further, the kangaroo talus lacks the head seen in the human talus. The sheep talus is different again and is distinct in being shaped like a 'knuckle bone' used in the children's game of the same name. The sheep talus is relatively rectangular in shape with distinct rounded and grooved articular areas on each end (trochlea).

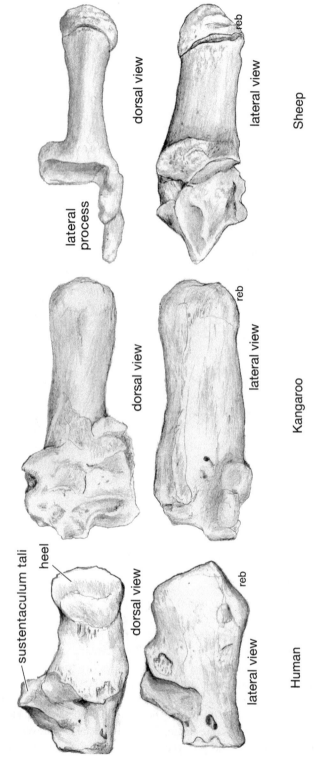

Plate 6.15

Calcaneus (foot bone). Left side shown: top and side (lateral) of human, kangaroo and sheep. The human calcaneus (which forms the bony part of the heel) is roughly rectangular with a very prominent medial (inner side) projection anteriorly called the sustentaculum tali. The kangaroo calcaneus is narrower and has bony projections on both sides (lateral and medial) towards the front of the bone. The sheep calcaneus is distinctive in having a very marked, blade-like projection anteriorly (toward the front) on the lateral (outer) side which is labelled the lateral process here.

References

Croker, S., & Donlon, D. (2006, April). *Human or non-human: Possible methods for the identification of bone fragments.* Poster presented at Conference Proceedings of the 18th International Symposium of the Forensic Sciences, Fremantle, Australia.

Dewey, T., & Yue, M. (2001). *Macropus rufus* (Online), Animal Diversity Web. Available at http://animaldiversity.ummz.umich.edu/site/accounts/information/Macropus_rufus.html.

Reavill, C. (2000). *Ovis aries* (Online), Animal Diversity Web. Available at http://animaldiversity.ummz.umich.edu/site/accounts/information/Ovis_aries.html

2

Techniques of Human Identification

Forensic Anthropology in Australia: A Brief History and Review of Casework

Denise Donlon

While forensic anthropology has been practiced as a sideline by many anatomists and anthropologists in Australia for many years, it is now on the cusp of being recognised as a discipline in its own right. As well as dealing with the 'normal forensic cases', that is, those that probably involve a suspicious death, forensic anthropology in Australia also includes the investigation of suspected Indigenous remains and, increasingly, the investigation of those killed in wars and in terrorist actions, both within Australia and offshore.

This chapter provides a brief outline of the history of forensic anthropology in Australia, as it has been dealt with in more detail elsewhere (Donlon, in press), followed by comments on the present role of the forensic anthropologist in forensic approaches to death and disaster. Also described are examples of casework to illustrate historical aspects of forensic anthropology, as well as recent forensic cases, World War II war dead and mass disasters. Suggestions for future areas of research in forensic anthropology in Australia will be discussed.

History

The history of forensic anthropology in Australia is short and the development slow. Forensic anthropology in Australia, as in the United States, has its roots in the anatomical sciences. Throughout Australia, anatomists were called on by coroners and the police to give opinions of the identification of skeletonised remains. These very early anatomists were Neil Macintosh (Elkin, 1978; Macintosh, 1952, 1965, 1972) and Stan Larnach (Larnach & Freedman, 1964; Larnach & Macintosh, 1967, 1970; Oettle & Larnach, 1974) of the University of Sydney, Les Ray at the University of Melbourne (Ray, 1959), Fredrick Wood Jones (1931) and Andrew Arthur Abbie (1976) of the University of Adelaide, David Allbrook (1961) and Len Freedman (1964) of the University of Western Australia and Walter Wood of the University of Queensland (Wood, 1968, 1993; Wood, Briggs, & Donlon, 2002).

These anatomists shared a common interest in the osteology of the Australian Aborigines. They also had access to large collections of (mainly) Aboriginal skeletal remains for research and the training of students. Some students of these anatomists became forensic anthropologists and many of them are currently training students. There are currently many university courses available in forensic science, although not so many in forensic anthropology. This may be because of the lack of resources (i.e., skeletal collections) necessary for training in this discipline. Aboriginal remains that were once used by the anatomists are being repatriated from museums or are difficult to gain access to (Donlon, 1994). There is also a lack of collections of non-Aboriginal skeletal remains in Australia and so we depend on research on those assemblages from the United States as they include large collections of Caucasoids (Iscan, 1988).

Many American anthropologists have benefited from the experience of identifying the war dead following their repatriation to the United States (Joint POW/MIA Accounting Command, JPAC). These skeletonised remains are often examined by physical anthropologists for the purpose of identification, but in addition, much research has been carried out on those remains as they are of known age, ancestry, sex and stature thus providing an excellent source of data for forensic research (e.g., McKern & Stewart, 1957; Trotter & Gleser, 1958). Australian legislation, on the other hand, has meant that identification and reburial of their war dead of World Wars I and II were all made in the theatre of war in which they died. Since the Vietnam War all Australian war dead have been repatriated. Anthropologists in Australia have been involved in the identification of Australians involved in terrorist acts, such as the Bali Bombing. The associated Australian deaths have resulted in the production of the Australasian Disaster Victim Identification (DVI) Procedures (*Australasian DVI Standards Manual*, 2004) by a combination of Australian government agencies. It includes protocols for anthropologists (Buck, 2004) in the specialist team in the mortuary.

Of importance for the growth of forensic anthropology in Australia has been an increasing representation of practitioners at conferences of forensic associations since the late 1990s. There are three main associations to which those practicing forensic anthropology belong: The Australian Academy of Forensic Science (AAFS), The Australian and New Zealand Forensic Science Society (ANZFSS) and The Australasian Society for Human Biology (ASHB).

The AAFS, formed in 1967, includes lawyers, medical practitioners, scientists, sociologists, police officers and government officials. Today the academy publishes a journal entitled *Australian Forensic Science*. They do not hold a conference but do hold a few lectures per year. The ANZFSS was formed in 1971 with the aim of bringing together scientists, police, criminalists, pathologists, and members of the legal profession actively involved with the forensic sciences. The society's objectives are to enhance the quality of forensic science providing symposia and lectures encompassing the various disciplines within the science (ANZFSS, n.d.). The first symposium to include a session on forensic anthropology was in Sydney in 1996 when American anthropologists William Bass and Diane France were invited keynote speakers. All symposia since (except for 2002 in Canberra) have held an anthropology session with the most recent symposium in Fremantle in April 2006 holding the largest session yet (ANZFSS, 2006). The ASHB has some forensic anthropologists as members but they are primarily biological anthropologists. It was formed in 1996 by Charles Oxnard, then head of the School of Human Biology at the University of Western Australia. However, it is a very small society of around a few hundred members and it is only in the last three or four years that forensic sessions have been included in their conferences (e.g., *Proceedings*, 2005).

Unlike the United States (see Reichs, 1998), Australia does not have a truly professional organisation for forensic scientists. Neither does it have 'Sections' within the forensic organisations devoted to specific disciplines of forensic science, nor a Board of Forensic Anthropology, as does the United States. The American Board collects data on casework done in the United States, providing a nice overview of the state of the discipline in the United States (Reichs, 1998).

Few full-time forensic anthropologists are employed in Australia, with approximately one per state or territory (Donlon, in press). A few are employed on a full-time or part-time basis in institutions of forensic medicine or with the police and most remain strongly linked with university departments of anatomy.

Casework

Casework in Australia is normally done in close association with forensic pathologists and forensic dentists. The forensic anthropologist may thus be involved in the assessment of trauma and determination of time of death as well as identification. Some anthropologists are also trained in archaeology and may be involved in the search and recovery of the dead. This combination of training makes them well placed in disaster victim identification.

I now present a summary of 15 years of casework in the state of New South Wales. The purpose of this summary is to attempt to throw light on any trends that may be occurring in the discipline, on the assumption that NSW reflects the situation of the country as a whole. While New South Wales is the fifth largest state in Australia, it is the most heavily populated state with almost 7 million people. The following aspects of casework will be examined: caseload, the type of agency that commissioned the work, the geographic source of the casework, a breakdown of the nature of the cases, condition of the remains and appearances in court.

All of the cases in this survey were examined by myself and took place mainly at two institutions in Sydney, the capital of New South Wales: the NSW Department of Forensic Medicine in Glebe and the Department of Forensic Medicine in Westmead. A few were examined at country mortuaries attached to hospitals in New South Wales and interstate, while a few were examined in neighbouring countries such as Indonesia and Papua New Guinea. All cases from 1992 to 2006 inclusive were chosen, as I have been doing casework in New South Wales for this period of time. A few cases have been done by other anthropologists and archaeologists in country areas. These have not been included in this survey. Also not included were nonhuman cases, but not because they were few — quite the contrary. In many of such nonhuman cases no records have been kept. In forensic institutions, the pathologist is often able to distinguish nonhuman from human bone if the bones are reasonably complete. The most commonly mistaken bones for human bones in New South Wales are those of sheep and kangaroo (Croker & Donlon, 2006; see also Oxenham and Barwick, Chapter 6).

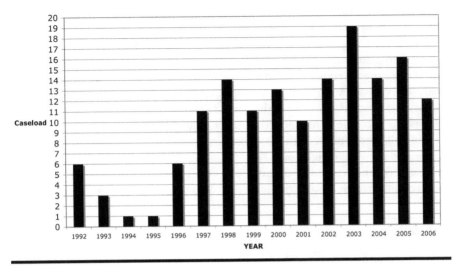

Figure 7.1
Forensic anthropology caseload in NSW over 15 years.

Caseload

In New South Wales the number of cases investigated has increased steadily over the last 15 years (Figure 7.1). The total number is 153 cases. This increase is probably more a reflection of the increasing value seen in the contribution of the forensic anthropologist than in other factors such as a possible increase in murder rate. In the last 10 years in New South Wales the murder rate has actually decreased, with an average annual percentage change of –1.2% (NSW Bureau of Crime Statistics, n.d.). The caseload is small (an average of 10 per year) and can easily be completed by one anthropologist on a contract basis. Another factor probably contributing to the increase in caseload is the increasing use of the anthropologists in cases of recovery of the war dead and in mass disasters.

Case Study: Possum Brush

A typical case, in some respects but not in others, was that of case number 87/1223. In 1987 skeletonised remains were found in the bushland near Possum Brush on the mid-north coast of New South Wales. Most of the long bones, pectoral girdle, pelvic girdle and vertebral column were represented, while most of the bones of the hands and feet were absent. The skull was complete except for one missing tooth. An unusual feature was a button osteoma located on the frontal bone near the coronal suture. However, this would most likely have been hidden behind the hairline and so could not be used in identification. Associated with the skeleton were jewellery and women's clothing; nevertheless the bones were initially identified by a pathologist as that of a male transvestite. This was probably because of the poor condition of the pelvis and the rather robust nature of the skull and large, deep palate. In 1998 with a pathologist I examined the remains and we concluded they were female, aged 20 years to 30 years old when she died and 154 cm to 162 cm in height (Donlon, 1999). DNA analysis later confirmed these

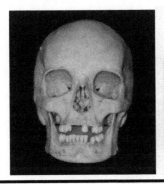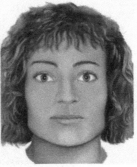

Figure 7.2
The skull, reconstruction and photograph of the woman found at Possum Brush.

remains were those of a female. She also had a possible perimortem fracture to the side to the cranium. A computerised facial image was produced (thought worthwhile because of the hair preserved with the body) and widely publicised (Figure 7.2). In 2003 a relative came forward after reading the police missing person's website and in 2004 a DNA match was made. This young woman was 22 years old when she disappeared. This case unfortunately took 17 years to identify because of the mistaken sex determination.

Type of Agency Requesting the Work

The agency most commonly requesting the services of a forensic anthropologist is the Coroner's Office and its associated Department of Forensic Medicine (64%) (Figure 7.3). In most cases a forensic pathologist would contact the anthropologist to ask for a report on the bones, which have already been delivered to the forensic institution by the police. They may arrive skeletonised, burned or in the process of decomposing. Reporting usually includes an inventory, description of the condition and completeness of the bones, the ancestry, sex, age and height. Any features that might assist in identification, such as healed fractures or unusual nonmetric variants are also included.

The next largest agency requesting work is that of the police at 18% of cases. Requests directly from the police mainly involve the search for and recovery of remains, including excavation and exhumation from cemeteries. Police are also increasingly requesting the anthropologist (often in conjunction with a forensic odontologist) to assist in facial recognition cases. Requests from the Australian Defence Forces make up only 7% of cases and include excavation and recovery and identification of those missing in action from World War II in Papua New Guinea and Christmas Island and those killed as a result of accidents while assisting victims of mass disasters in Indonesia, such as Nias Island near Sumatra. The ADF employs its own forensic anthropologist who is a reservist in the RAAF.

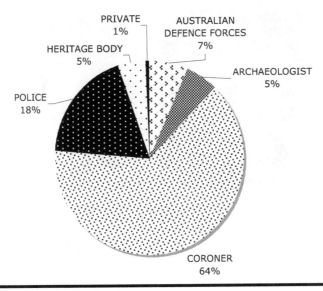

Figure 7.3
Type of agency commissioning cases in NSW over the 15 year period (1992–2006).

Archaeologists and heritage bodies such as the Department of Environment and Conservation each make up 5% of requests and almost all of these cases involve the recovery, excavation and/or identification of prehistoric Aboriginal remains. In very rare cases (1%) a private institution requires the services of an anthropologist — usually in the recovery of prehistoric Aboriginal remains.

In NSW, and in some other Australian states, it is not always clear which legislation applies when skeletal remains are found. Problems occur because of the difficulty of determining time elapsed since death of some remains. The two heritage bodies that deal with prehistoric (Department of Environment and Conservation) and historic cases (The Heritage Office of NSW) each have guidelines on how to manage such remains (Bickford et al., 1999; Thorne & Ross, 1986). The following case study illustrates some of the problems and overlap in agencies involved in the discovery of skeletal remains in New South Wales.

Case Study: Aboriginal Remains in the Eastern Suburbs of Sydney

In 2003 a construction worker using a backhoe found human bones in a large sand body in the eastern suburbs of Sydney. The police were called and they in turn called the Department of Forensic Medicine at Glebe. The forensic pathologist suspected the bones were Aboriginal and of some antiquity and asked me to examine them. I established they were indeed Aboriginal and on the basis of a combination of the weathered condition of the bone and severe tooth wear, combined with the presence of dental caries, suggested they were from the early period after European settlement of Sydney. The police had called the National Parks and Wildlife Service (NPWS now the Department of Environment and Conservation) and they in turn contacted the appropriate Local Aboriginal Land Council. It was the decision of the Land Council

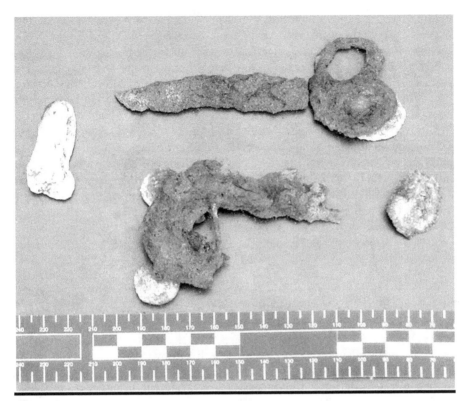

Figure 7.4
Metal grave goods from Aboriginal burial. Photo courtesy of Dr Mary Casey.

and NPWS that there should be a salvage excavation of the remains as they had been highly disturbed from the building process and the remainder of the bones were located under an old, and unstable, pier and footings.

The NPWS of New South Wales issued me with a permit to carry out a salvage excavation. The excavation and analysis were carried out in 2 days and the skeleton and grave goods were buried the third day. During the excavation, metal grave goods including very corroded scissors and lead musket balls were found (Figure 7.4; see also Oxenham et al., Chapter 2). As these were suspected of being more than 50 years old they could be considered a 'relic' under the Heritage Act of New South Wales. It was necessary then to get approval from the Heritage Office to remove the metal grave goods.

The skeleton was buried in a traditional flexed position and was of an Aboriginal woman in the age range of 30 years to 40 years and 171.5 cm ± 4.41 cm tall. She had a nonunited fracture of the left radius with a large callus formation. The left ulna had two old healed fractures. The position of these fractures in the radius and ulna suggest parry fractures. This woman's right clavicle had been badly broken during life and had healed in such a way that it became foreshortened. There were 11 old healed depressed fractures on the skull and a possible perimortem fracture of the frontal bone involving a hinge fracture — this was possibly related to the cause of her death. There was a large carious lesion present on the left third maxillary molar. This strongly suggests this woman was eating some sugars and refined carbohydrates. On the other hand, the moderate to severe attrition on all teeth suggest she was also eating a traditional diet containing rare meat, fibrous plant food and grit. The presence of metal grave goods indicates this woman was buried in the period after European contact. Grave goods included musket balls from the Long Land Service musket, also known as the Brown Bess, which was used by the Royal Marines of the British Army who accompanied the First Fleet in 1788. This gun was used in the Colony up until the mid-1880s. The musket balls cannot be used to date the remains except to say they are definitely after 1788. The musket balls may have been prized objects and used by this woman as weights or sinkers on a fishing line. She probably lived and died during the early time of European settlement of Sydney (Donlon, 2003) and the presence of dental caries, uncommon in precontact Aboriginal populations, supports this conclusion. This time period is supported by Attenbrow's (2002) conclusion that the precolonial way of life for Aboriginals had disappeared from the Sydney region by about the 1830s.

Geographic Source of the Casework

As might be expected the majority of casework comes from the state of New South Wales (Figure 7.5). The percentage of cases from the cities (48%) and the country (47%) are almost identical. It is not surprising that many cases are coming from the country as they mainly consist of skeletonised bodies found in bushland. A small number of cases originated from other states or offshore in countries close by such as PNG and Indonesia. Those from PNG were all war dead from World War II while those from Indonesia were more recent military cases.

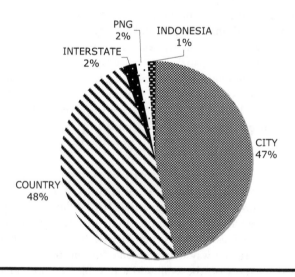

Figure 7.5
Geographical sources of casework in NSW over 15 years (1992–2006).

Case Study: Beaufighter Crash in East New Britain

During World War II an Australian RAAF Beaufighter A19–97 crashed near a village called Wokrice in East New Britain, Papua New Guinea. This aircraft (known as A19–97) from 30 Squadron went missing following operations on October 12, 1943, while engaged on a mission to strafe the airfield at Rabaul. Allied and Japanese air activity in the area was intense on the day. Following its discovery in 1999, an ADF Investigation Team consisting of members of the Specialist Reserve proceeded to the site in 2000 for the purposes of identification of the aircraft, recovery of the remains of the crew, and identification of the recovered bodies. The team consisted of a forensic dentist, a forensic pathologist and a forensic anthropologist. The dentist and pathologist also had expertise in modern aircraft accidents.

Logistic support was provided by the RAAF and PNG Government monitoring and oversight was provided by the PNG National Museum — as such crash sites are protected by the heritage legislation of Papua New Guinea. Medical and dental records of the two aircrew were provided by the Department of Veterans Affairs. The villages provided labour and assisted in clearing and excavating the site. The terrain consists of gently sloping land that at the time of the crash was covered by primary jungle, but which is presently part of a neglected copra plantation. According to the villagers, during the wet season the site becomes a swamp that empties into this stream. Thus we were not too optimistic about finding intact remains. Wreckage was limited to two Bristol-Hercules engines in close proximity and sections of undercarriage, both showing evidence of salvaging numerous pieces of molten aluminium, and fragments of aircraft. There was evidence of previous digging at the site, and two timber crosses with the names of the presumed dead were located near the engines. Sectors were examined using different screening techniques, depending on the perceived likelihood

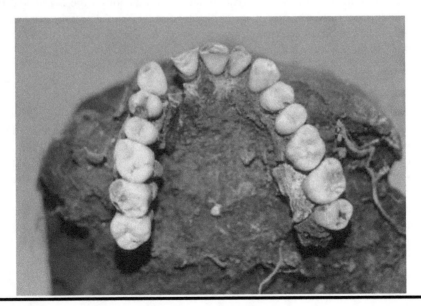

Figure 7.6
Dentition of the pilot from the Beaufighter A19-97.

of recovering remains. Some areas required visual surface search and use of metal detector while others required removal of soil and debris down to the level of the deposit from the reported 1937 volcano eruption, followed by wet sieving.

A relatively intact skeleton and dentition were found, along with personal items suggesting we had found the pilot (Figure 7.6). Many of the epiphyses were damaged but there was no sign of animal interference. The skeleton was clearly that of a Caucasoid male. Age was determined from the closure of epiphyses and was consistent with the pilot's age of 28 years. The pilot was identified on the basis of dental records (Griffiths et al., 2000). Later, severely burnt bone fragments were located, predominantly using wet sieving. The head of a humerus was found among these burnt bones. As two humeral heads were found with the skeleton of the pilot then, by elimination, the burnt bones were 'identified' by exclusion to be the radio operator/navigator. Additionally, a nonhuman bone and tooth, probably pig, were recovered from the site. Various personal effects, including ammunition, stainless steel D-shackles and safety harness materials were located in this area, as well as cockpit instrumentation. No 'dog tags' were located. The two individuals were buried in separate graves at the Bitta Paka Commonwealth War Cemetery near Rabaul.

The Nature of the Cases

This section describes whether the cases were of a recent nature, historic or prehistoric. The majority (57%) were recent and possibly suspicious (Figure 7.7). In NSW such remains fall under the *Coroners Act 1980*. In some cases the remains have not yet been identified and remain as 'cold cases' to be further investigated using DNA analysis. The next largest group were prehistoric Aboriginal skeletons at 18%. This reflects the very long occupation (c. 60,000 years) of Aboriginal people in Australia. Aboriginal remains that are more than 100 years old come under the jurisdiction of the *National Parks and Wildlife Act 1974*. The percentage of historic cases (17%) is almost the same as that of prehistoric remains. Under the legislation in NSW (the *Heritage Act 1977*) these historic cases include any remains that date to more than 50 years.

Condition of the Remains

This section describes the proportion of cases that are fleshed, decomposed, skeletonised, or burned. By far the majority of remains examined were skeletal (84%). Those fleshed remains (4%) required the services of an anthropologist because they were dismembered and determination of height, age and ancestry was difficult. Of the decomposed bodies (10%) a small number had been exhumed at the request of the coroner and most had formed adipocere.

Bodies consisting of burned bones were rare (2%). However, these may increase with more involvement in military cases and those involving mass disasters. An example of a case involving comingled burned bones was that of the Sea King helicopter crash in Indonesia.

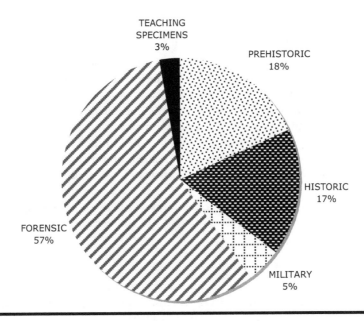

Figure 7.7
The nature of cases in NSW over 15 years (1992–2006).

Appearances in Court

In most cases of identification of ancestry, age, sex, and stature the evidence of forensic anthropologists is accepted and rarely goes to court. Cases involving facial recognition are not so readily accepted and have been increasingly seen in the courts. It has been rare for forensic anthropologists to appear in court in New South Wales. Of course many of their cases are not of a suspicious nature. Of the 153 cases cited here only five have required a court appearance and most have been in the Coroner's Court. Two of the court appearances were to give evidence on identification, two to give evidence on trauma versus taphonomic changes and one on the unsuccessful search for skeletal remains. This probably reflects the established roles of the forensic odontologist in identification and the forensic pathologist in trauma analysis. In all five cases the anthropologist was called by the prosecution. The possible contribution of the forensic anthropologist/osteologist as an expert witness has been described in an article by Walter Wood and colleagues (Henneberg, Chapter 21; Wood et al., 2002).

A possible stimulus for the involvement of forensic anthropologists in NSW was the shocking case of serial murders known as the 'Backpacker Murders'. In 1992 the bodies/skeletal remains of seven young people, mainly backpacking tourists from Europe, were found in the Belanglo State Forest south west of Sydney. Ivan Milat was found guilty of these murders and police speculate that he may also be responsible for more murders and disappearances of young people in the regions close to Sydney. As a result of these murders skeletal remains have been taken more seriously by the police and the coroner. The increase in terrorist activities and natural disasters in neighbouring regions have also resulted in greater involvement by anthropologists from around the country.

Forensic anthropology is on its way to being an established forensic discipline in Australia, albeit at a slow pace. Casework will increase, but so will the number of those trained in the area — far outnumbering the jobs in the field. The small caseload compared with that of the United States will mean jobs will be limited. The types of casework will probably include more work for the military and work related to antiterrorism. Identification of prehistoric Aboriginal remains and historic remains will always be required. Anthropologists will be called to appear in court more often as they gain expertise and will be asked to comment on trauma as well as identification. There has been very little published casework in Australia possibly because of the recent nature of many of the cases as well as the sensitivities and ethical issues involved in the reporting of both forensic cases and those of Aboriginal skeletal remains. Hopefully this chapter goes some way to addressing this issue.

Acknowledgments

Thanks to the following people for providing information and useful discussion: Catherine Bennett, Soren Blau, Chris Briggs, Alanah Buck, Maciej Henneberg, Colin Pardoe, Ellie Simpson, Alan Thorne, Darryl Tuck, Wally Wood, Richard Wright and particularly Ann Macintosh and Sarah Magnell.

References

Abbie, A.A. (1976). Morphological variation in the adult Australian Aboriginal. In R.L. Kirk & A.G. Thorne (Eds.), *The origin of the Australians* (pp. 211–214). Canberra, Australia: Australian Institute of Aboriginal Studies.

Allbrook, D. (1961). The estimation of stature in British and east African males. *Journal of Forensic Medicine, 8*, 15–28.

Australian and New Zealand Forensic Science Society. (n.d.) Retrieved December 6, 2006, from http://www.anzfss.org.au/history.htm

ANZFSS. (2006, April). *Conference proceedings of the 18th International Symposium of the Forensic Sciences, Fremantle, Australia.*

Attenbrow, V. (2002). *Sydney's Aboriginal past: Investigating the archaeological and historical records.* Sydney, Australia: UNSW Press.

Australasian DVI standards manual 2004. (Draft). Adelaide Research and Innovation Pty Ltd, Australasian Disaster Victim Identification Committee, Emergency Management Australia and the Commonwealth of Australia.

Bickford, A., Donlon, D., & Lavelle, S. (1999). *Skeletal remains: Guidelines for the management of human skeletal remains under the Heritage Act.* Sydney, Australia: NSW Heritage Office.

Buck, A. (2004). DVI forensic anthropology procedures (Appendix K). In *Australasian DVI Standards Manual* (pp. 127–130). Canberra, Australia: Emergency Management Australia and the Commonwealth of Australia, Canberra.

Croker, S., & Donlon, D. (2006, April). *Human or non-human: possible methods for the identification of bone fragments.* Poster session presented at the 18th International Symposium of the Forensic Sciences, Fremantle, Australia.

Donlon, D. (1994). Aboriginal skeletal collections and research in physical anthropology: An historical perspective. *Australian Archaeology 39*, 1–10.

Donlon, D. (1999). *Report on the examination of unknown skeletal remains from Possum Brush near Taree, NSW PM Number: 87/1223 (E29205).* Unpublished report for the National Parks and Wildlife Service, NSW.

Donlon, D. (2003). *Report on excavation and examination of unknown skeletal remains from NPWS Site #45–6–2665.* Unpublished report for the National Parks and Wildlife Service, NSW.

Donlon, D. (in press). The development and current state of forensic anthropology: An Australian perspective. In S. Blau & D. Ubelaker (Eds.), *Handbook of forensic anthropology and archaeology.* Walnut Creek, CA: Left Coast Press.

Elkin, A.P. (1978). N.W.G. Macintosh and his work. *Archaeology and Physical Anthropology in Oceania, 13,* 85–142.

Freedman, L. (1964). Metrical features of Aboriginal crania from coastal New South Wales Australia. *Records of the Australian Museum, 26,* 309–325.

Griffiths, C., Duflou, J., & Donlon, D. (2000). *Report on operation Ganae: Recovery of aircrew from Beaufighter A19–97.* Unpublished report for the Australian Department of Defence.

Isçan, M.Y. (1988). Rise of forensic anthropology. *Yearbook of Physical Anthropology, 31,* 203–230.

Joint POW/MIA Accounting Command, JPAC. Retrieved December 6, 2006, from *http://www.jpac.pacom.mil*

Larnach, S., & Freedman, S.L. (1964). Sex determination of Aboriginal crania from coastal New South Wales. *Records of the Australian Museum, 26,* 295–308.

Larnach, S., & Macintosh, N.W.G. (1967). The use in forensic medicine of an anthropological method for the determination of sex and race in skeletons. *Archaeology and Physical Anthropology in Oceania 2,* 155–161.

Larnach, S.L., & Macintosh. N.W.G. (1970). The craniology of the Aborigines of Queensland. *Oceania Monographs,* No. 15.

Macintosh, N.W.G. (1952). Stature in some Aboriginal tribes in south-west Arnhem Land. *Oceania 22,* 208–215.

Macintosh, N.W.G. (1965). The physical aspects of man in Australia. In R. Berndt & C. Berndt (Eds.), *Aboriginal man in Australia* (pp. 29–70). Sydney, Australia: Angus and Robertson.

Macintosh, N.W.G. (1972). The recovery and treatment of bone. In D.J. Mulvaney, (Ed.), *Australian archaeology: A guide to field and laboratory techniques* (pp. 77–85). Canberra, Australia: Australian Institute of Aboriginal Studies.

McKern, T.W., & Stewart, T.D. (1957). *Skeletal age changes in young American males, analyzed from the standpoint of identification* (Technical Reports EP–45). Natick, MA: Headquarters Quartermaster Research and Development Command.

NSW Bureau of Crime Statistics. (n.d.). Retrieved November 22, 2006, from *http://bocd.lawlink.nsw.gov.au/bocd/cmd/crimetrends/DateInput*

Oettle, T.H.G., & Larnach, S.L. (1974). The identification of Aboriginal traits in forensic medicine. In A.P. Elkin, & N.W.G. Macintosh (Eds.), *Grafton Elliot Smith: The man and his work.* (pp. 103–108). Sydney: Sydney University Press.

Proceedings of the Australasian Society for Human Biology, Sydney. (2005). *Homo-Journal of Comparative Human Biology, 57,* 219–244.

Ray, L.J. (1959). Metrical and non-metrical features of the clavicle of the Australian Aboriginal. *American Journal of Physical Anthropology 17,* 217–226.

Reichs, K, (Ed.). (1998). *Forensic osteology: Advances in the identification of human remains.* Springfield, IL: Charles C. Thomas.

Thorne, A.G., & Ross, A. (1986). *The skeleton manual.* Sydney, Australia: NPWS and Police Aborigine Liaison Unit.

Trotter, M., & Gleser, G.C. (1958). A reevaluation of estimation based on measurements of stature taken during life and of long bones after death. *American Journal of Physical Anthropology, 16,* 79–123.

Wood, W.B. (1968). An Aboriginal burial ground at Broadbeach Queensland: Skeletal material. *Mankind, 6,* 681–686.

Wood, W.B. (1993). Forensic osteology. In I. Freckelton & H. Selby (Eds.), *Expert evidence.* (pp. 3/601–3/797). Sydney, Australia: The Law Book Company.

Wood, W., Briggs, C., & Donlon, D. (2002). Forensic Osteology. In I. Freckelton & H. Selby. (Eds.), *Expert evidence.* (pp. 3/601–3/802). Sydney, Australia: Thomson Lawbook Co.

Wood-Jones, F. (1931). The non-metrical character of the skull as criteria for racial diagnosis. *Journal of Anatomy, 68,* 323–330.

Detection of Likely Ancestry Using CRANID

Richard Wright

This chapter describes a method for determining likely ancestry from a freely distributable computer program called CRANID. The name is an abbreviation of 'cranial identification'. The chapter first outlines some cases where CRANID has been used. It then discusses its multivariate statistical methods, some objections that have been raised to deriving ancestry from cranial morphology, and the underpinning of the method by the correlation between geography and cranial form. What the user must do to get a result is then outlined. Finally, the chapter discusses some more advanced methods that are not included in the distributable version of CRANID.

Identification of ancestry from measured cranial morphology (see also Littleton & Kinaston, Chapter 11) makes use of geographically patterned variation in cranial size and shape in our species *Homo sapiens*. Identification is made in the context of the 'ethnographic present', that is, the time prior to great mass movements of people between continents, for example, slaving out of Africa and European settlement of Australia.

The program assumes that the user is studying a skull of unknown ancestry or one for which a surmised ancestry needs to be verified. The program reports where the unknown person's ancestors were likely to have been living in the ethnographic present.

After analysing a series of measurements, the likelihood of correct identification of the unknown skull with one of the samples in the database is expressed as a probability. The output is a series of probabilities, in descending order of likelihood, of the unknown being a member of each of the 66 samples of skulls in a database made up of 2870 skulls from around the world.

This chapter discusses some assumptions underlying this type of identification, how the usefulness of the method can be validated, what measurements are used and how the results are presented.

Why Try to Identify Ancestry from Cranial Morphology?

Three areas of study in which CRANID has proved useful are summarily illustrated here: the forensic, repatriation, and general investigations in anthropology and archaeology. Details of the forensic and repatriation analyses by CRANID remain confidential to clients.

Two Forensic Examples

Forensic Case 1

Skeletonised female remains were found under floorboards in Britain in 1990. The skull looked to local forensic anthropologists as not being typically British and the teeth showed restorative dentistry not done according to British practice. The investigators wondered whether the remains were those of a British person of Afro–West Indian ancestry, many of whom lived in the area. Ancestry was sought for facial reconstruction, in order to determine the likely shape of the lips, colour of skin and form of the hair.

A CRANID result, obtained by the Natural History Museum in London using an earlier version of CRANID, unambiguously identified the unknown as of European ancestry. The subsequent display of facial reconstruction showed thin lips of European type, pale colour of skin, and straight form of hair. The display brought forward a claim from a member of the public (subsequently proved) that the reconstruction resembled a young woman who had once lived in a street near the place where the remains were discovered. She was from the Basque country of Spain.

Forensic Case 2

A skull was suspected as being that of a Japanese soldier killed in WWII. There were, however, suggestions that it might be that of a European person. CRANID classified the skull as coming from an Asian sample.

Two Examples From Repatriation Cases Relating to Skulls in Museums

Repatriation Case 1

A skull carried the label 'Indian'. Did the label imply an origin in the Indian sub-continent or in the Americas? The CRANID result indicated a skull from the Americas.

Repatriation Case 2

A skull carried a label 'Aboriginal', but two experts who had previously studied it concluded that it was of mixed Aboriginal/European ancestry. CRANID gave no support to any claim for Aboriginal ancestry. The skull had overwhelming probabilities of European ancestry. Subsequent historical enquiry proved that the person was of English ancestry, and had committed suicide in the early 19th century.

An Example From a Study in Prehistory

Thorne and Wolpoff claimed in situ evolution of Asiatic people from *Homo erectus*. The morphology of the late Pleistocene Upper Cave skull from Beijing (UC101) was said to support this case for in situ evolution (Thorne & Wolpoff, 1992). NonCRANID analysis (Kamminga & Wright, 1988) had already led to the conclusion that the Upper Cave skull was more like non-Mongoloid groups. CRANID, using an expanded set of data, confirmed the non-Mongoloid appearance of the Upper Cave skull (Wright, 1992). See also Wright (1995) for yet another approach.

Some of these questions about unknown crania can be settled by DNA analysis. So does not DNA make CRANID redundant? No, because:

(a) DNA may not survive in buried bone

(b) DNA analyses may take some weeks to complete, an initial CRANID result can be obtained within 15 minutes from start to finish (including the taking of measurements, entering data into the program and the computation)

(c) DNA is beyond the budget of many research investigations.

Methodological Background

Identification by CRANID is based on size and shape of crania, using what are known in statistics as multivariate methods of analysis. To understand the basic principle of analysis we must conceive of an unknown skull being examined in the multivariate space of 29 variables. This section is devoted to three examples that illustrate the phrase 'in the space of'.

In the Space of Two Variables

We start by considering a common aspect of older anthropological research: the examination of skulls in the space of two variables. The two variables were normally cranial length and breadth, a pair much loved by previous generations of biological anthropologists wanting to classify crania in a range from dolichocephalic (long headed) to brachycephalic (short headed).

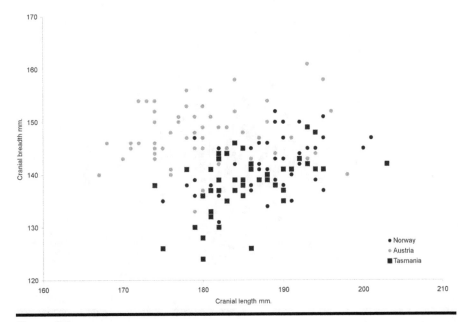

Figure 8.1
Crania shown in the space of two variables.

For descriptive purposes, anthropologists often reduced the two variables to a single dimension: the ratio of the breadth of a skull to its length. For the purpose of exposition we can create a scattergram (Figure 8.1) in which crania are shown in the space of the two dimensions, or variables, of length and breadth. Note that an unknown skull, for which we have measurements of length and breadth, may be placed in this space and conclusions about its similarity to the other samples inferred.

In the Space of Three Variables

The two variables of length and breadth provide a paltry description of such a complicated geometry as the human skull. What do we do if we want to enhance our description by adding a third dimension, for example, cranial height? Representation of the crania in the space of three dimensions can be done by a chart that simulates the third dimension by projection (Figure 8.2). Alternatively, the distribution of the skulls can be studied in a three-dimensional block that can be rotated by software such as a CAD package. Again the unknown can be placed within this 3D space, but interpreting its similarity to other samples is often difficult because of visual complexity.

In the Space of More Than Three Variables

Even the three dimensions of length, breadth and height may be brushed aside as an inadequate suite of variables for describing the human skull. So suppose we want to add a fourth dimension to length, breadth and height, for example, width of the nasal aperture. How do we visually represent the crania in the space of the resulting four dimensions?

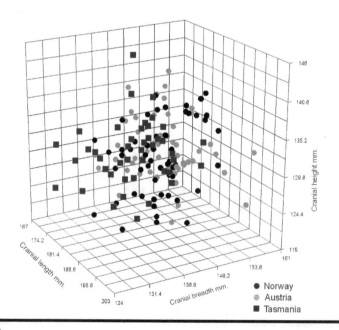

Figure 8.2
Crania shown in the space of three variables. Such 3D diagrams are intrinsically difficult to interpret.

The answer is that we cannot visualise a skull in the space of more than three dimensions. We come up against an aspect of what Bellman called the *curse of dimensionality* (Bellman, 1961). The implication of the word 'curse' is that as soon as we start to use a substantively adequate description then our efforts are doomed because we cannot represent the results.

Four variables cannot be visualised, yet CRANID uses 29 dimensions on 2870 crania from around the world. So how do we represent the similarities between these crania in such a manner that we can conclude 'what is like what' and 'what is not like what' morphologically? Examining multidimensional space is what multivariate statistics are all about. They get around the curse of dimensionality by what are known as methods of data reduction.

There are several methods of data reduction. The method used in the standard distributable method of CRANID is *linear discriminant analysis* (LDA). LDA has a 70-year-old history in multivariate analysis. The first application ever of LDA was on sorting out Egyptian crania (Barnard, 1935). LDA is a topic of current texts (Huberty & Olejnik, 2006). It has considerable advantages in the cranial analysis of groups, some of which are set out in a paper that applies the method to the recently discovered small hominin skull from Flores (Argue et al., 2006). There are two distributed packages that use LDA to examine the ancestry of an unknown skull: CRANID (described in this chapter) and FORDISC (Ousley & Jantz, 1996).

Various Objections to Inferring Ancestry from Craniometrics

Is there inheritance of cranial form or is cranial form plastic in response to environmental influences? Various objections have been made against the use of craniometrics to determine ancestry. Discussion of them could be the subject of a chapter in its own right. This chapter briefly examines four objections.

Boas's Influence

Many anthropologists believe that Boas has shown the plasticity of the human cranium in the face of environmental change. Specifically he claimed to have shown that descendents of immigrants to the United States in the early part of the 20th century had changed their cranial index of length and breadth towards the American norm. The change was claimed as a response to the new environment (Gravlee, Bernard, & Leonard, 2003; Sparks & Jantz, 2003).

If Boas' conclusions of plasticity applied to all measured variables (i.e., to multivariable analysis, not just to length and breadth) then the theoretical assumptions of approaches like CRANID would be undermined. However the statistical significance of Boas' use of even length and breadth has been questioned (Sparks & Jantz, 2003). Boas was not of course, in precomputer days, able to handle more than the two dimensions of length and breadth, so his morphological description of skulls is unacceptably meager when compared with the 29 variables of CRANID. Yet many accounts of Boas boldly characterise his two variables as representing 'cranial form'.

For a discussion of Boas' cranial index and its low relevance to multivariate analysis see Relethford (2004). Roseman (2004) also presents an important discussion of the general correlation between cranial morphology and molecular characteristics.

Use of Length and Breadth to Determine Ancestry

Related to Boas' approach is the once frequent obsession with cranial length and breadth to examine skulls. Texts of the 1920s and 1930s almost invariably emphasise this pair of measurements (e.g., Coon, 1939; Stibbe, 1930; Wilder, 1921). The fundamental problem of this descriptively meagre approach is that it produces seriously counter-intuitive results when it comes to evaluating ancestry. An example is shown in Figure 8.1. Here we see that European individuals from Norway are more like Aboriginal individuals from Tasmania than they are like European individuals from Austria.

This result is derived from the two variables of length and breadth. If taken literally it shows an otherwise unsuspected, and one would have to say historically dubious, affinity between certain long-headed north-western Europeans and Australian Aborigines, while denying a clear affinity between those long-headed north-west Europeans and other Europeans with short heads. To jump ahead a little, the multivariate resolution of these affinities, using 29 variables, can be seen on Figure 8.4. Here the results for the samples from Norway, Austria and Tasmania are intuitively acceptable.

In retrospect, the obsession with the cranial index did tend to throw the whole of craniometrics into disrepute. But that obsession was with a demonstrably inadequate bivariate description of skulls. Examining cranial form by multivariate descriptions of large samples had to await the use of computers.

Nonmetric Statistics

In the middle of the 20th century there developed an interest in nonmetric (or epigenetic) traits (Berry & Berry, 1967; Hauser & De Stefano, 1989). Analyses of nonmetric traits for determining ancestry were often presented with a rhetorical preamble that claimed them to be reliable (in an ancestral sense) in a way that metric traits were not.

It is the author's opinion that nonmetric traits, when used to determine ancestry, have not kept the promise of exclusive usefulness that was often made on their behalf. However, a recent study by Hanihara, Ishida and Dodo (2003) produces a chart based on nonmetric traits that shows a worldwide coherence of the sort that we see in Figure 8.4 of this chapter. Interestingly, the authors do not claim an exclusive usefulness for nonmetrics, but note that 'the clustering pattern is similar to those based on classic genetic markers, DNA polymorphisms, and craniometrics' (Hanihara et al., 2003: 241). Their work suggests to the author that an identification system of an unknown skull, using the multivariate approaches to classification of CRANID and Fordisc, may yet be possible for nonmetric data.

Correlation Between Geography and Cranial Form

A lack of correlation between cranial form and geography would clearly undermine the approach used by CRANID. Because of the importance of establishing such a correlation the author published an analysis of cranial form and geography for an earlier version of CRANID. This version used principal components analysis and not the LDA used in CRANID5. A good correlation was found (Wright, 1992).

A correlation resulting from the current version of CRANID5 is shown as Figure 8.4, described below under validation. The result of this cranial analysis produces a good correlation between cranial form and geography. Nevertheless the possibility of there being no correlation is sometimes revisited (e.g., Williams, Belcher, & Armelagos, 2005). The authors attempted a classification of some Nubian skulls by the FORDISC2 program. The author cannot in this chapter do this article critical justice, but it has several obvious weaknesses. For example, the authors use only 12 measurements, instead of the 21 that are available in FORDISC. So the analysis is based on an unnecessarily inadequate metrical description. The authors attribute their problematical results to FORDISC itself (as though the 11 variables they chose to use are as good as the 21 that FORDISC encourages). They then challenge the concept of there being a relation between cranial form and ancestry. Indeed, they boldly conclude from their single experiment: '[w]e suggest that skeletal specimens or samples cannot be accurately classified by geography ... [and] the attempt to classify populations into natural geographic groups ... will continue to fail' (Williams et al., 2005: 345).

This author contends that CRANID5 refutes the argument that samples cannot be accurately classified by geography and that attempts to classify populations have failed. If Williams et al. (2005) were correct then a scattergram such as Figure 8.4 could not be generated.

Properties of CRANID

What does CRANID actually do and how do you get it to do what it does?

The Database

The scope of the comparative database is worldwide. Most of the groups of crania come from the work of William White Howells (1996). In addition this author, with assistance from others, has expanded the database to fill in some gaps. Figure 8.3 shows the groups in the database of the current version, which is CRANID5. Most of the groups on the map include separate female and male samples. There are in all 66 samples in the database.

Variables Used

All 2870 crania in this database are described by 29 measurements. These are simply achieved measures that do not need fancy and expensive craniometric equipment. The instruments required are spreading, sliding and coordinate calipers (the manual that accompanies the program suggests a simple way of improvising coordinate calipers).

The necessary 29 variables (Table 8.1) are described in detail in the manual. To make use of CRANID5 the values for these 29 variables are entered into a spreadsheet. The program then reads this spreadsheet and saves the results of the linear discriminant analysis to disk as a text file.

Various alternatives to measured variables have been proposed, in particular the 3D approach of what has been called the *new morphometry*. The limitation of these interesting approaches is not their methodology but the lack of a comparative worldwide database of any substance. For example, Ross, McKeown and Konigsberg (1999) rely

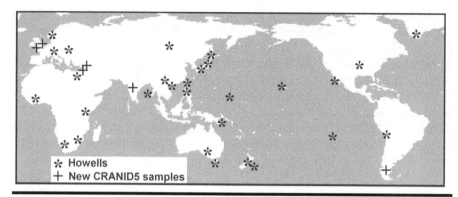

Figure 8.3
The origin of groups in the CRANID5 database. Most groups have separate female and male samples, which results in 66 samples in the database.

for their exposition of the new morphometry on merely 32 skulls of American black and white males. One can also note that the resulting linear discriminant analyses of both the 'old' and the new morphometry were little different in this study.

Validation Checks

Before we start using the database we need to be sure that the results for 2870 crania in the database make patterned sense. To this end there are several validation checks available. A basic test is to resubstitute each of the 2870 skulls into the LDA classification rules established by CRANID. The strict classification success rate is 70.3%. This rate is strict, in that classifying a male Norse skull as female is counted as an error, also counted as an error is classifying a male Norse skull as a Patagonian female. So, in a substantive sense the success rate is higher; the amount of success depending on how the user weights minor and major errors. In passing it is interesting to note that the classification success rate using only the two variables of length and breadth is a low 10.2%.

Table 8.1
Variables Used in CRANID

Measurement	Code	Measurement	Code
Glabello-occipital length	GOL	Palate breadth, external	MAB
Nasio-occipital length	NOL	Bimaxillary breadth	ZMB
Basion-nasion length	BNL	Zygomaxillary subtense	SSS
Basion-bregma height	BBH	Bifrontal breadth	FMB
Maximum cranial breadth	XCB	Nasio-frontal subtense	NAS
Maximum frontal breadth	XFB	Biorbital breadth	EKB
Biauricular breadth	AUB	Interorbital breadth	DKB
Biasterionic breadth	ASB	Cheek height	WMH
Basion-prosthion length	BPL	Frontal chord	FRC
Nasion-prosthion height	NPH	Frontal subtense	FRS
Nasal height	NLH	Parietal chord	PAC
Orbital height	OBH	Parietal subtense	PAS
Orbital breadth	OBB	Occipital chord	OCC
Bijugal breadth	JUB	Occipital subtense	OCS
Nasal breadth	NLB		

A different approach to validation is to plot the samples in the space of the first two canonical variates (or discriminant functions) shown in Figure 8.4. The results can then be examined for a correlation between cranial form and geographical origin.

This scattergram uses much less information than the full LDA that uses all 29 discriminant functions. It pools the results for both sexes of each group. The result is by no means a perfect map of the world; the placing of the Eskimo sample is counterintuitive. Nevertheless, even this limited information validates the CRANID approach by showing a high degree of correlation between cranial form and geography.

Output of Results (Distributable Version of CRANID)

The distributable version of CRANID, using LDA of size and shape, outputs a list of all the samples in decreasing order of the likelihood of the unknown coming from each sample. The following list is for the supposed Aboriginal skull intended for repatriation and discussed above. The list is abbreviated by showing only samples that have probabilities of 0.10 or greater. The probabilities indicate that the skull has a high likelihood of being that of a person with European ancestry. Furthermore, no Aboriginal samples are represented. In fact in the remainder of the list (not shown) the first Aboriginal sample does not appear until number 54 in the list of 66 samples. So the probability of the skull being Aboriginal is vanishingly small.

Order	Sample	Probability
1	Lond. Medvl. M	0.54
2	Norse Norway M	0.19
3	Berg Austria M	0.12

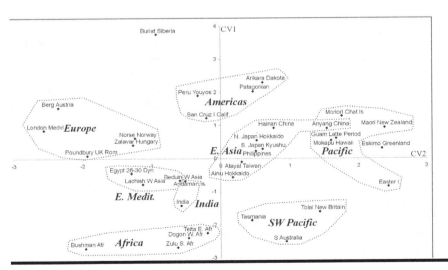

Figure 8.4

Samples in the CRANID5 database plotted in the space of the first two canonical variates (discriminant functions). The pattern, which is derived solely from cranial morphology, shows a reasonable resemblance to the world map. It thereby demonstrates that there is a correlation between cranial form and geography.

Analyses Beyond LLD of Size and Shape

The results of the distributable version of CRANID can be taken as reliable if both of the following conditions are met: (a) the most likely sample has a high probability, (b) the samples that immediately follow are consistently from contiguous geographical areas. It is not possible to define a priori what is a sufficiently high probability for acceptance, because there is a tradeoff between it and geographical consistency in the leading results. However, in general, any leading result with a probability of < 0.5 should be treated with care.

If the highest probability is low and the leading results geographically inconsistent then the CRANID database does not cater for the unknown cranium. It does not fit with the database. This lack of fit to the database may be due to one or more of several unrelated reasons, including (a) the measurements of the unknown have been wrongly made or entered, (b) the geographical area from which the person came is poorly represented in the database, (c) the person is morphologically atypical of their group, because of unusual growth or artificial deformation, and (d) the person is of mixed ancestry.

Unclear results (except for those due to erroneous measurement) require additional analysis that is not available in the distributable version of CRANID. These additional analyses, which may be carried out by the author on request, can include LDA by shape alone, where absolute size differences are excluded from the database.

There is an even more radical approach available, which ignores the parametric assumptions about the data underlying LDA. The approach was not possible until high speed computing became available. This intuitively appealing approach is called *nearest neighbour analysis*. Whereas LDA deals with proximity to sample mean values, nearest neighbour analysis deals individually with the 2870 crania in the database. It examines the location of an unknown skull in the 29 dimensional space of the discriminant functions and identifies which of the 2870 individuals are closest to the unknown in that multidimensional space. It then analyses the sample membership of these nearest neighbours.

This approach gave plausibility to the identification of a skull from WWII as Japanese (the case mentioned as forensic case 2). It was suspected as being that of a Japanese soldier. However, linear discriminant analysis classified the skull as Berg (Europe) by FORDISC 2.0 and Buriat (Siberia) by CRANID5. Admittedly the first eight preferred samples in the CRANID results were all Mongoloid in the broad sense, but a Japanese sample did not appear until the seventh sample was reached.

By contrast, nearest neighbour analysis of the CRANID database found that the actual nearest neighbour of the WWII skull was an individual from Howells' South Japanese male sample. The lesson to be learned from this discrepancy is that some individuals (in this case among the South Japanese males) may deviate in a non-normal manner from their sample mean and such deviation is ignored by linear discriminant analysis but detected by nearest neighbour analysis.

Access to CRANID

The freely distributable CRANID package, which includes the program and a manual, can be freely downloaded from http://www.box.net/shared/static/n9q0zgtr1y.EXE

Contact the author with questions and for information about updates at richwrig@tig.com.au or richwrig@hotmail.com.

Acknowledgment

I thank Mary Dallas for commenting on an earlier draft of this chapter.

References

Argue, D., Donlon, D., Groves, C., & Wright, R. (2006). Homo floresiensis: Microcephalic, pygmoid, Australopithecus, or Homo? *Journal of Human Evolution, 51,* 360–374.

Barnard, M.M. (1935). The secular variations of skull characteristics in four series of Egyptian skulls. *Annals of Eugenics, 6,* 352–371.

Bellman, R. (1961). *Adaptive control processes: A guided tour.* Princeton, NJ: Princeton University Press.

Coon, C.S. (1939). *The races of Europe.* New York: Macmillan.

Gravlee, C.C., Bernard, H.R., & Leonard, W.R. (2003). Boas's changes in bodily form: The immigrant study, cranial plasticity, and Boas's physical anthropology. *American Anthropologist 105,* 326–332.

Hanihara, T., Ishida, H., & Dodo, Y. (2003). Characterization of biological diversity through analysis of discrete cranial traits. *American Journal of Physical Anthropology, 121,* 241–251.

Hauser, G., & De Stefano, G.F. (1989). *Epigenetic variants of the human skull.* Stuttgart: E. Schweizerbart'sche Veerlagsbuchhandlung.

Howells, W.W. (1996). Howells' craniometric data on the nternet. *American Journal of Physical Anthropology, 101,* 441–442.

Huberty, C.J., & Olejnik, S. (2006). *Applied MANOVA and discriminant analysis.* (2nd ed.). Hoboken, NJ: John Wiley & Sons.

Kamminga, J., & Wright, R.V.S. (1988). The upper cave at Zhoukoudian and the origins of the Mongoloids. *Journal of Human Evolution, 17,* 739–767.

Ousley, S.D., & Jantz, R.L. (1996). *FORDISC 2.0: Personal computer forensic discriminant functions.* Knoxville, TN: University of Tennessee, Department of Anthropology.

Relethford, J.H. (2004). Boas and beyond: Migration and craniometric variation. *American Journal of Human Biology, 16,* 379–386.

Roseman, C.C. (2004). Detecting interregionally diversifying natural selection on modern human cranial form by using matched molecular and morphometric data. *Proceedings of the National Academy of Sciences of the United States of America, 101*(35), 12824–12829.

Ross, A.H., McKeown, A.H., & Konigsberg, L.W. (1999). Allocation of crania to groups via the 'new morphometry'. *Journal of Forensic Sciences, 44,* 584–587.

Sparks, C.S., & Jantz, R.L. (2003). Changing times, changing faces: Franz Boas's immigrant study in modern perspective. *American Anthropologist, 105,* 333–337.

Stibbe, E.P. (1930). *An introduction to physical anthropology.* London: Edward Arnold & Co.

Thorne, A.G., & Wolpoff, M.H. (1992). The multiregional evolution of humans. *Scientific American, 266,* 28–33.

Wilder, H.W. (1921). *A laboratory manual of anthropometry.* Philadelphia: P. Blakiston's Son & Co.

Williams, F.L., Belcher, R.L., & Armelagos, G.J. (2005). Forensic misclassification of ancient Nubian crania: implications for assumptions about human variation. *Current Anthropology 46,* 340–346.

Wright, R.S. (1992). Correlation between cranial forma and geography in *Homo sapiens*: CRANID — a computer program for forensic and other applications. *Archaeology in Oceania*, *27*, 105–112.

Wright, R.V.S. (1995). The Zhoukoudian Upper Cave Skull 101 and multiregionalism. *Journal of Human Evolution*, *29*, 181–183.

Identifying Child Abuse in Skeletonised Subadult Remains

Hallie R Buckley

Kelly Whittle

Child abuse is a distressing social phenomenon in which the young and defenceless are maltreated by those close to them. The abuse can manifest in several forms: *physical abuse* (nonaccidental injury), *sexual abuse, emotional abuse,* and *neglect* (Blumenthal, 1994). The physical abuse of children produces distinctive patterns of soft tissue and skeletal injuries that have been thoroughly documented in the clinical and forensic literature (Table 9.1). The motivation of biological and forensic anthropology investigations are essentially the same, both attempting to build a profile of a deceased person's life, and sometimes their death from bones and teeth. Therefore, with investigations of the skeletonised remains of the recently deceased, the methods of biological anthropology are applied in the medico–legal arena. In this chapter, the characteristic skeletal injuries observed clinically in child abuse victims will be reviewed, drawing on biological anthropology literature, in an attempt to provide a protocol for application on skeletonised subabult remains. Table 9.2 summarises the skeletal manifestations of child abuse discussed in the text.

Skeletal Manifestations of Child Abuse

The physical abuse of children was first described by Caffey in 1946 when he recognised the association of subdural haematomas and long bone fractures in children as most likely caused by nonaccidental injury. In 1962 Kempe, Silverman, Steele, Droegmueller, and Silver coined the term 'battered child syndrome' referring to the characteristic pattern of skeletal trauma that was apparent in deceased abused children (Kempe et al., 1962). Subsequently, a substantial amount of literature has amassed documenting the characteristic pattern of skeletal trauma in child abuse

Table 9.1
General Osteological Characteristics Pathognomic of Child Abuse

Bilateral fractures
Symmetrical periosteal lesions
Fractures in different stages of repair
Metaphyseal fractures
Fractures with no plausible origin
Fractures accompanied by other tell-tale soft tissue trauma (i.e., haematoma or brain injury)

Table 9.2
Summary of Skeletal Manifestations of Child Abuse

Injury	Age of victim	Mechanism of injury	Skeletal manifestation	Perimortem appearance	Antemortem appearance	Reference
Cranial fracture	Any	Blunt force impact (compression)	• bilateral • asymmetric • span sutural boundaries • basilar fractures • complex, stellate or depressed • growing fracture (i.e. wide linear instead of a simple line fracture)	• fracture lines (radiating or concentric) evident • breaks have sharp, jagged, irregular edges • haematoma staining may be apparent at fracture site. • cranial bone displacement along suture lines	• evidence of healing. • blunting of fracture edges • breaks have rounded edges • porosity indicating bone remodelling	Crist Washburn, Park, Hood, & Hickey (1997) Carty (1999)
Rib fracture	Any, but predominantly < 1 year	Anterior–posterior thoracic compression (during violent shaking) or via direct blunt force trauma	• fracture at the costovertebral angle • fracture at costochondral junction • fractured angle of rib • bilateral	• jagged and irregular fracture margins	• callous formation 1–2 weeks posttrauma	Walker, Cook, & Lambert (1997) Bulloch (2000)
Scapular fracture	Any	Blunt force trauma (compression)	• compression infraction of scapular blade • fracture of acromion or coracoid processes • fracture of scapular spine	• visible fracture lines with irregular and sharp margins • potential displacement of fractured bone	• blunt fracture margins • callous formation • remodelling and porosity • may have disfigurement if callous forms without realignment of fracture	Carty (1993)
Clavicular fracture (acromial end)	Any	Blunt force trauma, compression, torsion, bending forces	• oblique, greenstick or linear fracture of clavicle			Caffey (1972)
Vertebral fracture	Any	Hyperflexion and extension of vertebrae due to violent shaking	• usually thoraco–lumbar fractures • fracture of neurocentral synchondrosis • anterior or posterior subluxation of vertebrae	• malalignment of vertebral bodies • irregular and sharp fracture lines		Vialle, Mary, Schmnider, Ducou le Pointe, & Damsin (2006)
Phalangeal fracture	Nonambulatory infants	• twisting, pulling or compression force • crushing digits	• linear, oblique or spiral fracture of phalanges	• sharp fracture boundaries, jagged and irregular • bone displacement		Thompson (2005)

Table 9.2 (continued)
Summary of Skeletal Manifestations of Child Abuse

Injury	Age of victim	Mechanism of injury	Skeletal manifestation	Perimortem appearance	Antemortem appearance	Reference
Long bone fracture (particularly femur, tibia and humerus)	Any — particularly < 3 years	• twisting, pulling, bending or shearing forces • falling awkwardly • warding off blows • child pulled forcefully • shaking with limbs hanging	• linear, spiral or oblique fractures • proximal or distal metaphyses • mid-diaphysis • greenstick fractures	• sharp fracture boundaries, jagged and irregular • bone displacement	• evidence of healing • blunting of fracture edges • callous formation • breaks have rounded edges • porosity indicating bone remodelling	Carty (1999) Schwend et al. (2000) Thomas, Rosenfield, Leventhal, & Markowitz (1991)
Metaphyseal fracture	< 3 years	• proximal or distal metaphyses • transverse 'corner' or 'bucket handle' fracture	• separation of metaphysis from epiphyses; however, may not be apparent macroscopically; histological examination shows corner fractures through metaphysis	• difficult to view, no callous is formed as fracture heals through the growth plate cartilage		Kleinman, Nimkin, Spevak, Rayder, Madansky (1995) Thompson (2005)
Subperiosteal lesions	Any	• blunt force trauma causing superiosteal bleeding • acceleration/deceleration forces • repetitive trauma • rough handling	• rough areas of new bone deposition • raised • porous • delineated margins • symmetrical lesions	• porous lesions, vascular in appearance • defined margins	• rounded margins integrating into cortex • lessened porosity, indicating bone remodelling	Walker, Cook, & Lambert (1997) Carty (1999) Buckley (2000)

cases (e.g., Carty, 1993; Kleinman, Marks Jr, Richmond, & Blackbourne, 1995a; Meservy, Towbin, McLaurin, Myers, & Ball, 1987; Sawyer, Flynn, Dormans, Catalano, & Drummond, 2000; Strait, Siegal, & Shapiro, 1995; Thomas, Rosenfield, Leventhal, & Markowitz, 1991; Thompson, 2005; Williams & Hardcastle, 2005; Worlock, Stower, & Barbor, 1986).

Epidemiology of Abuse

Victims of child abuse are predominantly between birth and 3 years of age (Suggs, Leichenstein, McCarthy, & Jackson, 2001). As children become older the rate of victimisation decreases, as they have increased mobility and more ability to defend themselves. Any fractures seen in children less than 3 years of age should be treated with caution by the forensic pathologist or medical professional (Blumenthal, 1994), as at this age the development of their locomotion is not usually sufficient to sustain limb fractures via accidents (Suggs et al., 2001).

Bone lesions characteristic of abuse are multiple asymmetrical long bone fractures, in different stages of healing, metaphyseal fractures, subdural haematoma and fracture of the skull bones. In cadaveric material with well-preserved soft tissues, bone lesions caused by physical abuse can usually be determined by the presence of cutaneous injuries such as bruising, especially if the bruise mimics the shape of a weapon or a handprint (Thompson, 2005). However, in fully skeletonised material, cutaneous injuries and other signs such as subdural haematomas will not be preserved. The following outlines the characteristic skeletal pattern of 'battered child syndrome' and discusses whether these would be readily identifiable in skeletonised remains.

Bone Fractures

Carty (1993) summarises the types of fractures deemed pathognomonic of child abuse. Digital fractures in nonwalking children and complex fractures of the skull are both considered indicative of nonaccidental injury. Postcranial fractures commonly seen in child abuse are observed in the metaphyses of limb bones, ribs, scapulae, acromial aspect of the clavicle and vertebrae. Bilateral fractures and periosteal new bone lesions in different stages of remodelling also have a high specificity for child abuse (Carty, 1993).

Head and Thorax

Head trauma is the leading cause of mortality in child abuse cases (Suggs et al., 2001). Accidental skull trauma usually manifests as a simple, unilateral parietal fracture (Crist, Washburn, Park, Hood, & Hickey, 1997; Suggs et al., 2001). Cause for suspicion arises when children present with multiple and/or complex fractures that span sutural boundaries. Complex skull fractures are defined as those that are bilateral, stellate or depressed and are usually a result of inflicted injury on children. Suggs et al. (2001) state that significant force would be required to produce stellate, depressed, complex, bilateral or basilar skull fractures in children. Accidents such as falls from beds, couches and suchlike are not thought to result in serious skeletal trauma, so any patient presenting with a history of a fall and a complex skull fracture needs to be thoroughly examined to ensure their history corresponds with the presenting injury (Thompson, 2005).

The most common cranial bone for children to fracture is the parietal bone; however, this includes accidental and nonaccidental injuries (Suggs et al., 2001). In skeletonised remains, differentiating perimortem fractures from postmortem damage to fragile subabult bones is difficult, particularly if the skeleton is incomplete. However, Walker, Cook and Lambert (1997) report three cases of skeletonised child remains with cranial fractures associated with subtle subperiosteal changes in various stages of remodelling, which they attribute to abuse.

Thoracic compression and blunt force trauma is often the cause of rib and spinal fractures in child abuse cases, and are rarely the result of an accident (Suggs et al., 2001; Vialle, Mary, Schhmider, Ducou le Pointe, Damsin et al., 2006). Usually fractures are concentrated on the posterior aspect of the ribs, the costovertebral angles, the lateral aspect of the ribs and at the costosternal junction (Bulloch, Schubert, Brophy, Johnson, Reed et al., 2000; Suggs et al., 2001). If the child has been picked up and squeezed, the fractures are typically bilateral and multiple (Thompson, 2005). Worlock et al. (1986) state that in the absence of any history of chest trauma, the presence of multiple rib fractures is indicative of abuse. Children under 2 years old frequently exhibit fractures of the costal skeleton if they have been physically abused (Suggs et al., 2001).

Appendicular Skeleton

Fractures of the metaphysis–epiphysis of long bones are also indicative of child abuse (Blumenthal, 1994; Carty, 1993). These lesions are predominantly found in the proximal humerus, knee and distal tibia and fibula (Carty, 1993). They are caused by twisting or wrenching of the extremities that can occur when picking up a child by the torso and shaking them with limbs dangling, or forcefully grabbing and pulling a child by the limbs (Thompson, 2005).

The fracture occurs when the fragile metaphysis is pulled from the primary spongiosa of the growth cartilage where it attaches to the epiphysis (Thompson, 2005). In cadaveric material, radiographs will show a radiolucent line on the metaphysis and a metaphyseal chip fracture of the bone known as the classic 'bucket-handle tear' (Blumenthal, 1994). These lesions are difficult to identify on radiographs, as they heal within the cartilage of the growth plate and no bony callus forms. The fracture could also occur without disrupting the periosteum, thus periosteal new bone may not be evident radiographically (Carty, 1999). These fractures are pathognomonic of child abuse when multiple sites in different stages of repair are affected. However, because these lesions primarily affect the soft tissues of the growing bones, they will be difficult to identify in fully skeletonised remains.

If suspicious that long bone fractures in children are a result of physical abuse, one needs to complete a skeletal survey to see if the patient displays any characteristic patterns of inflicted trauma: multiple injury sites, healing fractures or lesions in different stages of repair (Kleinman, Nimkin, Spevak, ayder, Madansky et al., 1996; Thomas, Rosenfield, Leventhal, & Markowitz, 1991).

Inflicted long bone fractures frequently affect the proximal or distal metaphyses or mid-diaphysis of the bone (Thomas et al., 1991). The fractures are usually transverse, spiral or oblique (Thompson, 2005). A transverse fracture is caused by a direct blow, or bending of the bone to the point of fracture (Blumenthal, 1994). Spiral or oblique fractures are the result of twisting forces or a direct blow (Blumenthal, 1994). These injuries are caused by torsion to the bone, and when seen in children less than 3 years of age, are usually products of child abuse (Williams & Hardcastle, 2005).

Long bone fractures are not necessarily a result of abuse. Depending on their location, they could be the consequence of accidental trauma. For example, a supra-condylar fracture of the humerus is the classic result from an accidental fall onto the elbow or outstretched hand (Thomas et al., 1991). A nondisplaced oblique fracture of the distal tibia is commonly known as a 'toddler's fracture', acquired by children who are learning to walk (Carty, 1999; Thompson, 2005). In skeletonised remains it is often impossible to differentiate perimortem fractures from postmortem damage, although histological examinations may aid in identifying bone response to trauma not able to be detected with the naked eye or radiography (e.g., Klotzbach, Delling, Richter, Sperhake, & Puschel, 2003).

Trauma and Healing

In a forensic setting, medico–legal teams usually require the age determination of any fracture, to determine inconsistency (or concurrence) with the history of the victim (Carty, 1999). While dating fractures cannot be completed with total accuracy, a range of dates have been established according to the phase of fracture healing evident (Osier, Marks Jr, & Kleinman, 1993; Phillips, 2005). Thus, an understanding of the processes involved in fracture healing is imperative to the forensic anthropologist.

Carty (1999) summarises the healing phases following fractures of immature bones: associated periosteal new bone formation begins 4 to 21 days postinsult; the fracture line diminishes from radiographic view 10 to 21 days after trauma, which also denotes the time when a soft callous develops around the trauma site. The callous calcifies after 2 to 12 weeks, and remodelling takes place approximately 3 months postinsult. This time line depends on several factors: the health of the victim, immobilisation and medical intervention, the angle of fracture, and location of fracture on the bone (Carty 1999). Walker et al. (1997) also outline the timing of periosteal lesion remodelling and their expected macroscopic appearance.

Remodelling occurs at a faster rate in children compared to adults (Glencross & Stuart-Macadam, 2000). Immature bone has greater osteogenic activity and vascular supply than adult bone, making it easier to repair bone that has been subject to insult (Plunkett & Plunkett, 2000). However, if the injury occurs many months before death, the rate of repair may be sufficient to erase all evidence of trauma by the time of death. Remodelling is quickest in the following circumstances: when the bone has at least 2 years of growth remaining, when the fracture is close to the end of the bone and when fracture angulation occurs in the plane of motion (Glencross & Stuart-Macadam, 2000).

Periosteal Reactions and Traumatic Injury

Another common skeletal lesion seen in child abuse cases is that of periosteal strip-ping or 'bone bruising' (Blumenthal, 1994). Subperiosteal bleeding follows a physical insult that strips the periosteum from the bone surface (Plunkett & Plunkett, 2000). The subsequent inflammatory response invokes the deposition of new bone by osteoblasts within the periosteum. This enlarges the cambium layer of the perios-teum, and creates an area of radiolucency when examined radiographically (Plunkett

& Plunkett, 2000). This 'callous' of new bone forms approximately 1 to 2 weeks postinsult and may occur in conjunction with, or independent of, skeletal fractures (Walker et al., 1997).

Physiological vs. Pathologic Periosteal New Bone

Physiologic, bilateral, and symmetrical periosteal reactions are part of normal bone growth in infants aged 1 to 6 months and are characterised by the uniform periosteal elevation of long bone diaphyses (Blumenthal, 1994; Plunkett & Plunkett, 2000). Carty (1999) notes that the bone deposition is smooth and lamellar in appearance. The exact aetiology of the condition is unknown. It is imperative to recognise the difference between normal, physiologic periosteal new bone and pathologic periosteal new bone when examining children for skeletal markers of abuse (Prosser, Maguire, Harrison, Mann, Sibert et al., 2005). As the periosteum is loosely attached to the bones of infants, mild unintentional trauma may also be sufficient to pull the tissue off bone and stimulate an osteoblastic reaction (Carty, 1999).

Pathologic periosteal new bone can be a result of nonaccidental trauma and is usually asymmetric in distribution and associated with long bone metaphyses and diaphyses. Following trauma, osteoblasts are stimulated to deposit new bone under the periosteum in an excessive and nonuniform manner (Blumenthal, 1994). Physiologic periosteal reaction seldom extends to the end of the metaphysis, however, it is on the shaft of the long bones that periosteal reactions are primarily observed in physical abuse cases (Kleinman, 1990; Osier et al., 1993). Periosteal new bone in response to infection will affect multiple bones, and may not be symmetrical. However, it can usually be distinguished from trauma by the absence of soft tissue injury, multiple fractures and haematoma formation (De Silva, Evans-Jones, Wright, & Henderson, 2003).

A number of subadult skeletons from forensic cases were reported by Walker et al. (1997), which constitutes the only published account of physical abuse in skeletonised subadult remains. Because of the absence of soft tissue in most of these cases, subtle changes on the subperiosteal surfaces, not observable by radiography, were able to be identified. The authors argue that a pattern of multiple, asymmetric, radiographically undetectable periosteal reactions (less than 0.5 mm thick) in different stages of repair are diagnostic of severe and prolonged abuse.

The occurrence of subperiosteal new bone and abnormal porosity is one of the most frequent observations in prehistoric skeletal material (Lewis, 2000). Therefore, it is important that a differential diagnosis is made of skeletal lesions in immature skeletonised remains. Infection, inflammation, and accidental trauma can all cause similar pathological responses in bone and a careful examination must be carried out to determine the correct aetiology.

For example, infections such as congenital syphilis (*Treponema pallidum*), yaws (*Tr. pertenue*), metabolic diseases, and genetic diseases can all cause skeletal changes similar to those observed in child abuse (Blondiaux, Secousee, Cotton, Danze et al., 2002; Buckley & Tayles, 2003; Miller & Hangartner, 1999; Taitz, 1987).

While Walker et al. (1997) state that skeletal evidence of child abuse was absent in the thousands of prehistoric children they have examined and argue for the specificity of healed periosteal reactions to physical abuse, the multifactorial aetiology of periosteal lesions and porosity is well recognised in palaeopathology. Sometimes diagnosis of the underlying disease causing the lesions is not possible, especially in subadults (Buckley 2000a; Buckley and Tayles 2003; Lewis 2000).

Lewis (2000) states that for an accurate diagnosis to be made from subadult skeletal lesions, the skeleton needs to be complete and well preserved. Furthermore, she concludes that differentiating skeletal lesions pathognomonic of infection, inflammation or trauma in the archaeological record is very difficult, as they all occur commonly in newborns and infants. Furthermore, these immature skeletons are the least likely to survive internment and the loss of small bones from disturbance of remains by animals and other taphonomic processes may cause evidence for the lesions to be lost (Lewis, 2000).

Despite these problems, Blondiaux et al. (2002) claim to document the first case of prehistoric child abuse in a 2-year-old girl from a burial site in 4th century AD Lisieux, Normandy. The remains expressed bilateral, yet asymmetric, injuries to the cranium that were in different stages of repair, implying that her injuries were sustained at different intervals prior to her death. Concurrent indications of rickets in the bones of this child complicated the interpretation of traumatic lesions and serve to remind us that concurrent metabolic or infectious disease may also be present in abuse cases. It is well documented that physically abused children are invariably also neglected, leaving them vulnerable to infections and metabolic disease, hindering the accurate identification of abuse as the cause of the lesions (Kempe & Goldbloom, 1987; Walker et al., 1997). Other literature documenting trauma in prehistoric subadult bones provides useful comparative data for differentiating prolonged physical abuse from accidental injury (Glencross & Stuart-Macadam, 2000) and traumatic injury related to single catastrophic events, such as warfare (Buckley, 2000b).

Conclusions

Literature detailing the skeletal manifestations of child abuse in modern cases stress that skeletal lesions cannot tell the whole story. One needs to carefully examine the whole skeleton for markers of trauma, and then compare it with patient history to identify any inconsistencies (Blumenthal, 1994; Suggs et al., 2001; Thompson, 2005). Thus, a meticulous examination of subadult skeletonised remains for the possibility of child abuse, without corroborating personal testimony, can only ever become an educated prediction.

References

Blondiaux, G., Blondiaux, J., Secousee, F., Cotton, A., Danze, P. & Flipo, R. (2002). Rickets and child abuse: The case of the two year old girl from the 4th Century in Lisieux (Normandy). *International Journal of Osteoarchaeology, 12*, 209–215.

Blumenthal, I. (1994). *Child abuse: A handbook from health care practitioners*. London: Edward Arnold.

Buckley, H.R. (2000a). Subadult health and disease in prehistoric Tonga, Polynesia. *American Journal of Physical Anthropology, 113*, 481–505.

Buckley H. (2000b). A possible fatal wounding in the prehistoric Pacific Islands. *International Journal of Osteoarchaeology, 10*, 135–141.

Buckley, H.R., & Tayles, N. (2003). Skeletal pathology in a prehistoric Pacific Island sample: Issues in lesion recording, quantification and interpretation. *American Journal of Physical Anthropology, 122*, 303–324.

Bulloch, B., Schubert, C.J., Brophy, P.D., Johnson, N., Reed, M.H., & Shapiro, R.A. (2000). Cause and clinical characteristics of rib fractures in infants. *Pediatrics* 105, 48–52.

Caffey, J. (1946.) Multiple fractures in the long bones of infants suffering from chronic subdural hematoma. *American Journal of Roentgenology, 56*(2), 163–173.

Carty, P.R.H. (1993). Fractures caused by child abuse. *Journal of Bone and Joint Surgery, 75*–B, 849–857.

Carty, P.R.H. (1999). Non-accidental injury: Review of the radiology. *European Radiology, 7*, 1365–1376.

Crist, T.A.J., Washburn, A., Park, H., Hood, I., & Hickey, M.A. (1997). Cranial bone displacement as a taphonomic process in potential child abuse. In W.D. Haglund & M.H. Sorg (Eds.), *Forensic taphonomy: The post-mortem fate of human remains*. Boca Raton, FL: CRC Press.

De Silva, P., Evans-Jones, G., Wright, A., & Henderson, R. (2003). Physiological periostitis: A potential pitfall. *Archives of Disease in Childhood, 88*, 1124–1125.

Glencross, B., & Stuart-Macadam, P. (2000). Childhood trauma in the archaeological record. *International Journal of Osteoarchaeology, 10*, 198–209.

Kempe, R.S. & Goldbloom, R.B. (1987). Malnutrition and growth retardation ('Failure to thrive') in the context of child abuse and neglect. In R.E. Helfer & R.S. Kempe (Eds.), *The battered child* (pp. 313–335). Chicago: University of Chicago Press.

Kempe, C.H., Silverman, F.N., Steele, B.F., Droegmueller, W., & Silver, H.K. (1962). The battered child syndrome. *Journal of the American Medical Association, 181*, 17–24.

Kleinman, P.K. (1990). Diagnostic imaging of infant abuse. *American Journal of Roentgenology, 155*, 703–712.

Kleinman, P.K., Marks Jr, S.C., Richmond, J.M., & Blackbourne, B.D. (1995). Inflicted skeletal injury: A post-mortem radiologic-histopathologic study in 31 infants. *American Journal of Roentgenology, 165*, 647–650.

Kleinman, P.K., Nimkin, K., Spevak, M.R., Rayder, S.M., Madansky, D.L., Shelton, Y.A. et al. (1996). Follow-up skeletal surveys in suspected child abuse. *American Journal of Roentgenology, 167*, 893–896.

Klotzbach, H., Delling, G., Richter, E., Sperhake. J.P., & Puschel, K. (2003). Post-mortem diagnosis and age estimation of infants' fractures. *International Journal of Legal Medicine, 117*, 82–89.

Lewis, M. (2000). Non-adult paleopathology: current status and future potential. In M. Cox & S. Mays (Eds.), *Human osteology* (pp. 39–58). London: Greenwich Medical Media.

Meservy, C.J., Towbin, R., McLaurin, R.L., Myers, P.A., & Ball, W. (1987). Radiographic characteristics of skull fractures resulting from child abuse. *American Journal of Roentgenology, 149*, 173–175.

Miller, M.E., & Hangartner, T.N. (1999). Temporary brittle bone disease: Association with decreased fetal movement and osteopenia. *Calcified Tissue International, 64*, 137–143.

Osier, L.K., Marks, Jr S.C., & Kleinman, P.K. (1993). Metaphyseal extensions of hypertrophies chondrocytes in abused infants indicate healing fractures. *Journal of Pediatric Orthopedics, 13*, 249–254.

Phillips, A.M. (2005). Overview of the fracture healing cascade. *Injury, 36*, S5–S7.

Plunkett, J., & Plunkett, M. (2000). Physiologic periosteal changes in infancy. *American Journal of Forensic Medicine and Pathology, 21*, 213–216.

Prosser, I., Maguire, S., Harrison, S.K., Mann, M., Sibert, J.R., & Kemp, A.M. (2005). How old is this fracture? Radiologic dating of fractures in children: A systematic review. *American Journal of Roentgenology, 184*, 1282–1286.

Sawyer, J.R., Flynn, J.M., Dormans, J.P., Catalano, J., & Drummond, D.S. (2000). Fracture patterns in children and young adults who fall from significant heights. *Journal of Pediatric Orthopedics, 20*, 197–202.

Schwend, R.M., Werth, C., & Johnston, A. (2000). Femur shaft fractures in toddlers and young children: Rarely from child abuse. *Journal of Pediatric Orthopedics, 20*(4), 475–481.

Strait, R.T., Siegal, R.M., & Shapiro, R.A. (1995). Humeral fractures without obvious etiologies in children less than 3 years of age: When is it abuse? *Pediatrics, 96*, 667–671.

Suggs, A., Leichenstein, R., McCarthy, C., & Jackson, M.C. (2001). Child abuse/assault — general. In J.S. Olshaker, M.C. Jackson & W.S. Smock (Eds.), *Forensic emergency medicine* (pp. 151–172). Philadelphia: Lippencott, Williams and Wilkens.

Taitz, L.S. (1987). Child abuse and osteogenesis imperfecta. *British Medical Journal, 295,* 1082–1083.

Thomas, S.A., Rosenfield, N.S., Leventhal, J.M., & Markowitz, R.I. (1991). Long-bone fractures in young children: Distinguishing accidental injuries from child abuse. *Pediatrics, 88,* 471–476.

Thompson, S. (2005). Accident or inflicted? Evaluating cutaneous, skeletal, and abdominal trauma in children. *Pediatric Annals, 34,* 373–381.

Vialle, R., Mary, P., Schhmider, L., Ducou le Pointe, H., Damsin, J., & Filipe, G. (2006). Spinal fracture through the neurocentral synchondrosis of battered children. *Spine, 31,* E345–349.

Walker, P.L., Cook, D.C., & Lambert, P.M. (1997). Skeletal evidence for child abuse: A physical anthropological perspective. *Journal of Forensic Sciences 42,* 169–207.

Williams, R., & Hardcastle, N. (2005). Best evidence topic report. Humeral fractures and non-accidental injury in children. *Emergency Medical Journal, 22,* 124–125.

Worlock, P., Stower, M., & Barbor, P. (1986). Patterns of fractures in accidental and non-accidental injury in children: A comparative study. *British Medical Journal, 293,* 100–102.

Methods of Facial Approximation and Skull-Face Superimposition, With Special Consideration of Method Development in Australia

Carl N. Stephan

Ronn G. Taylor

Jane A. Taylor

Methods of craniofacial identification comprise two techniques: (a) the comparison of a face to a skull to determine whether a match exists (skull-face superimposition), and (b) the prediction of the face from a skull (facial approximation). In skull-face superimposition, an antemortem photograph of a person to whom the skeletal remains are expected to belong is used, and the face image overlaid with an image of the skull to enable evaluation of the degree of anatomical match. In the case of facial approximation, the constructed face is advertised in the public arena, via newspaper or television or other media, with the hope that somebody may recognise the face or the other information presented along with the approximation. Although these methods can be used to help contribute to the identification of a set of skeletal remains, it should be recognised they may not, and in many cases do not, enable positive identifications to be established.

Superimposition and facial approximation both depend on the hypothesis that the anatomy of the skull is intimately associated with the surface anatomy of the face (Krogman & Iscan, 1986; Stewart, 1979). Such a relationship clearly exists at a gross level as human skulls must fit beneath their soft tissue facial profiles (Schaeffer, 1942; Williams, 1995). It is in this sense that the commonly quoted phrase 'skulls are to faces what tent poles are to tents or walls to houses' is valid (e.g., Prag & Neave, 1997). However, care should be taken not to place too much emphasis on this saying, as soft tissues of the body are not merely draped over bones, nor are the bones so significantly responsible for the outward appearance of the body. The relationships between bones and the external appearance of the body are complicated by muscle, fat, vasculature, and connective tissue (Schaeffer, 1942; Williams, 1995) and the degree of information evident from the skull is incompletely known at this time.

Irrespective, it is the face, the bodily feature key to characterising our identities and personalities in everyday life (Bruce & Young, 1998), which gives these methods their identification value. The almost unique configuration of the human face (except perhaps in identical twins and probably a few individuals out of the 6.5 billion world-wide who share similar facial appearances to any one individual) clearly plays a role in the success of superimposition and facial approximation, although the latter may be complicated by other factors (see Haglund, 1998; Stephan, 2003a; and below).

Skull-face Superimposition

Generic Principles and Method Overview

Comparisons of skulls to faces can, and have, been made via side-by-side evaluations (e.g., Lander, 1918; Webster, Murray, Brinkhous, & Hudson, 1986). However, superimposition of images holds the advantage that anatomies from both pieces of evidence can be directly compared and visualised one on top of the other (see Figure 10.1). Since an antemortem photograph is used for comparison, not all shape information displayed by the skull can be used in the evaluation of the degree of fit of the skull to a face and thus comparisons are complicated by the two dimensional nature of the procedure.

Images can be superimposed using a variety of methods, such as tracings from photographs, photographs alone, or video footage (Figure 10.1). Video super-imposition has become the most popular in recent times as it enables real time visu-alisation of the superimposed structures, speeding up methods. In this process two video cameras are usually used; one focused on the skull, the other on the ante-mortem photograph and the two resultant images mixed together. Whatever the method used, be it photographic or video, some core principles underpin the methods.

Quality of Images and Their Display

Good quality antemortem face images (i.e., with high resolution, precise focus, good lighting and so on) must be sought so the facial anatomy can be clearly seen — the more detail evident the more robust the comparison will be. Ideally at least two images from different viewpoints should be used, they should be as recent as possible and should display anterior dentition on the skull (Austin-Smith & Maples, 1994; Glaister & Brash, 1937; Taylor & Brown, 1998). During superimposition the entire photo-graph should be parallel to the image-forming plane of the lens of the camera to prevent additional distortions being introduced (Taylor & Brown, 1998).

Photographic Conditions

Attempts should be made to replicate the photographic conditions of the ante-mortem photograph when recording images of the skull, as any deviations can impact on the comparison (Iten, 1987; Taylor & Brown, 1998). For example, subject distance from the camera impacts on perspective and magnification (e.g., Taylor & Brown, 1998), viewpoint impacts on perspective, and focal length of the camera lens impacts on magnification (and of lesser importance field of view). While these factors may be approximated to some degree from the antemortem photo-graph, enquiries should be made to determine these factors as precisely as possible (e.g., to the photographer who shot the original photograph). If the antemortem photographic conditions are replicated then adjustments in the magnification of one

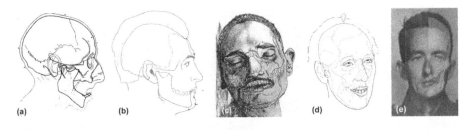

Figure 10.1

Examples of superimposition: (a) superimposition of face and skull outlines of Kant conducted by Welcker (1883), image reproduced from Grunner (1993: 33), with permission from John Wiley & Sons; (b) superimposition by Stadtmuller (1932) using skull and face outlines, image reproduced from Gruner (1993: 36), with permission from John Wiley & Sons; (c) superimposition using a skull outline conducted by Pearson and Morant (1934); (d) superimposition using skull and face outlines conducted by Glaister and Brash (1937); (e) video superimposition of a skull and face showing a right-side half-face wipe.

image, to match the other, will not be required. If the face in the antemortem photograph is small, dual-scaling of the images to a larger size will facilitate comparisons; however, no 'hard and fast' rules exist for this process. Life-size images have been seen as favourable (Glaister & Brash, 1937; Taylor & Brown, 1998), but images of sufficiently large size that are 'convenient for work' seem appropriate (Prinsloo, 1953). If photographic conditions cannot be precisely replicated some adjustments to the magnification of one of the images, while not favourable, will be required so that the two approximate similar size and thus become 'comparable' (Taylor & Brown, 1998).

Skull Orientation

Orientation of the skull to match the face in the antemortem photograph is crucial. Poor correspondence of the skull position to the face will result in significant inconsistencies even if the two are a match in reality. While most practitioners use trial and error for determining correct skull orientation (Austin-Smith & Maples, 1994; Bastiaan, Dalitz, & Woodward, 1986; Brocklebank & Holmgren, 1989; Brown, 1983; Glaister & Brash, 1937; Gordon & Drennan, 1948; Loh & Chao, 1989; McKenna, 1988; Sen, 1962; Taylor & Brown, 1998; Ubelaker, Bubniak, & O'Donnell, 1992; Webster, 1955; Webster et al., 1986), some have suggested using measurements to determine alignment (Iten, 1987; Janssens, Hansch, & Voorhamme, 1978), and complex mathematical formula have also been proposed (Chai & Lan, 1993; Chai et al., 1989; Sekharan, 1973; Sekharan, 1993). Numerous mounts have also been invented to hold the skull during orientation. The most basic is the skull or donut ring (Austin-Smith & Maples, 1994; Ubelaker et al., 1992), but more sophisticated systems have been developed that record the position either of the skull to the camera (Brocklebank & Holmgren, 1989; Taylor & Brown, 1998), or the camera to the skull (McKenna, 1988).

Historical Development

Superimposition originally developed out of attempts to verify the identities of skeletons thought to represent well-known historical figures (e.g., Welcker, 1883, 1888; and Figure 10.1). The method received some investigation prior to being employed in a forensic context, however, this research was minimal (see Pearson & Morant, 1934; Stadmuller, 1932). With little prior research findings on which to base the methods, Glaister & Brash were especially meticulous when first implementing the method to corroborate the identity of two individuals in 1937. This was a landmark case and set the standard for superimposition use in forensic casework. Glaister and Brash (1937) used tracings of the skulls and facial photographs similar to earlier authors (see Figure 10.1). Methods later evolved for the use of photographs alone; the first reported use is by Webster (1955), but see also Sen (1962). In the 1970s video equipment became widely available and motion picture cameras replaced the still frame cameras previously employed. Video superimposition was first reported by Clyde Snow in 1976; however, others were also using essentially identical methods at similar times (e.g., Brown, Hollamby, Clark, & Reynolds, 1978; Helmer & Gruner, 1977). The use of video superimposition became widespread in the 1980s (Bastiaan et al., 1986; Brown, 1983; Delino, Colonna, Potente, & Introna, 1986; Iten, 1987; Koelmeyer, 1982) and it has essentially carried through, unchanged, to recent times.

Australian Method History, Developments and Contributions

Still-image photographic superimposition has been used in an Australian setting at least since the 1960s (Brown, personal communication, 2006; for examples see Cocks, 1970; and Dalitz, 1971) and became replaced by video in the late 1970s. The exact number of cases in which superimposition has been used and/or resulted in positive results within Australia is unknown, but would appear to be in the hundreds. For video superimposition, the latest count indicates that it has been used in over 150 cases since 1977 (Brown, personal communication, 2006).

The development and first use of video superimposition in Australia was by Kenneth Brown, Cecil Hollamby, Barry Clark and Leslie Reynolds for use in a 1977 forensic case (Brown, 1983; Brown et al., 1978). Unknown at the time was its roughly 1-year earlier employment by Clyde Snow in America, and roughly 2-week earlier employment by Richard Helmer in Germany. In Australia, it was Cecil Hollamby, a South Australian police officer, who first suggested using a video camera to speed up the process of superimposition (Brown, personal communication, 2006). Video cameras enabled Brown and colleagues to achieve a superimposition for their case within approximately 15 minutes (Brown, personal communication, 2006). Soon after this case, video superimposition was employed in the 'Truro murders' case and it was these successes that prompted the establishment of the Forensic Odontology Unit at The University of Adelaide in 1980 (Brown, 1993).

A subsequent presentation of the method by Brown at an Australian conference inspired Tim Koelmeyer of New Zealand to use the method and publish a paper in 1982. Brown promptly followed by publishing a summary of his methods in 1983. In 1987, Jane Taylor and Kenneth Brown developed permanent and dedicated superimposition equipment at the Forensic Odontology Unit. The equipment included a specialised skull mount capable of movement in 6° of freedom (i.e., three perpendicular planes and three axes of rotation) and cameras mounted on fixed tracks enabling easy and precise adjustment of camera distance (Taylor & Brown, 1998). In 1988 Taylor used this equipment to conduct a Masters research project on the effects of camera distance on the superimposition method (Taylor, 1988).

The Forensic Odontology Unit has since been the centre for superimposition within Australia over the past 26 years and has assisted in several interstate and international cases. While methods have been used nationlly (e.g., by Alex Forrest and John Garner from Brisbane, Chris Griffiths from Sydney, and Clement and Hill from Melbourne) the Forensic Odontology Unit at The University of Adelaide has contributed most to the literature on the topic (see Brown, 1983, 1993; Brown et al., 1978; Taylor & Brown, 1998).

Current Approaches and Method Essentials

Skull-face superimposition is presently dominated by video comparison techniques and modern setups use digital devices. Equipment requirements begin at the image and skull mounts. Image mounts should be designed so that photographs are held flat and their plane parallel to the image forming plane of the lens of the camera (Taylor & Brown, 1998). Use of a camera lens diaphragm with a small aperture and a mirror placed in the position that the face would occupy in the photograph on the mount enables this to be evaluated (see Taylor & Brown, 1998). The skull mount can be as simple as the ring or donut type, but more sophisticated systems that record skull position hold major advantages (see above).

Photographic lights should be used to provide good illumination to the photograph and those used to illuminate the skull should possess the flexibility to closely approximate conditions evident in the antemortem photograph. Video cameras should be of professional quality, of the same make and type, and specifically ordered and bought in pairs to reduce any inconsistencies (Helmer, 1984; Taylor & Brown, 1998). Attachment of video cameras to mounts fixed to the floor but enabling accommodation of different subject-camera distances is favourable (Taylor & Brown, 1998). Video output, for both cameras, should be fed into a quality video mixer that maintains image quality and provides flexibility for effects; the Panasonic AG-MX70 is well suited to the task. One to three display monitors can be used to view the superimposition (three enable the skull alone, the face alone, and the superimposition to be viewed) and the entire superimposition process can be recorded onto digital video discs. The possibility also exists for video signals to be feed directly into a computer where they can be mixed and viewed directly within a computer environment.

Degree of match between the face and the skull should be assessed using established anatomical criteria. In general, soft tissue profiles should encompass the entirety of the skull without the protrusion of any bony margin; note that this has been an issue in some previously superimpositions that have claimed success (Taylor & Brown, 1998). Clearly, other general relationships, such as lips over teeth, eyes within orbits, nose over nasal aperture and so on, should also be evident, and use of other more specific criteria used will depend on the view and head position displayed in the antemortem photograph (Table 10.1 lists criteria that have been reported as useful in the past). Soft tissue depths may also be used to evaluate the fit of the skull to the face (Helmer, 1984) and for Caucasoid Australians pooled data seem most useful (see Domaracki & Stephan, 2006; Stephan, Norris, & Henneberg, 2005a). Note here that computer based quantitative methods for assessing the degree of fit of a skull to a face have also been reported by Nickerson, Fitzhorn, Koch and Charney (1991).

Table 10.1

Criteria Available for Matching Soft Tissue to the Skull in Skull-face Superimposition

Author	Frontal view
Webster (1955)	Length of skull from nose to chin Length of skull from top to chin or nose Margin of eye-sockets Bi-temporal width Width of face, as measured from one cheek bone to the other Position of the mastoid process Position of the mid-point of the upper jaw between the sockets for the central incisor teeth, and its relation to the nose Position of the teeth in the upper jaw on the left side Position of the angle of the jaws
Austin-Smith and Maples (1994)	Length of skull from bregma to menton fits within the face Width of cranium fills the forehead area of the face Temporal line of skull corresponds to the temporal line on face Eyebrow follows the upper edge of the orbit over the medial two-thirds Orbits completely encase the eye, including medial and lateral folds. Points of palpebral ligament attachment on the skull align with the folds of the eye. If visible, the lacrimal groove of the face aligns with that of the skull Breadth of bony nose bridge is similar to that of soft tissue and the two should align Opening of external auditory meatus lies medial to the tragus of the ear The nasal aperture falls inside the borders of the nose The anterior nasal spine lies superior to the inferior border of the medial crus of the nose When visible, the oblique line of the mandible corresponds to the line on the face The curve of the mandible is similar to that of the face jaw. Rounded, pointed, or notched chins will be evident in the mandible.
	Profile view
Austin-Smith and Maples (1994)	Vault of the skull and head height must be similar Glabella outline of skull and face should be similar although may not be exactly the same Lateral angle of eye lies in bony orbit Nasal bones fall within nose and shapes of each should correspond Zygomatic bones and their prominence on the face should correspond The anterior nasal spine lies posterior to the base of the nose Porion aligns just posterior to the tragus, slightly inferior to the curs of the helix Prosthion lies posterior to the anterior edge of the upper lip Pogonion lies posterior to the indentation observable in the soft tissue chin The mental protuberance of the mandible lies posterior to the point of the chin. The shape of the bony chin (rounded or pointed) corresponds to the shape of the overlying soft tissue The occipital curve lies within the outline of the back of the head

Despite the broad use of craniofacial superimposition little research has been conducted on the methods (McKenna, 1985; Ubelaker, 2002). One of the most comprehensive is by Austin-Smith & Maples (1994). These authors compared three skulls to 98 frontal and 97 lateral facial images of nontarget individuals and found that some false positive matches were obtained. In the case of frontal images the rate of incorrect matching was 8.5%, while for profile views it was 9.5%, and for both views combined it was 0.6% (note that anterior dentition was not considered). These authors thus concluded that without anterior dentition analysis craniofacial superimposition is reliable when two photographs, taken from different angles, are used.

In 1992 Ubelaker and colleagues conducted a study employing collections at the Department of Anthropology at the National Museum of Natural History. A single skull accompanied by an antemortem image was used for the study and after comparing anthropometric data from the reference skull to that of skeletons contained within the collections (representing more than 30,000 skeletons) four were identified as possible matches. When skulls of these four individuals were superimposed on the photograph of the missing woman, inconsistencies were found for all four skulls that were, therefore, excluded as matches.

Chai and Lan (1993) and Chai et al. (1989) tested the accuracy and reliability of superimposition methods using a complex system of landmarks and 'examining lines'. In essence, their method involves comparing lines drawn through similar landmarks on the face and skull after accounting for head position (e.g., face rotation, lateral tilt and anteroposterior pitch). In their study they compared 10 skulls to 1000 nontarget images and when using a total of eight examining lines found the rate for false positive identifications to be 0.05% (Chai et al., 1993, 1989).

It is important to reiterate at this point that only few investigators have regarded skull-face superimposition powerful enough to establish positive identification of skeletal remains (for authors that do regard it as an identification method see Sen, 1962; Chai & Lan, 1993; Chai et al., 1989). Most investigators use the methods in a less-absolute corroborative context and give heavier weighting to exclusions (Austin-Smith & Maples, 1994; DeVore, 1977; Dorion, 1983; Glaister & Brash, 1937; McKenna, 1985; Prinsloo, 1953; Simpson, 1943). With visible anterior dentition on the antemortem image and on the skull it has, however, been proposed that positive identifications can be established (Austin-Smith & Maples, 1994; McKenna, Jablonski, & Fearnhead, 1984; Webster et al., 1986). One case has been reported in the literature of a false positive identification using superimposition methods (Dorion, 1983).

Facial Approximation
Generic Principles and Method Overview
In forensic contexts, facial approximation is conducted under blind conditions (i.e., not knowing the facial appearance of the individual to whom the skull belongs). The faces can be constructed by drawing (Cherry & Angel, 1977; Taylor, 2001b), sculpting (Gatliff, 1984; Gerasimov, 1971; His, 1895; Kollman & Buchly, 1898; Krogman, 1946; Merkel, 1900; Prag & Neave, 1997; Stephan & Henneberg, 2006; Taylor & Angel, 1998; von Eggeling, 1913; Ullrich, 1958, 1966; Wilkinson, 2004) or using computer generated methods (Evison, 2001; Nelson & Michael, 1998; Quatrehomme et al., 1997; Tu et al., 2005; Turner et al., 2005; Vanezis et al., 1989; Vanezis, Vanezis, McCombe, & Niblett, 2000). Sculpting is by far the most common method currently employed, principally because skulls lend themselves to 3-dimensional build-ups, being themselves 3-dimensional structures, and because these methods give practitioners total control over construction of the face without software limitations.

Some practitioners undertake the task of manual sculpting directly on top of the skull (Gatliff & Taylor, 2001; Gerasimov, 1955; Ullrich, 1958); however, this carries the danger of damaging more delicate specimens either by direct physical trauma or absorption of materials from sculpting products (e.g., water or oils). Most practitioners, therefore, conduct facial approximation on a plaster skull where such damage is of little concern (Prag & Neave, 1997; Stephan & Henneberg, 2001; Taylor & Angel, 1998; Wilkinson, 2004). The plaster replica, usually cast from an alginate mould (see below and Figure 10.2), is an accurate and cost-effective method that enables the original skull to be used as a reference during the face construction process.

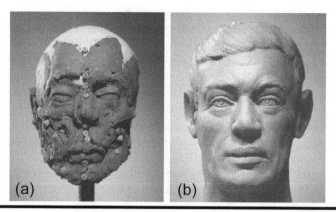

Figure 10.2
Day and English's (1991) facial approximation of a male skull: (a) skull cast with average soft tissue depths in place, note merging of Gatliff and Neave type styles (see e.g., Prag & Neave, 1997; Snow et al., 1970); (b) the completed facial approximation. Reprinted with permission from News Corporation.

Although methods of facial approximation are highly varied between practitioners, they all depend on face anatomy and average soft tissue depths to some degree (Stephan, 2006). Methods, therefore, differ as a result of different emphases placed on either one of these components. Average soft tissue depths are employed in all methods for the same purpose; to help determine the amount of soft tissue cover over the skull. Average soft tissue depths have been collected using a variety of methods, for example, needle puncture of cadavers (Domaracki & Stephan, 2006; Simpson & Henneberg, 2002; Suzuki, 1948), ultrasound (Aulsebrook, Becker, & Iscan, 1996; De Greef et al., 2006; El-Mehallawi & Soliman, 2001; Helmer, 1984; Manhein et al., 2000; Wilkinson, 2002), X-ray (Garlie & Saunders, 1999; Ogawa, 1960; Smith & Buschang, 2001; Williamson, Nawrocki, & Rathbun, 2002), computed tomography (Phillips & Smuts, 1996) and magnetic resonance imaging (Sahni, Jit, Gupta, Singh, & Suri, 2002). They have also been represented over the skull using slightly different methods, such as using rubber cylinders (Gatliff, 1984), match sticks (Taylor & Angel, 1998), or wooden pegs (Prag & Neave, 1997).

Soft tissue features that are evident from the skull are also used by practitioners to construct the face, but again approaches are varied. For example, Taylor & Gatliff (see Taylor, 2001a) do not directly represent muscles on the skull but take them into account during face construction; Gerasimov (1955, 1971) and Ullrich (1958, 1966, 1967, 1972) represent the large superficial masticatory muscles on the skull, but not to represent the finer muscles of facial expression as they are considered not to be evident; and Neave (Prag & Neave, 1997), Wilkinson (2004) and Taylor (Taylor & Craig, 2005) represent both the muscles of mastication and those of facial expression on the skull.

Once the face has been constructed it is photographed, the image converted to greyscale if it is not already in that format, and placed in a public advertisement to accompany a written case description. The aim of the advertisement is to prompt recognition of the person described, by somebody who previously knew this individual.

Historical Development

Like superimposition, facial approximation also developed out of attempts to verify the identities of skeletons thought to represent well-known historical figures (e.g., His, 1895). In early times, facial approximation methods were couched with a cautious regard to what they could be expected to achieve; that is, a similar face type was expected but not correct face recognition or clear resemblance (Kollman & Buchly, 1898; Merkel, 1900; von Eggeling, 1913). Some also doubted the value of the methods for forensic investigations (von Eggeling, 1913). Over time these views changed, at least in part, because of successful outcomes produced when methods were employed in forensic contexts — facial approximation is reported to have achieved its first case success in 1913 (Wilder & Wenworth, 1918). Since this case, facial approximation methods has been used to generate many other successful case outcomes (e.g., Gatliff & Snow, 1979; Gerasimov, 1971; Prag & Neave, 1997; Suzuki, 1973; Taylor, 2001a; Taylor & Craig, 2005).

From their origin, facial approximation methods heavily relied on average soft tissue depth data (His, 1895; Kollman & Buchly, 1898) and it was this aspect that received considerable research focus early on (e.g., Czekanowski, 1907; Edelman, 1938; Martin, 1957; Stadtmuller, 1922) and more recently (e.g., De Greef et al., 2006; Domaracki & Stephan, 2006; Manhein et al., 2000; Sahni et al., 2002; Simpson & Henneberg, 2002; Smith & Buschang, 2001; Wilkinson, 2002; Williamson et al., 2002). Manual sculpting methods have largely dominated at all times (e.g., Gatliff & Taylor, 2001; Gerasimov, 1955; Prag & Neave, 1997; His, 1895; von Eggeling, 1913; Wilkinson, 2004).

Basic principals of the traditional sculpting method have remained essentially unchanged over the life of the method although some soft tissue prediction methods have been refined and additional data collected (e.g., Ryan & Wilkinson, 2006; Stephan, 2002b, 2002c, 2003c; Stephan & Henneberg, 2003; Stephan, Henneberg, & Sampson, 2003; Wilkinson & Mautner, 2003; Wilkinson, Motwanu, & Chiang, 2003; and below). Mean soft tissue depths continue to be widely used, although some consideration has been given to use of medians and modes (Domaracki & Stephan, 2006).

Australian Method History, Developments and Contributions

Facial approximation was first used in forensic investigations in Australia in 1975. Since this time facial approximation appears to have been formally recorded in 20 instances. The method, therefore, receives an average forensic use of once every 1.5 years for a population approximately sized 20.5 million and four have ultimately proved to be useful.

The first use of facial approximation methods in Australia was in 1975 when Warren Day and Harold English built the face of a man who had been shot in the head (Safe, 1991). Despite extensive public advertisement, this facial approximation did not produce a successful identification result. In 1976, Day and English undertook another reconstruction, this time of a female, which was also advertised without result (Safe, 1991). After a readvertisement in a newspaper 14 years later, a tentative identification was made by a close associate (stepsister) and was verified through fingerprint comparison and dental records (Safe, 1991). A third facial approximation was constructed by Day and English in 1991 (Safe, 1991) but results of its advertisement are unknown to us. The methods of Day and English were strongly influenced by both American and UK sources

(Figure 10.2), which is not surprising given that Day travelled to both locations in 1983 under a Churchill Fellowship to study the method. It is evident that Day and English were principally concerned with casework application of methods since no published contributions to the professional literature were made.

From 1989 Ronn Taylor was also working on the construction of faces for police investigations. Over a period of 17 years Taylor has constructed 14 faces for the police, with three contributing to correct identifications. Taylor's work, therefore, accounts for the largest portion of Australian-made facial approximations (~70%). Examples of Taylor's work include the 'Nhill Man' constructed in 1989, which has not been identified (Safe, 1991; Figure 10.3), the 'Silvan Dam Man' also constructed in 1989 and unidentified (Safe, 1991); a male face, constructed in 1990, which was correctly recognised in 1991 from a television advertisement (Taylor & Craig, 2005; Figure 10.4); and a male face, constructed in 2002, which was recognised in 2003 from a newspaper advertisement (Taylor & Craig, 2005). Taylor's technique was based on that of Neave's (Prag & Neave, 1997), with the added component that after face construction a police computer graphics specialist (Adrian Paterson) adds skin tone/texture, eyebrows, hair and other features to the image to enhance it (Hayes et al., 2005). Taylor has contributed to the professional literature on facial approximation with particular regard to general overviews of the method (Taylor & Angel, 1998; Taylor & Craig, 2005), details of his personal methods (Hayes, Taylor, & Paterson, 2005; Taylor & Craig, 2005), average soft tissue depths of Australian samples (Taylor & Angel, 1998) and precision skull casting (Taylor & Angel, 1998).

In 1994 Meiya Sutisno constructed a facial approximation for the NSW Police, followed by another in 1999. Sutisno's other contribution to the field was a PhD thesis on human facial soft-tissue thickness (Sutisno, 2003).

In 1996, Maciej Henneberg at The University of Adelaide began conducting and supervising Australian research in craniofacial identification and started with research on the relationships between average soft tissue depths and head size (Anderson, 1996). Several years later Henneberg's team was associated with facial approximations produced for the South Australian Police concerning the 'Lower Light case'

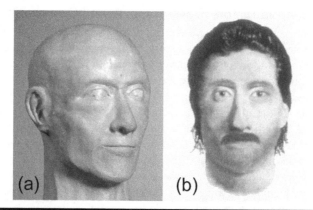

Figure 10.3
Ronn Taylor's 1989 facial approximation of the 'Nhill Man'. (a) clay facial approximation before computer enhancement, (b) facial approximation after computer enhancement. (The skeletal remains of this individual have not been identified.)

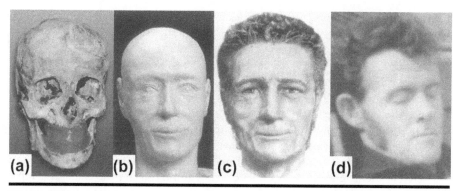

Figure 10.4

Ronn Taylor's 1990 facial approximation: (a) skull, (b) facial approximation before computer enhancement, (c) facial approximation after computer enhancement by Adrian Patterson, (d) target individual, image reprinted from Taylor and Craig (2005: p. 49), with permission from Elsevier.

that were advertised without result. In 1998, Ellie Simpson joined Henneberg's team and continued research on head size and facial soft tissue depths, producing in 2002 a formal published study (Simpson & Henneberg, 2002).

In 1998, Carl Stephan also joined the Henneberg team and a year later produced, on request from the Forensic Odontology Unit, a new facial approximation concerning the 'Lower Light case' that was not advertised before an identification was established through other methods (Stephan & Henneberg, 2006). In conjunction with Henneberg, Stephan also established research and teaching collaborations with Ronn Taylor and John Clement at The University of Melbourne. Stephan and colleagues' research has been published in leading forensic science journals and has examined a variety of method aspects including average soft tissue depths (Domaracki & Stephan, 2006; Stephan et al., 2005a), overall accuracy of methods and how to assess it (Stephan & Arthur, 2006; Stephan & Henneberg, 2001, 2006; Stephan, 2002a; Stephan, Penton-Voak, Clement, & Henneberg, 2005c), accuracy of specific soft tissue prediction guidelines and their improvements (Stephan, 2002b, 2002c, 2003b, 2003c; Stephan & Henneberg, 2003; Stephan, Henneberg, & Sampson, 2003), theoretical underpinnings of methods and conceptual method overviews (Stephan, 2003a, 2005, 2006), and standardised photography and average face generation (Stephan, Clement, Owen, Dobrostanski, & Owen, 2004; Stephen, Penton-Voak, Clement, & Henneberg, 2005b).

In Brisbane, Alex Forrest and John Gardener have also conducted a number of facial approximations related to forensic casework (up to approximately 14; Forrest personal communication, 2006).

Current Approaches and Method Essentials

The complex arrangement of the soft tissue face over the skull, the innumerable approaches to how it could be constructed and/or represented, and the relatively few scientific investigations examining these approaches, means that no one approach of facial approximation has been identified as being empirically any better than any other. Given space restrictions it is not possible to present all methods that are currently used;

instead, relatively common approaches used within Australia will be presented, and, where possible, findings from scientific investigations presented.

The first step of the facial approximation process is to cast the skull (see above for justification). The mandible is set in the glenoid fossa in a position representative of the living body with simulation of the interarticular disc of the temporomandibular joint (e.g., Schaeffer, 1942; Williams, 1995) and a free-way space of 2 mm to 3 mm between the anterior teeth (Pleasure, 1951). Undercut bony regions of the skull are filled in so the skull can be easily removed from the mould at a later stage. A split-mould casting technique, similar to that of Neave, is used (Prag & Neave, 1997). A clay table is first built around the inferior portion of the skull, essentially at its largest diameter, at the height of the zygomatic arches and traversing the cranium (Figure 10.5: after Taylor & Angel, 1998). Location marks are made on the superior surface of the table at the periphery. Dental alginate material is then poured over the top to form a layer approximately 20 mm thick. Once set, location marks are made in the alginate by cutting out triangular lugs, and plastic food wrap is spread over the alginate (pressing it into the location marks), on which plaster is poured to form a backing shell. Once dry, the plaster backing and skull is upturned, the clay table removed and the process repeated to form the second half of the mould. When completed, the skull is removed and the alginate in each half of the mould cleaned with water and a soft brush. A fresh batch of dental plaster is then made, and each half of the mould exactly filled to its brim. The plaster is briefly allowed to cure in the mould (but remains fluid) and one half of the mould quickly and precisely placed on the other. The mould is then left in place for approximately an hour while the cast sets.

Once hardened, the plaster cast is removed and the join line trimmed. Average soft tissue depths are then selected from the literature and holes drilled in the skull cast at appropriate anatomical landmarks to glue in place small diameter wooden dowels to mark the soft tissue depth (Prag & Neave, 1997). As for superimposition methods, pooled data reported by Domaracki & Stephan (2006) are recommended for Caucasoid Australians. The dowels can be precut 5 mm longer than required and glued at the appropriate depth using two-part epoxy resin and a metal rule with a 0.5 mm scale (Figure 10.6).

Prosthetic eyeballs can be placed in the orbit and should project approximately 16 mm from the lateral orbital wall (Stephan, 2002b; Swan & Stephan, 2005; Wilkinson & Mautner, 2003). In the coronal plane it is said that they should also be centrally positioned (e.g., Gatliff & Snow, 1979); however, the validity of this guideline is suspect (Stephan & Davidson, in press). The muscles of mastication that leave clear markings on the skull can be built (Gerasimov, 1955; Gerasimov, 1971; Ullrich, 1958, 1966, 1967). Muscles of facial expression can also be added (Prag & Neave, 1997; Taylor & Craig, 2005; Wilkinson, 2004; Figure 10.7), however, their determination from the skull is controversial (Gerasimov, 1955; Stephan, 2003a; Ullrich, 1958, 1966).

As with the muscles, the remaining soft tissues of the face must also be built with regard to the robustness of the skull. Nose projection appears to be best estimated by using the method of George (1987); see also Ryan and Wilkinson (2006), and Stephan et al. (2003); and nose width according to Hoffman, McConathy, Coward and Saddler (1991). The shape of the bridge of the nose can be estimated from the shape of the nasal bones (George, 1987). Mouth width can easily be approximated by using canine width as 75% of the mouth width (Stephan & Henneberg, 2003)

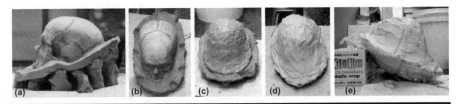

Figure 10.5

Skull casting sequence: (a) lateral view of 'clay table' constructed about skull, (b) superior view showing location marks placed in the 'clay table', (c) superior view with layer of dental alginate added, (d) superior view with plaster backing added over plastic wrap covering alginate, (e) lateral view of mould during skull cast production (plaster has been added in place of skull and entire assemblage set aside in order for cast to dry before mould is removed).

and it is reported that lip height can be determined from tooth enamel height (Wilkinson et al., 2003). The ears are known to be larger than the nose for the majority of the population (Farkas, Forrest, & Litsas, 2000) and their inclination is known not to equal that of the nose (Farkas, Forrest, & Litsas, 2000; Farkas, Sohm, Kolar, Katic, & Munro, 1985; Skiles & Randall, 1983). Few other tested guidelines are known. While general positions of the eyebrows are evident a priori from living faces, precise details of relationships to skulls are not known. The superciliare landmark appears to fall close to the lateral aspect of the iris, while for males it appears to be more lateral (Stephan, 2002c), but these characteristics are highly variable (e.g., Rozprym, 1934). Many other soft tissue prediction guidelines have been proposed, however, they are not discussed here since they have not been subject to empirical tests (for further discussion see Stephan, in press).

Accuracy of facial approximation methods has been an issue at the forefront of the field, particularly since claims of method abilities have changed from a reserved and cautious approach (Gatliff & Snow, 1979; Kollman & Buchly, 1898; Merkel,

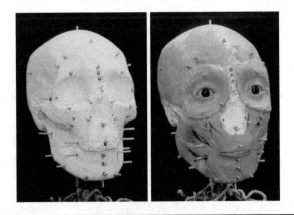

Figure 10.6

An example of a partially completed facial approximation following methods most similar to Neave (Prag and Neave, 1997). Left image shows the plaster skull replica with soft tissue depths markers attached (here according to Helmer, 1984). Right image shows the partially completed face with prosthetic eyes in place, and muscles of mastication and facial expression modelled.

1900; Neave, 1979; von Eggeling, 1913) to more recent bolder claims of purposeful face recognition (e.g., Gerasimov, 1971; Prag & Neave, 1997; Wilkinson, 2004), despite few changes to methods.

Accuracy of facial approximation was first assessed by the comparison of constructed faces to a death mask of the person to whom the skull belonged (von Eggeling, 1913). Clearly, this approach was limited as death masks do not well represent an individual in life, and resemblance was gauged; not recognition (see for further discussion Haglund, 1998; Stephan, 2002a). A landmark paper by Snow and colleagues in 1970 rectified these problems by using, for the first time, an antemortem face array. Individuals assessing the facial approximation had to pick a corresponding face from the face array (with all faces presented at the same time). Results were statistically compared against the chance rate for selecting any face (14%) and it was found that both facial approximations were recognised above chance rates (one facial approximation at a success rate of 68% the other 26%).

It was not until 1993 that the next face array test was conducted. Van Rensberg (1993) tested 15 facial approximations using death masks and thus the findings of this study have limitations as highlighted above (average success rate was 26%; chance rate = 7%; statistical tests unreported). In 2001, Stephan and Henneberg conducted an antemortem face array test that examined 16 facial approximations and presented all faces in the face array simultaneously. In contrast to Snow and colleagues' study, where a forced choice protocol was used (assessors had to select a face from the face array), Stephan and Henneberg allowed assessors to select an option of not identifying any face (i.e., if assessors thought that no face was worth nominating based on the appearance of the facial approximation). Recognition rates were not as high as those found by Snow and colleagues, with only 1 of 16 facial approximations recognised above chance rates at statistically significant levels (mean rate across all facial approximations = 8%; chance rate = 5%). In 2002, Wilkinson and Whittaker (2002; see also Wilkinson, 2004) conducted an antemortem face array test of five 'juvenile' facial approximations, but since the face array included all target individuals, which were also of disparate ages (8–18 years), results must be held with caution (mean recognition rate of 44%). Collectively these results do not appear to offer any definitive answer regarding the accuracy of facial approximation methods, except perhaps that recognition rates may in general be less than those first reported by Snow and colleagues.

Despite the introduction of more rigorous testing methods by Snow and colleagues (1970), practitioners continued to look to inferior methods for assessing facial approximation accuracy. This included reliance on reported casework success (Gerasimov, 1971; Prag & Neave, 1997), and comparisons of resemblance or similarity between a facial approximation and antemortem appearances of the target individual (Helmer, Rohricht, Petersen, & Morr, 1993; Krogman, 1946; Prag & Neave, 1997; Suzuki, 1973). The former method is now known to be unreliable for at least two reasons: (a) other case specific information contained in public case advertisements may be responsible for casework recognition (Haglund, 1998), and (b) practitioners seem predisposed to reporting casework success in the best possible light (Clement & Marks, 2005; Stephan, 2003a). The latter method is also recognised to be an unreliable measure of facial approximation accuracy because: (a) it does not account for nontarget faces who may bear closer resemblance to the facial approximation (Stephan, 2002a; Stephan & Henneberg, 2006), and (b) it tests for similarity of faces not the ability to recognise them (Stephan, 2002a; Stephan & Henneberg, 2006).

These aspects have been clearly demonstrated by a study examining both resemblance ratings and recognition tests on the same facial approximation (Stephan & Henneberg, 2006). Resemblance ratings showed the facial approximation to possess good resemblance to the target individual (~ 7 out of 10), but when recognition tests were conducted the facial approximation performed poorly (mean success rate = 20%; chance = 10%). In fact, recognition results were better when assessors did not use the facial approximation but merely guessed who the 'murder victim' was (Stephan & Henneberg, 2006). In addition to highlighting the potential for bias in face arrays used for facial approximation testing, this study was also the first to employ simultaneous and sequential face arrays in a facial approximation setting and demonstrated that, as previously found for eyewitness identification tests (Gonzalez, Ellsworth, & Pembroke, 1993; Malpass & Devine, 1983; Wells, 1993), sequential arrays significantly reduce the number of false positive identifications while not significantly effecting true positive identifications.

Although face array tests have been a significant step forward in facial approximation identification, they remain limited as they test people who are unfamiliar with, or do not closely know, the target individual. This is not representative of real life facial approximation casework, as it is usually a family member or close associate who comes forward with a suggested identity. Similar to unfamiliar face array studies, a number of tests have been conducted where a practitioner has blindly approximated a face of a living person from their skull (e.g., using a laser sintered skull from computed tomography data) to see if that practitioner can recognise the correct person. For example, Neave constructed a head-on-a-skull replica, and found it to be sufficiently similar to the target individual for him to recognise the target in a room full of people (Prag & Neave, 1997). While such tests also offer some insight into the abilities of the method, testing practitioner recognition (that is based in an unfamiliar context) seems several times removed from familiar recognition that is frequent in forensic casework. Thus, the ultimate facial approximation test is one where familiar recognition is assessed.

Stephan and colleagues (2005c) circumvented the problems above by warping average human faces to exact face shapes of living target individuals, thus enabling close associates of the living targets to be surveyed for their recognition responses. Note here that no skulls were used so that the facial approximations produced had the exact same two-dimensional face shapes as their target individual; something that is not possible in current forensic casework. Successful recognition rates were found to average approximately 43%, suggesting that recognition rates in real life casework, where it is unlikely for exact face shapes to be replicated, are less.

Conclusions

The methods of skull-face superimposition and facial approximation have a proven track record in assisting casework success and are thus indispensable tools for aiding in the identification of human skeletal remains. Skull-face superimposition is particularly useful for excluding individuals to whom the skeletal remains do not belong, however, with two or more different facial views and anterior dentition comparison, evidence of a match can be strong. Facial approximation is a more inaccurate and unreliable method but continues to hold an important role, which is especially pronounced when other identification methods cannot be used. With increased research and empirical testing both methods of craniofacial identification may come to carry more weight in skeletal remains investigations of the future.

Acknowledgments

Special thanks are extended to: Kenneth Brown for sparing the time to discuss invaluable information concerning the history and development of craniofacial superimposition methods in Australia, and to the Discipline of Anatomical Sciences at The University of Adelaide for the use of the skull and antemortem photographs displayed in Figure 10.1. Thanks also go to Alex Forrest who was able to provide information in regards to the facial approximation casework he has conducted and to Grant Townsend for the clarification of a practitioner's name.

References

Anderson, W. (1996). *The correlation between soft tissue thickness and bony proportions of the skull and how they relate to facial reconstruction.* Unpublished manuscript (3rd year project), The University of Adelaide, Australia.

Aulsebrook, W.A., Becker, P.J, & Iscan, M.Y. (1996). Facial soft-tissue thickness in the adult male Zulu. *Forensic Science International, 79,* 83–102.

Austin-Smith, D., & Maples, W.R. (1994). The reliability of skull/photograph superimposition in individual identification. *Journal of Forensic Sciences, 39,* 446–455.

Bastiaan, R.J., Dalitz, G.D., & Woodward, C. (1986). Video superimposition of skulls and photographic portraits: A new aid to identification. *Journal of Forensic Sciences, 31,* 1373–1379.

Brocklebank, L.M., & Holmgrn, C.J. (1989). Development of equipment for the standardization of skull photographs in personal identifications by photographic superimposition. *Journal of Forensic Sciences, 34,* 1214–1221.

Brown, K.A. (1983). Developments in cranio-facial superimposition for identification. *The Journal of Forensic Odonto-Somatology, 1,* 57–64.

Brown, K.A. (1993). The Truro murders in retrospect: A historical review of the identification of the victims. *Annals/Academy of Medicine, Singapore, 22,* 103–106.

Brown, K.A., Hollamby, C., Clark, B.J., & Reynolds, L. (1978). *Abstract. A video technique of cranio-facial photo-superimposition for identification* (pp. 22–26). 8th Meeting of the International Association of Forensic Sciences.

Bruce, V., & Young, A. (1998). *In the eye of the beholder.* New York: Oxford University Press.

Chai D-S, & Lan, Y-W. (1993). Standards for skull-to-photo superimposition. In M.Y. Iscan & R. Helmer (Eds.), *Forensic analysis of the skull* (pp: 171–181). New York: Wiley-Liss.

Chai, D.-S., Lan, Y.-W., Tao, C., Gui, R.-J., Mu, Y.-C., Feng, J.-H., Wang, W.-D., & Zhu, J. (1989). A study on the standard for forensic anthropologic identification of skull-image superimposition. *Journal of Forensic Sciences, 34,* 1343.

Cherry, D.G., & Angel, J.L. (1977). Personality reconstruction from unidentified remains. *FBI Law Enforcement Bulletin, 46,* 12–15.

Clement, J.G., & Marks, M.K. (2005). Introduction to facial reconstruction. In J.G. Clement & M.K. Marks (Eds.), *Computer-graphic facial reconstruction* (pp. 3–13). Boston: Elsevier: Academic Press.

Cocks, F.B. (1970). The Barkly highway murder. *The Australian Police Journal, 24,* 173–185.

Czekanowski, J. (1907). Untersuchungen uber das Verhaltnis der Kopfmafse zu den Schadelmafsen. *Archiv fur Anthropologie, 6,* 42–89.

Dalitz, G.D. (1971). *Abstract. Superimposition as an aid to identification.* National Symposium on the Forensic Sciences.

De Greef, S., Claes, P., Vandermeulen, D., Mollemans, W., Suetens, P., & Willems, G. (2006). Large-scale in-vivo Caucasian soft tissue thickness database for craniofacial reconstruction. *Forensic Science International, 159S,* S126–S146.

Delino, V.P., Colonna, M., Potente, F., & Introna, F.J. (1986). Computer-aided skull/face super-imposition. *The American Journal of Forensic Medicine and Pathology, 7,* 201–212.

DeVore, D.T. (1977). Radiology and photography in forensic dentistry. *Dental Clinics of North America, 21,* 69–83.

Domaracki, M., & Stephan, C.N. (2006). Facial soft tissue thicknesses in Australian adult cadavers. *Journal of Forensic Sciences, 51,* 5–10.

Dorion, R.B.J. (1983). Photographic superimposition. *Journal of Forensic Sciences, 28,* 724–734.

Edelman, H. (1938). Die profilanalyse: Eine studie an photographischen und rontgenographischen durchdringungsbildern. *Zeitschrift fur Morphololgie und Anthropologie, 37,* 166–188.

El-Mehallawi, I.H., & Soliman, E.M. (2001). Ultrasonic assessment of facial soft tissue thickness in adult Egyptians. *Forensic Science International, 117,* 99–107.

Evison, M.P. (2001). Modeling age, obesity, and ethnicity in a computerized 3-D facial reconstruction. *Forensic Science Communications 3.* Retrieved June 15, 2006, from http://www.fbi.gov/hq/lab/fsc/backissu/april2001/evison.htm

Farkas, L.G., Forrest, C.R., & Litsas, L. (2000). Revision of neoclassical facial canons in young adult Afro-Americans. *Aesthetic Plastic Surgery, 24,* 179–184.

Farkas, L.G., Sohm, P., Kolar, J.C., Katic, M.J., & Munro, I.R. (1985). Inclinations of the facial profile: art versus reality. *Plastic and Reconstructive Surgery, 75,* 509–519.

Garlie, T.N., & Saunders, S.R. (1999). Midline facial tissue thicknesses of subadults from a longitudinal radiographic study. *Journal of Forensic Sciences, 44,* 61–67.

Gatliff, B.P. (1984). Facial sculpture on the skull for identification. *The American Journal of Forensic Medicine and Pathology, 5,* 327–332.

Gatliff, B.P., & Snow, C.C. (1979). From skull to visage. *The Journal of Biocommunication, 6,* 27–30.

Gatliff, B.P., & Taylor, K.T. (2001). Three-dimensional facial reconstruction on the skull. In K.T. Taylor (Ed.), *Forensic art and illustration* (pp. 419–475). Boca Raton, FL: CRC Press.

George, R.M. (1987). The lateral craniographic method of facial reconstruction. *Journal of Forensic Sciences, 32,* 1305–1330.

Gerasimov, M. (1955). *Vosstanovlenie lica po cerepu.* Moskva: Izdat. Akademii Nauk SSSR.

Gerasimov, M. (1971). *The face finder.* London: Hutchinson & Co.

Glaister, J., & Brash, J.C. (1937). *Medico-legal aspects of the Ruxton Case.* Baltimore, MD: William Wood and Co.

Gonzalez, R., Ellsworth, P.C., & Pembroke, M. (1993). Response biases in lineups and showups. *Journal of Personality and Social Psychology, 64,* 525–537.

Gordon, I., & Drennan, M.R. (1948). Medico-legal aspects of the Wolkersdorfer case. *South African Medical Journal, 22,* 543–549.

Gruner, O. (1993). Identification of skulls: A historical review and practical applications. In M.I. Iscan & R.P. Helmer (Eds.), *Forensic analysis of the skull* (pp. 20–45). New York: Wiley-Liss.

Haglund, W.D. (1998). Forensic "art" in human identification. In J.G. Clement & D.L. Ranson (Eds), *Craniofacial identification in forensic medicine* (pp. 235–243). London: Arnold.

Hayes, S., Taylor, R., & Paterson, A. (2005). Forensic facial approximation: An overview of current methods utilised at the Victorian Institute of Forensic Medicine/Victoria Police Criminal Identification Squad. *The Journal of Forensic Odonto-Somatology, 23,* 45–50.

Helmer, R. (1984). *Schadelidentifizierung durch elekronicshe bildmischung: Sugl el beitr zur konstitutionsbiometrie U Dickermessung d Gesichtsweichteile.* Heidelberg: Krminalistik-Verlag.

Helmer, R.P., & Gruner, O. (1977). Vereingachte schadelidentifiziening nach dem super projektionsver fahren mit Hilfe einer video-anlage. *Sectschrift Rectsmedizin, 80,* 183–187.

Helmer, R.P., Rohricht, S., Petersen, D., & Mohr, F. (1993). Assessment of the reliability of facial reconstruction. In M.Y. Iscan & R.P. Helmer (Eds.), *Forensic analysis of the skull* (pp. 229–246). New York: Wiley-Liss.

His, W. (1895). Anatomische Forschungen uber Johann Sebastian Bach's Gebeine und Antlitz nebst Bemerkungen uber dessen Bilder. *Abhandlungen der mathematisch-physikalischen Klasse der Königlichen Sachsischen Gesellschaft der Wissenschaften, 22,* 379–420.

Hoffman, B.E., McConathy, D.A., Coward, M., & Saddler, L. (1991). Relationship between the piriform aperture and interalar nasal widths in adult males. *Journal of Forensic Sciences 36,* 1152–1161.

Iten, P.X. (1987). Identification of skulls by video superimposition. *Journal of Forensic* Sciences, *32,* 173–188.

Janssens, P.A., Hansch, C., & Voorhamme, L.L. (1978). Identity determination by superimposition with anthropological cranium adjustment. *OSSA, 5,* 109–122.

Koelmeyer, T.D. (1982). Videocamera superimposition and facial reconstruction as an aid to identification. *The American Journal of Forensic Medicine and Pathology, 3,* 45–48.

Kollman, J., & Buchly, W. (1898). Die persistenz der rassen und die reconstruction der physiognomie prahistorischer schadel. *Archives fur Anthropologie, 25,* 329–359.

Krogman, W.M. (1946). The reconstruction of the living head from the skull. *FBI Law Enforcement Bulletin, 17,* 11–17.

Krogman, W.M., & Iscan, M.Y. (1986). *The human skeleton in forensic medicine.* Springfield, IL: Charles C. Thomas.

Lander, K.F. (1918). The examination of a skeleton of known age, race and sex. *Journal of Anatomy LII,* 282–291.

Loh, F.C., & Chao, T.C. (1989). Skull and photographic superimposition: A new approach using a second party's interpupil distance to extrapolate the magnification factor. *Journal of Forensic Sciences, 34,* 708–713.

Malpass, R.S., & Devine, P.G. (1983). Measuring the fairness of eyewitness identification lineups. In SMA Lloyd-Bostock & B.R. Clifford (Eds.), *Evaluating witness evidence: Recent psychological research and new perspectives* (pp. 81–102). New York: John Wiley and Sons.

Manhein, M.H., Listi, G.A., Barsley, R.E., Musselman, R., Barrow, N.E., & Ubelaker, D.H. (2000). In vivo facial tissue depth measurements for children and adults. *Journal of Forensic Sciences, 45,* 48–60.

Martin, R. (1957). *Lehrbuch der Anthropologie.* Stuttgart: Gustav Fischer Verlag.

McKenna, J.J.I. (1985). Studies of the method of matching skulls with photographic portraits using landmarks and measurements of the dentition. *The Journal of Forensic Odonto-Somatology,* 3: 1–6.

McKenna, J.J.I. (1988). A method of orientation of skull and camera for use in forensic photographic investigation. *Journal of Forensic Sciences, 33,* 751–755.

McKenna, J.J.I., Jablonski, N.G., & Fearnhead, R.W. (1984). A method of matching skulls with photographic portraits using landmarks and measurements of the dentition. *Journal of Forensic Sciences, 29,* 787–797.

Merkel, F. (1900). Reconstruction der buste eines Bewohners des Leinegaues. *Archives fur Anthropologie, 26,* 449–457.

Neave, R.A.H. (1979). Reconstruction of the heads of three ancient Egyptian mummies. *Journal of Audiovisual Media in Medicine, 2,* 156–164.

Nelson, L.A., & Michael, S.D. (1998). The application of volume deformation to three-dimensional facial reconstruction: a comparison with previous techniques. *Forensic Science International, 94,* 167–181.

Nickerson, B.A., Fitzhorn, P.A., Koch, S.K., & Charney, M. (1991). A methodology for near-optimal computational superimposition of two-dimensional digital facial photographs and three-dimensional cranial surface meshes. *Journal of Forensic Sciences, 36,* 480–500.

Ogawa, H. (1960). Anatomical study on the Japanese head by X-ray cephalometry. *The Journal of the Tokyo Dental College Society [Shika Gakuho], 60,* 17–34.

Pearson, K., & Morant, G.M. (1934). The Wilkinson head of Oliver Cromwell and its relationship tobusts, masks and painted portraits. *Biometrika, 26,* 18–378.

Phillips, V.M., & Smuts, N.A. (1996). Facial reconstruction: utilization of computerized tomography to measure facial tissue thickness in a mixed racial population. *Forensic Science International, 83,* 51–59.

Pleasure, M.A. (1951). Correct vertical dimension and freeway space. *The Journal of the American Dental Association, 43,* 160–163.

Prag, J., & Neave, R. (1997). *Making faces: Using forensic and archaeological evidence.* London: British Museum Press.

Prinsloo, I. (1953). The identification of skeletal remains in Regina versus K and another: The Howick Falls murder case. *Journal of Forensic Medicine, 1,* 11–17.

Quatrehomme, G., Cotin, S., Subsol, G., Delingette, H., Garidel, Y., & Grevin, G. et al. (1997). A fully three-dimensional method for facial reconstruction based on deformable models. *Journal of Forensic Sciences, 42,* 649–652.

Rozprym, F. (1934). Eyebrows and eyelashes in man: Their different forms, pigmentation and heredity. *The Journal of the Royal Anthropological Institute, 64,* 353–395.

Ryan, C., & Wilkinson, C.M. (2006). Appraisal of traditional and recently proposed relationships between the hard and soft dimensions of the nose in profile. *American Journal of Physical Anthropology, 130,* 364–373.

Safe, M. (1991, January 19–20). Faceless no more: How an identity was given to a mystery skeleton. *The Australian,* pp. 14–20.

Sahni, D., Jit, I., Gupta, M., Singh, P., & Suri, S. (2002). Preliminary study on facial soft tissue thickness by magnetic resonance imaging in Northwest Indians. *Forensic Science Communications 4.* Retrieved June 15, 2006, from http://www.fbi.gov/hq/lab/fsc/backissu/jan2002/sahni.htm

Schaeffer, J.P., (Ed.). (1942). *Morris' human anatomy: a complete systematic treatise.* Philadelphia: Blakiston.

Sekharan, P.C. (1973). A scientifc method for positioning of the skull for photography in superimposition studies. *Journal of Police Science and Administration, 1,* 232–240.

Sekharan, P.C. (1993). Positioning the skull for superimposition. In M.Y. Iscan & R.P. Helmer, (Eds.), *Forensic analysis of the skull* (pp. 105–118). New York: Wiley-Liss.

Sen, N.K. (1962). Identification by superimposed photographs. *International Criminal Police Review, 162,* 284–286.

Simpson, K. (1943). The Baptist church cellar murder. *Police Journal, 16,* 270–280.

Simpson, E., & Henneberg, M. (2002). Variation in soft-tissue thicknesses on the human face and their relation to craniometric dimensions. *American Journal of Physical Anthropology, 118,* 121–133.

Skiles, M.S., & Randall, P. (1983). The aesthetics of ear placement: an experimental study. *Plastic and Reconstructive Surgery, 72,* 133–140.

Smith, S.L., & Buschang, P.H. (2001). Midsagittal facial tissue thickness of children and adolescents from the Montreal growth study. *Journal of Forensic Sciences, 46,* 1294–1302.

Snow, C.C. (1976, February). *A video technique for skull-face superimposition.* Paper presented at the 28th Annual Meeting of the American Academy of Forensic Sciences, Washington, D.C.

Snow, C.C., Gatliff, B.P., & McWilliams, K.R. (1970). Reconstruction of facial features from the skull: An evaluation of its usefulness in forensic anthropology. *American Journal of Physical Anthropology, 33,* 221–228.

Stadtmuller, F. (1922). Zur Beurteilung der plastischen Rekonstruktionsmethode der Physiognomie auf dem Schadel. *Zeitschrift fur Morphollologie und Anthropologie, 22,* 337–372.

Stadmuller, F. (1932). Identitatsprufung bei corliegendem Erkennungsdienst-Photogramm des vielleicht als ehemaliger Trager in Frage kommenden Individuum. *Deutsche Zeitschrift für die gesamte gerichtliche Medizin, 20,* 33–52.

Stephan, C.N. (2002a). Do resemblance ratings measure the accuracy of facial approximations. *Journal of Forensic Sciences, 47,* 239–243.

Stephan, C.N. (2002b). Facial approximation: Falsification of globe projection guideline by exophthalmometry literature. *Journal of Forensic Sciences, 47*, 1–6.

Stephan, C.N. (2002c). Position of superciliare in relation to the lateral iris: Testing a suggested facial approximation guideline. *Forensic Science International, 130*, 29–33.

Stephan, C.N. (2003a). Anthropological facial 'reconstruction' — recognizing the fallacies, 'unembracing' the error, and realizing method limits. *Science and Justice, 43*, 193–199.

Stephan, C.N. (2003b). Commentary on facial approximation: Globe projection guideline falsified by exophthalmometry literature. *Journal of Forensic Sciences, 48*, 470.

Stephan, C.N. (2003c). Facial approximation: An evaluation of mouth width determination. *American Journal of Physical Anthropology, 121*, 48–57.

Stephan, C.N. (2005). Facial approximation: A review of the current state of play for archaeologists. *International Journal of Osteoarchaeology, 15*, 298–302.

Stephan, C.N. (2006). Beyond the sphere of the English facial approximation literature: Ramifications of German papers on Western method concepts. *Journal of Forensic Sciences, 51*, 736–739.

Stephan, C.N. (in press). Craniofacial identification: Techniques of facial approximation and craniofacial superimposition. In S. Blau & D.H. Ubelaker (Eds.), *Digging deeper: Current trends and future directions in forensic anthropology and archaeology*. Walnut Creek, CA: Left Coast Press.

Stephan, C.N., & Arthur, R.S. (2006). Assessing facial approximation accuracy: How do resemblance ratings of disparate faces compare to recognition tests? *Forensic Science International, 159S*: S159–S163.

Stephan, C.N., Clement, J.G., Owen, C.D., Dobrostanski, T., & Owen, A. (2004). A new rig for craniofacial photography put to the test. *Plastic and Reconstructive Surgery, 113*, 827–833.

Stephan, C., & Davidson, P. (in press). The placement of the human eyeball and canthi in craniofacial identification. *Journal of Forensic Sciences*.

Stephan, C.N., & Henneberg, M. (2001). Building faces from dry skulls: Are they recognized above chance rates? *Journal of Forensic* Sciences, *46*, 432–440.

Stephan, C.N., & Henneberg, M. (2003). Predicting mouth width from inter-canine width: A 75% rule. *Journal of Forensic Sciences, 48*, 725–727.

Stephan, C.N., & Henneberg, M. (2006). Recognition by facial approximation: Case specific examples and empirical tests. *Forensic Science International, 156*, 182–191.

Stephan, C.N., Henneberg, M., & Sampson, W. (2003). Predicting nose projection and pronasale position in facial approximation: A test of published methods and proposal of new guidelines. *American Journal of Physical Anthropology, 122*, 240–250.

Stephan, C.N., Norris, R.M., & Henneberg, M. (2005a). Does sexual dimorphism in facial soft tissue depths justify sex distinction in craniofacial identification? *Journal of Forensic Sciences, 50*, 513–518.

Stephan, C.N., Penton-Voak, I.S., Clement, J.G., & Henneberg, M. (2005c). Ceiling recognition limits of two-dimensional facial approximations constructed using averages. In J.G. Clement & M. Marks (Eds.), *Computer graphic facial reconstruction* (pp. 199–219). Boston: Academic Press.

Stephan, C.N., Penton-Voak, I., Perrett, D., Tiddeman, B., Clement, J.G., & Henneberg, M. (2005b). Two-dimensional computer generated average human face morphology and facial approximation. In J.G. Clement & M. Marks (Eds.), *Computer graphic facial reconstruction* (pp. 105–127). Boston: Academic Press.

Stewart, T.D. (1979). *Essentials of forensic anthropology: Especially as developed in the United States.* Springfield, IL: Charles C Thomas.

Sutisno, M. (2003). Human facial soft-tissue thickness and its value in forensic facial reconstruction. Unpublished doctoral dissertation, the University of Sydney, Australia.

Suzuki, H. (1948). On the thickness of the soft parts of the Japanese face. *Journal of the Anthropological Society Nippon, 60*, 7–11.

Suzuki, T. (1973). Reconstitution of a skull. *International Criminal Police Review, 264*, 76–80.

Swan, L.K., & Stephan, C.N. (2005). Estimating eyeball protrusion from body height, interpupillary distance, and inter-orbital distance in adults. *Journal of Forensic Sciences, 50*, 1–3.

Taylor, J.A. (1988). The significance of distortion in craniofacial video superimposition. Unpublished master's thesis, The University of Adelaide, Adelaide, Australia.

Taylor, J.A., & Brown, K.A. (1998). Superimposition techniques. In J.G. Clement & D.L. Ranson (Eds.), *Craniofacial identification in forensic medicine* (pp. 151–164). London: Hodder Arnold.

Taylor, K.T. (Ed.). (2001a). *Forensic art and illustration*. Boca Raton, FL: CRC Press.

Taylor, K.T. (2001b). Two-dimensional facial reconstruction from the skull. In K.T. Taylor (Ed.), *Forensic art and illustration* (pp. 361–417). Boca Raton, FL: CRC Press.

Taylor, R., & Craig, P. (2005). The wisdom of bones: facial approximation on the skull. In J.G. Clement & M.K. Marks (Eds.), *Computer-graphic facial reconstruction* (pp. 33–55). Boston: Elsevier; Academic Press.

Taylor, R.G., & Angel, C. (1998). Facial reconstruction and approximation. In J.G. Clement & D.L. Ranson (Eds.), *Craniofacial identification in forensic medicine* (pp. 177–185). New York: Oxford University Press.

Tu, P., Hartley, R.I., Lorensen, W.E., Alyassin, A., Gupta, R., & Heier, L. (2005). Face reconstructions using flesh deformation modes. In J.G. Clement & M.K. Marks (Eds.), *Computer-graphic facial reconstruction* (pp. 145–162). Boston: Elsevier Academic Press.

Turner, W.D., Brown, R.E.B., Kelliher, T.P., Tu, P.H., Taister, M.A., & Miller, K.W.P. (2005). A novel method of automated skull registration for forensic facial approximation. *Forensic Science International, 154*, 149–158.

Ubelaker, D.H. (2002). Cranial photographic superimposition. In C.H. Wecht (Ed.), *Forensic sciences* (pp. 3–38). New York: Matthew Bender, Inc.

Ubelaker, D.H., Bubniak, E., & O'Donnell, G. (1992). Computer-assisted photographic superimposition. *Journal of Forensic Sciences, 37*, 750–762.

Ullrich, H. (1958). Die methodischen Grundlagen des plastischen Rekonstruktionsverfahrens nach Gerasimov. *Zeitschrift fur Morphollologie und Anthropologie, 49*, 245–258.

Ullrich, H. (1966). Kritische Bemerkungen zur plastischen Rekonstruktionsmethode nach Gerasimov auf Grund personlicher Erfahrugen. *Ethnographisch-archäologische Zeitschrift, 7*, 111–123.

Ullrich, H. (1967). Plastische Gesichtsrekonstructionen urgeschichtlicher Menschen nach der Methode von Gerasimov. *Neue Museumskunde, 10*, 456–475.

Ullrich, H. (1972). Plastische Gesichtsrekonstruktionen auf ur- und fruhgeschichtlichen Scadeln als wissenschaftliche Dokumente. *Zeitschrift für Archäologische, 6*, 91–103.

van Rensburg, J. (1993). Abstract. Accuracy of recognition of 3-dimensional plastic reconstruction of faces from skulls. *Anatomical Society of Southern Africa 23rd Annual Congress, Krugersdorp: Game Reserve*, 20.

Vanezis, P., Blowes, R.W., Linney, A.D., Tan, A.C., Richards, R., & Neave, R. (1989). Application of 3-D computer graphics for facial reconstruction and comparison with sculpting techniques. *Forensic Science International, 42*, 69–84.

Vanezis, P., Vanezis, M., McCombe, G., & Niblett, T. (2000). Facial reconstruction using 3-D computer graphics. *Forensic Science International, 108*, 81–95.

von Eggeling, H. (1913). Die Leistungsfahigkeit physiognomischer Rekonbstruktionsversuche auf Grundlage des Schadels'. *Archiv fur Anthropologie, 12*, 44–47.

Webster, G. (1955). Photography as an aid in identification: the Plumbago Pit case. *Police Journal, 28*, 185–191.

Webster, W.P., Murray, W.K., Brinkhous, W., & Hudson, P. (1986). Identification of human remains using photographic reconstruction. In K.J. Reichs (Ed.), *Forensic osteology: Advances in the identification of human remains* (pp. 256–276). Springfield, IL: Charles C. Thomas.

Welcker, H. (1883). *Schiller's Schadel und Todtenmaske, nebst Mittheilungen uber Schadel und Todtenmaske Kant's*. Braunschweig: Viehweg F. and Son.

Welcker, H. (1888). Zur Kritik des Schillerschadels. *Archives fur Anthropologie, 17*, 19–60.

Wells, G.L. (1993). What do we know about eyewitness identification? *American Psychologist, 48,* 553–571.

Wilder, H.H., & Wenworth, B. (1918). *Personal identification: Methods for the identification of individuals, living or dead.* Boston: Gorham Press.

Wilkinson, C. (2004). *Forensic facial reconstruction.* Cambridge: Cambridge University Press.

Wilkinson, C.M. (2002). In vivo facial tissue depth measurements for white British children. *Journal of Forensic Sciences, 47,* 459–465.

Wilkinson, C.M., & Mautner, S.A. (2003). Measurement of eyeball protrusion and its application in facial reconstruction [technical note]. *Journal of Forensic Sciences, 48,* 12–16.

Wilkinson, C.M., Motwani, M., & Chiang, E. (2003). The relationship between the soft tissues and the skeletal detail of the mouth. *Journal of Forensic Sciences, 48,* 728–732.

Wilkinson, C.M., & Whittaker, D.K. (2002). Juvenile forensic facial reconstruction: A detailed accuracy study. *Proceedings of the 10th Biennial Scientific Meeting of the International Association for Craniofacial Identification, Bari, Italy* (pp. 98–110).

Williams, P.L. (Ed.). (1995). *Gray's anatomy* (38th ed). New York: Churchill Livingstone.

Williamson, M.A., Nawrocki, S.P., & Rathbun, T.A. (2002). Variation in midfacial tissue thickness of African-American children. *Journal of Forensic Sciences, 47,* 25–31.

Ancestry, Age, Sex, and Stature: Identification in a Diverse Space

Judith Littleton

Rebecca Kinaston

In the last 10 years the number of forensic anthropology texts has been growing. While they expand in the range of techniques applied, the four basics of identification from human remains are always included: geographic ancestry, or what is sometimes termed race, or inappropriately, ethnicity; age; sex; and stature. Work in Kosovo (Rainio, Hedman, Karkola, Lalu, Petola et al., 2001) confirms that these basics are still required in modern practice, while the routine work that concerns many of us, distinguishing indigenous from nonindigenous, and historic from modern cases, frequently requires that such decisions are made quickly and often in the field.

There seem to be two problems: (a) the nature of the reference samples, and (b) the range of variation in the Asia–Pacific region. An ideal reference sample is, in itself, inherently biased. Due to the many types of variation, ontogeny (growth), sexual dimorphism, and individual variation the reference sample must typify the population that it was gleaned from (White, 2000). A large sample size, known context and a wide variety of known ages and sexes are the best way to combat this problem, but the variations between populations, due to the myriad of variables that can affect growth, is still a major issue hindering the accuracy of identification (Usher, 2002). As there is no way to circumvent the problem of a biased reference sample(s), the biological anthropologist must 'make do' with the resources available and use statistical methods to reduce error (see Hoppa & Vaupel, 2002, for a thorough overview of methods). Increasingly, however, it is being found these standards may not be particularly accurate outside their original geographic and temporal location (Komar, 2003; Ross & Kongisberg, 2002).

In the southern hemisphere the range of human variation is continuous and wide-ranging and this presents a further issue. Donlon's (2003; see also Chapter 7) summary of casework in New South Wales involved Aboriginal Australians, European Australians, Asians (Chinese and Vietnamese), and people from near and remote Oceania (Melanesians and Polynesians). Unfortunately most of these are also the populations not found in sufficiently high enough numbers in northern America or Europe from where most texts originate.

This chapter therefore is a brief introduction to the basic standards for the major population groups in the region; concentrating primarily on indigenous populations. It is not an exhaustive summary but rather a quick review of some of the most widely used standards and their applicability to issues of human identification.

Geographic Ancestry

Most forensic texts point out that assessing geographical ancestry is the most difficult aspect of human skeletal identification (Gill & Rhine, 1990; Stewart, 1979). There are several reasons for this: basic racial categories are culturally specific; geographical variation is continuous with no clear dividing lines; and morphology changes over time. At the same time, however, gaining some idea of the potential ancestry of remains continues to be a crucial underlay in other aspects of human identification. Assessments of sex, age and stature are all, to variable extents, dependent on understandings of the possible ancestry of the remains. Furthermore, circumstances may demand, particularly in mass disasters, the rapid separation of individuals from different possible origins. And finally, in both Australia and New Zealand identification of indigenous from nonindigenous remains has implications for jurisdiction (Masters, 2006) and equally, if not more importantly, for whom takes ultimate responsibility for the remains, their treatment, and final resting place (Cox et al., 2006. In other words, assessment of population affinity presents skeletal analysts with a cleft stick: an obligation to undertake some form of assessment if possible and yet a realisation that in many cases it may be an extremely difficult task.

Determination of geographic ancestry relies most heavily on characteristics of the cranium, whether identified through observation or by measurement. Forensic texts routinely define the markers of Whites, Blacks and Asians and American Indians (combined) or alternatively Caucasoid, Negroid and Mongoloid (Ubelaker, 1999). The source of these observations is often not made clear and the descriptions have become mutually reinforcing. Most of this work has originated in North America and therefore even the broad categorisations that are used have the potential to exclude part of the inherent variability encompassed by each category (Komar, 2003).

In the Asia–Pacific region, the range of populations that need to be considered is much larger. On the other hand, the area also encompasses groups that have been seen as morphologically and metrically distinct. Metrical analyses by Howells (1973, 1989, 1995) and Pietresewsky (1970, 1973, 1979, 1983, 1984, 1990a, 1990b, 2004) have shown that populations of the region tend to divide between a distinctive Australo–Melanesian and a larger branch encompassing peoples from remote Oceania ('Polynesia'), again distinct from Island South-East Asia. There is, of course, intergrading; particularly in the region of near Oceania. In Pietresewsky's successive analyses of cranial metrics a cline is visible in the Australo–Melanesian groups, with North Queensland and Torres Strait Islander remains resembling those from Papua New Guinea and with Fijian populations falling in with Polynesian populations (Pietrusewsky, 1990a; 1990b). Populations from individual islands in Micronesia also often fall (not uniformly) between Polynesian and Island South-East Asian populations, even in some cases grouping with Melanesians (Pietrusewsky, 1990a). While in large-scale comparisons, Asian populations tend to group together, there are differences between North and South-East Asian populations (Hanihara, 1994; Howells,

1995; Turner, 1989, 1990) None of this, of course, deals with populations of European origin resident in the area. The following discussion will focus primarily on morphological characters of the crania.

With respect to the two most distinct groups (Australian Aboriginal people and people from Polynesia) comprehensive lists of cranial characters have been made (e.g., Brown, 1973; Fenner, 1939; Houghton, 1980; Houghton, 1996; Larnach, 1978; Snow, 1974; Wood et al., 2002). Larnach (1978) and Larnach and MacIntosh (1970, 1971) approached the issue of distinguishing Aboriginal crania systematically. They recorded a large series of cranial traits among crania initially from New South Wales and then from eastern Australia, reducing the list to 20 characters that occurred in high frequency among their sample. These characters were each assigned a score that is 'in a sense, a measure of the expression of the pattern in the skull' (Larnach, 1978: 191). The averages of the scores for the NSW coastal sample (51.5, range 44–60) varied widely from that obtained from a small sample of 11 European male crania (26.3, range 14–32) and 17 male crania from East Asia (27.6, range 20–34). Twelve mandibular traits separating Aboriginal from Asian mandibles were also identified. While effectively this is a simplified form of discriminant function it does not have the statistical measures of probability attached. They did, however, apply the technique to a larger sample from across Australia with similarly successful results. There was, however, a substantial overlap between their initial sample and crania from New Guinea. In order to maximise discrimination between these two groups they distinguished a list of 12 traits that could be used to maximise discrimination. Unsurprisingly, the results still show clinal variation with remains from Cape York having the greatest resemblance to those from Papua New Guinea.

A description of a characteristic Holocene Aboriginal male crania was extrapolated from the results (Larnach, 1978: 190): a narrow skull with zygomatic arches visible from above, the vault keeled and long with a distinct occipital torus. The frontal inclines to flatness and palatine tori are common. The upper face is broad with distinct superciliary ridges and zygomatic trigones, and a marked glabella. Orbits are rectangular although with a possibly rounded lower margin. The malars are rugged and often have an everted lower margin. Interorbital breadth is broad and the nasal root may be depressed. The nasal sill is either rounded or shows a distinct depression. The lower face is distinctly projecting.

Remains from Papua New Guinea or the northern part of Australia tend to have a shorter cranial vault, be narrower in the supraorbital region (although still wide compared to other populations), have a broader nose and slightly longer upper face (Green, 1990; Howells, 1970; Pietrusewsky, 1990a; Swindler, 1991). In reality these distinctions are purely relative and highly variable.

A similar study has not been undertaken for remains from Polynesia but descriptions from specific places (New Zealand, Hawaii) are available and Houghton has summarised the overall picture (Houghton, 1996). Pietresewsky (1990a, 1990b, 1990c, 1997) has compared metrically crania from across the Pacific and while his study confirms the homogeneity of remains from Polynesia (including Fiji) he and Houghton both point out that in some characters Easter Island is distinct and also that there is geographical variation in the degree of brachycephaly (Houghton, 1996; Pietrusewsky & Ikehara-Quebral, 2001). This variation needs to be taken account of in terms of weighting individual characteristics.

The other issue requiring attention is the careful assessment of observations and methods of measurement. One characteristic, the rocker jaw, is often weighted in practice as the most useful determinant of Polynesian ancestry (Weisler & Swindler, 2002). This characteristic jaw formation is defined as: 'the inferior margin of the mandibular body is convex downward. As a result, the bone may teeter like a rocking chair if placed on a table top and depressed and released either on the chin or the top of the ramus' (Marshall & Snow, 1956: 414).

Kean and Houghton (1990) argue that it is a functional adaptation to the long flat face of people from the region and does occur, albeit in lower frequency (2–4%) among other populations. Data from Pietresewsky (1984, 1989) suggests much higher frequencies than 2% to 4% in surrounding populations but this is partly because his figures include 'partial rocker' jaw, that is, a jaw that 'rests squarely on a level surface posterior, while anteriorly the chin is elevated' (Weisler & Swindler, 2002: 29). Full 'rocker' morphology can occur in any individual who has the same relatively flat face, so the rocker jaw by itself needs to be considered in relation to other characteristics.

Most commonly human crania from remote Oceania are described as pentagonal when viewed from the back or from above. The temples are flat and the zygomatic arches are observable from above. The face is flat sided with the zygomatic arches turning at roughly 90 degrees at the face. Faces are flat without subnasal projection. The vault is high; but roundedness is a variable feature. The mandible is frequently of the rocker form and shovel shaped incisors are common (Houghton, 1978, 1980, 1996; Marshall & Snow, 1956).

Based on work by Howells (1989: 15) and Pietresewsky (1990b), Micronesians are variably intermediate in morphology between their eastern and western neighbours, although some characteristics are shared with populations to the south. Heathcote (1996), however, has described three hyperostotic traits that occur in high frequency in Oceania and particularly high frequency in the Mariannas: tubercles on the occipital torus; retromastoid processes; and posterior supramastoid tubercles as well as a 'downwardly convex inferior border of the malar, coupled with massive malar development and premature synostosis of the suture between the malar and temporal bone' (Heathcote, 1995: 6).

Asian skulls are generally described as brachycephalic, with a flat face. Facial width is greater than head width. The nose is moderately wide with a slightly pointed lower margin. Orbits are round and palates are wide. Shovel shaped incisors are common (Rhine, 1990; Ubelaker, 1999). There is, however, evidence of a north–south cline, described by Hanihara as a series of contrasts between north and south: 'short vs. long head; low vs. high head; flat vs. narrow head; high vs. low face; round vs. angular (high vs. low) orbit; and narrow vs. wide nose' (Hanihara 1994: 419).

The other set of characters, dental traits (both morphology and size) have largely been used to map patterns of geographical variation rather than as clusters indicative of geographic ancestry. However, among Asia–Pacific populations high rates of some characters, incisor shovelling and a 'Y' cuspal pattern on the upper first molar, for example, have been observed (Harris & Bailit, 1987; Harris et al., 1975). Similarly, Richards and Telfer (1979) identified variant characters among European, Asian, New Hebridean (Vanuatu) and Australian Aboriginal populations. Finally, Turner points out the difference between a sinodont (or North Asian dental morphology) and a sundadont pattern more representative of southern groups (Turner, 1989; 1990). These distinctive dental characters seem to be underused in terms of assessing geographic ancestry in view of their variation across space. One exception is Chiu and Donlon (2000) who studied tooth size differences in modern East Asian and European Australians developing discriminant functions. Brace (1980) also suggests clear gradients in molar size that could distinguish populations. Clearly in some disaster situations teeth are actually going to be the most useful indicator of ancestry. A second advantage (already demonstrated by Chiu and Donlon) is that such methods can be developed using dental casts of contemporary populations allowing for external validation of the discriminant function.

Cranial metrics beginning with the use of discriminant functions (Giles, 1976) is increasingly dominated by use of two computer programs: CRANID (Wright, 1992; Chapter 8), based on Howells' measurements of human remains from around the world and on subsequent museum specimen measurements and FORDISC (Ousley & Jantz, 1996). Both programs began with the Howells' measurements of 28 populations. FORDISC, however, has a separate data bank of identified forensic cases while CRANID has been added to with additional samples by Wright. Effectively, they both give the statistical likelihood of one individual skull belonging to one of the groups identified in the database; this is reliant on the museum labels, for example, the constitution of Howells' Tasmanian sample has been queried (Larnach, 1978: 88). As Williams et al. (2005) point out, it is striking that despite enthusiastic reports about both techniques there are very few published tests of their utility (although see Bulbeck 2005a, 2005b and discussion in Chapter 8). Interpretation of results requires knowledge of the samples used in the database and knowledge of a broad range of population characters so that anonmalous or nondistinct individuals can be interpreted in meaningful ways (e.g., Heathcote, 1995).

The above discussion is necessarily brief and does not include discussion of post-cranial variants or of cultural attributes useful in assessing ancestry. It confirms, however, that while geographic ancestry is difficult to assess, some useful areas (such as teeth) have not been adequately explored. There is no magic bullet to this situation and computer programs, while inherently useful, are doing the same thing statistically that people do when examining a skull morphologically: comparing the observations to a known database; in the case of observations a database of personal experience and expectation along with a published list. The most characteristic crania are most likely to be identified but crania that have a mixture of characters or fall outside the database (whether statistical or personal experience) are more likely to be misclassified. The situation is much more acute for juvenile remains and for remains that come from time frames outside the common databases, that is, older remains or recent remains. There are three solutions: more research, maintenance of more thorough databases, and caution in attribution.

Sex Identification

Sexual identification of skeletal material is an integral part of any anthropological investigation. The pelvic bones, followed by the skull and the long bones, are the most significant bones used for the sexual assessment of an individual. While these are the bones that display the greatest sexual dimorphism, it is recommended that the whole skeleton (or as much of the skeleton as possible) be assessed when possible, as multivariate techniques are more accurate than univariate techniques when sexing skeletal material (Mays & Cox, 2000).

As with geographic ancestry, many of the original sexing methods employ primarily American or European samples. Lorenzo, Carretero, Arsuaga, Gracia and Martinez (1998: 20) warns that sexual dimorphism is population specific 'not only in degree but also depending on what part of the body is analysed' and that 'sexual dimorphism has a genetic and an environmental component'. Past populations most likely developed differently from many populations of today, displaying dissimilar growth rates, and inviting a bias that could be crucial when using modern specimens to sex archaeological samples (Chamberlain, 1994). Therefore, the reference sample and the sample in question should, in ideal circumstances, be selected from a comparable background and the use of statistical methods to reduce error should be employed (Hoppa & Vaupel, 2002).

There has been very little literature published regarding population-specific sexing standards in the southern hemisphere. Over the years, many reports from archaeological digs record using 'the standard morphological criteria' (unspecified) but do specify that cranial, pelvic, and long bones were used in the analysis (Houghton, 1977; Katyama, 1985; Pietrusewsky, 1976; Snow, 1974; Sutton, 1979; Wiriyaromp, 1984). Other reports from these areas specify that the major standards for sexing, such as Bass (1987), Phenice (1969), and Ubelaker (1999) were employed, as regionally specific standards were not available.

Sexing techniques are either morphological (thus potentially subjective to the observer) or metric. The morphological sexually dimorphic traits are (most of the time) inherent to all humans, but the disparity between sexual dimorphism in today's populations and prehistoric ones is unknown. Though total accuracy of sex determination can never be achieved due to intrinsic variation between males and females, morphological techniques are less rigid than their metric counterparts. As it is well known that populations may vary in bodily proportions, the metric sexing standards available are largely only applicable for groups of people with a similar distribution of characters to the reference population.

Fortunately, researchers studying a wide range of populations from the southern hemisphere have assessed this metric dilemma. Australian anthropologists have published the largest amount of literature on the subject (Ray, 1959; Wood, 1920). Davivongs (1963a, 1963b) published papers assessing the degree of sexual dimorphism in the Australian Aboriginal femora and pelves. He measured 75 male and 55 female femora and concluded that the sex differences were so apparent that he could discriminate male and female Aboriginal Australians (Davivongs 1963a: 466). Contemporary work examining the bones of the shoulder girdle concluded that the head of the humerus was similarly discriminatory (van Dongen, 1963).

Larnach and Freedman (1964) described a technique for the sexing NSW coastal Aboriginal Australian crania and Larnach and Macintosh (1971) developed a method to sex eastern Australian Aboriginal mandibles using metric and nonmetric traits. The Larnach and Freedman technique was reassessed by Brown (1981: 53) on crania from the Murray River Valley. He found that there was a large overlap between male and female crania when assessed using this technique and suggested adjusting the criteria for more robust Australian groups.

Townsend, Richards and Carrol (1982) assessed the sexual differences of Australian Aboriginal crania by discriminant function analysis. They found that sex estimation using this technique was an accurate method to sex Aboriginal crania and provided an objective technique compared to that of Larnach and Freedman. In addition, studies focusing on the sexual features of Aboriginal teeth have been undertaken by Townsend and Brown (1979) and Barker (1973) to use in conjunction with cranial sexing techniques.

There are few studies of population specific sexing standards for the Pacific. Houghton and de Souza (1975) published a paper using discriminant function analysis to sex prehistoric New Zealand long bones. They found a high degree of accuracy for this method, increasing when more bones were present. In contrast, Dennison (1979) found that there was a large overlap in the size of male and female teeth from prehistoric New Zealand.

Due to interpopulation variation, studies using 'Mongoloid' skeletal remains should be metrically sexed using specific population standards when possible. Iscan, Yoshino and Kato (1995: 459) summarised the sexual dimorphism found in modern Japanese crania, highlighting morphological change in the last 50 years. Iscan, Yoshino and Susumu (1994) used discriminant function analysis to determine the sex from the tibia of the modern Japanese. Song, Lin and Jai (1992) calculated the sex of Chinese skulls using multiple stepwise discriminant function analysis, while Liu (1989) and Iscan and Shihai (1995) tested the sex determination of Chinese femur using the same technique. King, Iscan and Loth (1998) conducted a metric and comparative study of the sexual dimorphism in Thai femora and found that the difference between Thai and Chinese femora indicates a need for population specific standards. Lastly Iscan, Loth, King, Shihai and Yoshino (1998) compared the sexual dimorphism of the humerus between Chinese, Japanese, and Thais. The group concluded the same outcome as King et al. (1998), that though 'Mongoloid', the populations had significant differences between them that merited specific population standards.

While sex has been more extensively studied with an applied end in mind the same issues of reference sample identity and observer familiarity with regional variation still apply.

Age

Of all of the individual characters, age at death has been the most controversial, especially for adults (although it is not problem-free for children). Two major difficulties are the availability of collections of human remains of known age and sex covering the entire period of adult development and the impact of inter-individual variation in ageing (particularly when what is being recorded is the process of breaking down rather than development).

There has been, particularly in relation to adults, an assumption of uniformitarianism, that is, that the pattern of age changes observed in reference samples (based on modern populations) does not vary significantly from past populations. Furthermore, the assumption has also been made that there are no statistically significant differences in these patterns between populations. However, geographic and temporal differences have been noted (Hoppa, 2000). Nevertheless, most methods of ageing adults have not been systematically tested as to their appropriateness or usefulness for identifying people who do not conform in terms of ancestry or time period to the reference sample.

There is no current solution to this without further research; however, analysts probably require 'a reminder that mapping the physiological process of ageing on the bony skeleton is a difficult and challenging task' (Hoppa 2000: 190). With one exception (dental attrition) no specific methods of adult ageing have been developed or tested on Oceanic populations and normal practice is to follow the standard methods, of which there are many reviews (e.g., Buikstra & Ubelaker, 1994; Katzenberg & Saunders, 2000; Ubelaker, 1999).

The rate of dental wear is one character that is explicitly temporally bound and population specific. However, its usefulness as a predictor of age also seems to vary by population, giving highly variable results. Richards and coworkers examined the relationship between dental attrition and age in dental casts from three Aboriginal populations dating to the 1950s and 1960s and, in general, living on government settlements (Richards & Miller, 1991). They measured the area of exposed dentine relative to crown area of the first and second molars, finding a correlation between chronological age and attrition greater than 0.80 for the premolars and first molars. The authors suggest that age could be estimated from tooth wear with confidence limits of ± 10 years. The applicability of these formulae to other populations, however, is unknown.

A more recent study applies a similar method (although this time using ordinal scores for wear) to a forensic sample from northeastern China (Li & Ji, 1995). The authors suggest that the first or second molar (either upper or lower) is most inform-ative. They obtain much higher regression coefficients (ranging from 0.94–0.97) and suggest a maximum error for personal ageing of ± 4.53 years.

These two studies demonstrate the usefulness of tooth wear as an indicator of relative age (particularly when dealing with a known population), as well as the potential utility of other methods of adult ageing based on teeth, for example, root transparency and cementum annulation, since human teeth of known age are much easier to access than skeletal remains. It is also clear, however, that much more work remains to be done in this area.

In contrast to adults, ageing subadult human remains is based on 'more clock-like developmental events' (Konigsberg & Holman, 1999: 267). Therefore, children can often be aged with higher levels of accuracy, although not all methods of ageing are equal. Some (such as tooth emergence or eruption) increase in variability with age, others (such as long bone growth or epiphyseal fusion) are much more suscep-tible to environmental conditions. Of all of the most commonly used indicators (dental formation, dental eruption, ossification sequences, and long bone growth), dental development has been considered the least susceptible to environmental vari-ation. However, as Smith (1992) points out, most standards are based on serial radi-ographs of children of European ancestry. Smith (1991) suggests that sex-specific standards might prove more accurate though it is difficult to determine sex from subadult remains (Townsend, 2002).

In determining age based on dental formation and eruption schedules, one needs to be aware both of the nature of the reference sample and the method used in defining age stages and assigning children to them. The most widely used method based on dental formation has been developed by Moorees, Fanning and Hunt (1963) on the basis of serial X-rays of American children. The standards include separate age ranges for males and females. In the case of dental eruption the most widely used standards are Massler, Schour and Poncher (1941) and Ubelaker (1999). Massler et al.'s eruption charts are based largely on Logan and Kronefeld (1933), using 30 individuals (many suffering from chronic diseases). Ubelaker's (1999) chart is a revision of Massler and Schour's data, incorporating additional data from modern native Americans and other non-European populations. In it the ages at each stage of dental formation are slightly earlier than Massler et al.'s (1941) chart. One potential area of error is the difference between gingival and alveolar emergence: the latter preceding the former by a variable period of time, approximately 0.69 to 1.4 years (Haavikko, 1970).

In the Asia–Pacific region the most extensive set of studies on dental development have been those by Brown and colleagues based on the longitudinal data (both casts and X-rays) collected from the Yuendumu Aboriginal settlement, central Australia, in the 1950s and 1960s (Brown, 1978; Brown, Jenner, Barrett, & Lees, 1979; Fanning & Moorees, 1969). Their studies of dental eruption rely on gingival emergence (not full occlusion) as indicated by oral examination. Comparison with other populations suggests that deciduous dental development for these children tended to be delayed up to 12 to 18 months of age and then followed a similar timing. The authors, however, note a high level of individual variability.

Brown et al. (1979) uses a similar criterion of gingival emergence to determine the sequence and age of dental eruption among the permanent dentition. In this sample, initial emergence of the permanent dentition (the first 12 teeth or phase 1) appears to follow a similar pattern and age relationship to a European descended population from Western Australia. However, among the Yuendumu children the 'quiescent period' between eruption of these first teeth and the later teeth is shorter, so that the modal age of emergence for the 28th tooth was 0.4 to 0.8 years advanced of European norms. Third molars where observed to emerge in this population some years before the European comparison (approximately 16 years for girls, and 16.5 yrs for boys). Using the Massler et al. (1941) standard would consequently tend to overestimate the age of older Aboriginal children. Some of this difference is probably due to differences in the morphology of the jaw. The Aboriginal children studied had much more gingival space for the emergence of the latter teeth than European children of the same age. However, there are also some underlying differences in the formation of the later teeth at least (Fanning & Moorees, 1969).

A larger cross-sectional study by Abbie also on Aboriginal children from Central and Western Australia emerged with similar results (Abbie, 1975a). He used the criterion of full emergence of the crown that makes it easier to translate these results to dry bone remains. Abbie identified a similar pattern of early dental retardation; incisors not routinely appearing until 9 months compared to 6 months. His work, however, does not seem to indicate the early emergence or development of the third molars evident in the Yuendumu sample. The variability raises the need for cautious estimates if using the third molar as the basis for age.

More recently, Diamanti and Townsend have constructed a permanent dental eruption sequence based on radiographs of a large number (8676) of Australian children from a range of backgrounds and ancestries (Diamanti & Townsend, 2003).

They give median times of emergence plus the percentile ranges. In this series girls are 4.5 to 5.3 months advanced relative to boys. Most surprising, however, these emergence times are later than those previously reported for Australian children and are delayed relative to Massler et al. (1941) and Ubelaker (1999). They are also later than the times reported for Asian children and for Finnish children (Diamanti & Townsend, 2003). However, as the authors emphasise these are potentially the most valid standards to be using for recent Australians.

There have been several studies of dental eruption among children from Papua New Guinea. Brook and Barker's study of 4873 children from Eastern Papua New Guinea indicate no significant difference in deciduous eruption between their sample and children from the United States (Brook & Barker 1972). Eruption of the permanent dentition, on the other hand, is earlier than the United States average, with only relatively minor differences between the three populations studied. By the final stage of development recorded (incisors present and second molar erupted) girls from Papua New Guinea were around 1.37 to 2.17 years ahead of the United States counterparts. A similar pattern was observed by Friedlander and Bailit (1969).

One study (Ulijaszek, 1996) contradicts the finding of no significant difference between deciduous emergence times. Among Anga children in Papua New Guinea, deciduous dental emergence was delayed. This combined with the delay among Yuendumu children (Brown & Barrett, 1973) suggests that while the deciduous dentition may be under tighter genetic control, it may still be disrupted in some environmental circumstances.

Using the same criterion of gingival emergence among children from the Cook Islands, two studies found advanced dental emergence relative to European standards: by 0.76 years for the maxilla and 0.28 years for the mandible (Fry, 1976; Yamada, Kawamoto, Tairea, & Rere, 1999). These differences are of the same order of magnitude as for Aboriginal children and children from Papua New Guinea.

Asian populations (based on gingival emergence) tend to be intermediate between the Oceanic and Australian populations described above and European populations (Eveleth & Tanner, 1976; Halcrow, Tayles, & Bucklety, in press; Hoffding, Maeda, Yamaguchi, Tsuji, Kuwabara et al., 1984). However, the single South-East Asian population recorded (Thai) are relatively delayed to European standards, suggesting distinct East Asian and South-East Asian patterns (Kamalanathan, Hauck, & Kittiveja, 1960; Krailassiri, Anuwongnukroh, & Dechkunakorn, 2002). This slower eruption among South-East Asians corresponds to apparently slower formation (Halcrow et al., in press).

In Figure 11.1, these data are summarised using gingival emergence. The figure is indicative only given the different methods used between studies to calculate age at emergence. Compared to dental formation, eruption can be more variable as it is affected not just by the developmental environment but also the local oral environment. However, the differences are sufficiently systematic to suggest geographic diversity in developmental rates. It is striking that the recent Australian data, rather than suggesting a secular trend to faster development, suggest slower development (Diamanti & Townsend, 2003). This may well be because the composition of Australia's population has changed, although it also reflects changing dental hygiene. It serves to emphasise the overall requirement for conservatism in age estimates until more population and environmental specific data are gathered.

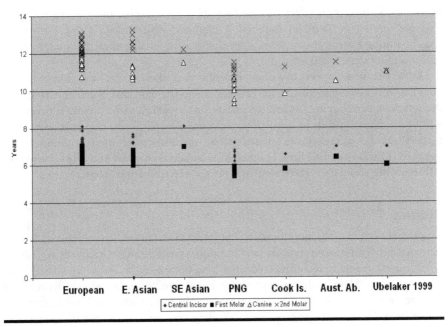

Figure 11.1
Summary of tooth emergence for various populations (based on: Eveleth & Tanner, 1990; Ubelaker, 1999; Yamada et al., 1999; Diamanti & Townsend, 2003).

The other well-researched measure of subadult age is the rate of ossification (particularly hand and wrist) and epiphyseal fusion. While the studies of the hand and wrist have been extensive and based on fairly large samples, other work on epiphyseal closure is commonly derived from very small samples and frequently from radiography rather than dry bone (Brickley, 2004).

The children from Yuendumu were compared to the Greulich-Pyle standards and found to be retarded on average 6 months for boys and 4 months for girls (Brown & Grave, 1976). Brown and Grave conclude, however, that the standard could be used if the age scale is adjusted to compensate for the delay. In contrast Abbie's larger study suggests very little difference in the times of ossification, although the children he recorded seem precocious in terms of foot development (Abbie, 1975b).

Wood undertook a similar study in Papua New Guinea (Wood, 1976). Here he found a similarity between coastal Papuan children and the Gruelich Pyle standards. However, the central highland population, the Bundi was markedly delayed. The inconsistency between these results and between the two Australian results further testifies to the significant impact of environment on skeletal growth rates.

The final measure of subadult age used is the diaphyseal lengths of bones. Scheuer and Black (2000) is the most comprehensive review of information on the development of the subadult skeleton. The British standards (Brickley, 2004) recommend that the measurements detailed in Buikstra and Ubelaker (1994) are used to measure younger children. However, they point out that the relationship between these lengths and modern reference samples is difficult to determine: archaeological remains may be the result of the child having had a debilitating illness, modern reference data are often based on radiographs, and modern reference data are often very small in number. A common observation is that long bone lengths among historical populations are significantly smaller than the modern comparisons (Saunders, 2000).

As for the other aspects of human identification, there is clearly a distinct lack of population or environment specific references and the data that is available (e.g., the data on dental emergence) indicate that caution in making age estimates is necessary. Part of the caution needs to apply to the selection of a particular standard, what population was the reference, and what precise methods were used to generate the standard. Obviously until further research is undertaken there is a requirement for full recording and a clear statement of how age determinations were reached.

Stature

As a marker of personal identification, height is an important characteristic. Its significance has been proven recently in excavations of mass graves (Rainio et al., 2001).

Stature is generally reconstructed from long bone length. There are several basic methods used. Most widely reported are regression formulae where (frequently) cadaveric stature as the dependent variable is regressed against dry bone length (see Konigsberg, Hens, Janta, & Jungers, 1998, for a critique of such inverse calibration). Infrequently stature/limb segment ratios have been derived from measurements of live people where the ratio of a long bone (extrapolated from live measurements) is calculated against living height. Increasingly in a forensic context, however, anatomical measurements are used where the bones contributing to height of the body are measured in anatomical position and added to a correction faction (comprising corrections for soft tissue and for anatomical positioning) to derive cadaveric height (Fully, 1956).

With the exception of the Fully method and formulae produced by Sjovold (1990, although see Formicola, 1993), the formulae are population and sex specific, as well as potentially time delimited. This is because limb proportions and their contribution to living height vary between populations and by sex within populations and are also subject to change over time. Hence Trotter and Gleser noted a difference between their estimates based on the World War II dead and the Korean dead — a difference they attribute to longer growth periods in the older population (Trotter & Gleser, 1958: 121–122). Secular changes in height have not only affected the length of the growth period and velocity of growth but also the proportionality of the body (Bogin, 1999; Frisancho, Gilding, & Tanner, 2001; Tanner, Hayashi, Preece, & Cameron, 1982).

The most widely used sets of standards are those of Trotter and Gleser that were derived from the macerated bones of World War II male personnel and the Terry skeletal collection and later, the Korean war dead (Trotter, 1970; Trotter & Gleser, 1952, 1958, 1977). Different error margins attend to different bones and the generally advised technique is to use the combination of long bone lengths in the regression equation resulting in the least error. A recent review by Konigsberg et al. (1998) indicates that the standard formulae can really only safely be used when there is prior knowledge of population affinity. Trotter (1970) sounded her own words of warning advising people not to combine formulae from different sources or based on different geographical or racial groups or generations. Furthermore, they warned against calculating an average stature from several separate formulae (e.g., from the femur and from the tibia).

In using regression formulae, therefore, accurate application standards rely in the first instance on an accurate judgment of population affinity and sex. Female stature estimates differ from males because the femoral angulation means that the femur comprises a different percentage of total height in the two sexes. In addition, however, the adjustments for age declines in height also need to be taken into account. These are, based on Trotter (1970), 0.06 times age in years minus 30 years (final height in centimetres) although such declines may not be linear (Cline, Meredith, Boyer, & Burrows, 1989).

In the southern hemisphere the range of populations is greater than that covered by Trotter and Gleser, and there has been a general awareness of the need to use population specific formulae. Comparisons between European males and the Trotter and Gleser formulae for white males (Konigsberg et al., 1998; Ross and Kongisberg, 2002) raise the possibility that even for 'Caucasians' in the region there is potentially a limited applicability of current formulae. Considering more broadly the range of potential points of origin the issue of variation in limb proportionality becomes even more acute (Table 11.1).

In Australia, for remains of Aboriginal origin, one practice has been to apply the Trotter and Gleser formulae for American blacks to long bone lengths (Donlon, personal communication, December 1998; Freedman, personal communication, December 1998). This is based on an overall similarity of proportion between the two populations, for example, tibial length contributes, on average, approximately 24% of living stature in Aboriginal populations and approximately 22% for American black populations — a much higher contribution to final height than other populations (Pretty et al., 1998). The exceptions are the arm proportions: Abbie (1957: 225) reported relatively short arm lengths among Aboriginal populations. The advantage of using the established Trotter and Gleser formulae (at least for the leg long bones) is that there is a recognised associated standard error and Krogman and Iscan (1986), for instance, recommend reporting heights with 2 SE thereby having a 1 in 22 chance of the height falling outside that range. However, because in this usage Trotter and Gleser formulae are being used on an unrelated population there is no external measure of the accuracy of such estimates. The only internal measure is the level of consistency between such estimates based on different long bones.

Table 11.1
Population Variation in Limb Proportionality

	Sitting height ratio	Tibia/femur	Source
Taiwan	53.9–55.1		
Thailand	50.6–52.9(m)		
South-East Asians		83.8–84.9	Biggs, 2003
Polynesian (average)		80.26–81.4	Biggs, 2003
Tonga		80.1–82.1	Biggs, 2003
Society Is	52.1–52.2		Eveleth & Tanner, 1990
New Zealand	54.0	80.4 (m+f)	Houghton, 1980
Papua New Guinea	52.2–53.1		Eveleth & Tanner, 1990
Australian Aborigine	47.3–48.1	84.3 (86.2)	Biggs, 2003; Eveleth & Tanner, 1990

Alternatively, in a recent comparison of South Australian human remains to modern populations, Pretty, Henneberg, Lambert and Prokopec (1998) suggested using the ratio of humeral, femoral or tibial length to overall living height. The ratios are based on Abbie's measurements of Aboriginal people, largely from central Australia. One difficulty is, however, that Abbie was not specific about which measurements he used so it cannot be assumed that there is an unproblematic translation of a living 'humerus length', for instance to the dry bone measurement of maximum humerus length (Biggs, 2003: 63). This partly explains why there are some consistent differences between estimates based on Trotter and Gleser and those based on a constant ratio (Pretty et al., 1998). The second difficulty with the use of the stature ratio as derived by Pretty et al. (1998) is the lack of a standard error or range that results in a single point estimate potentially misleading in forensic situations. Finally, Biggs noted that among Abbie's samples there was a slightly negative relationship between the crural index and total leg length (Biggs, 2003: 94). In other words, the longer the leg, the more the femur was contributing to total length, that is, the ratio of tibial length to height (via leg length) is not consistently linear (see also Duyar & Pelin, 2003).

In New Zealand, Houghton, Leach and Sutton (1975) also derived stature estimates based on data from living individuals, in this case the men of the Maori Battalion returning from World War I (recorded by Sir Peter Buck). They used an iterative procedure whereby linear regression equations linking height with living thigh length and lower leg length were derived. The equations were then adjusted to account for the difference between living length and dry bone length (not undertaken in the Pretty et al. 1998 example above), including femoral physiological length to femoral maximum length. Female equations were then derived from male equations using a constant difference; there is a problem here in that there has been no allowance made in the preceding step for sex differences in the ratio of femoral physiological to maximum length. Side specific formulae were also derived using a constant from the formulae for the right side. Furthermore, using the assumption that these proportions of long bones to height were constant across time, the statures of skeletal remains were calculated and then this estimated value used as the independent value to derive long bone lengths for the humerus, ulna and fibula (Houghton, 1980).

The method incorporates several levels of error: the derivation of dry bone measurements from live measurements; the extrapolation from males to females; the extrapolation to side; and the extrapolation from femur, tibia and radius measurements to humerus, ulna and fibula. Partly this iterative procedure explains why the standard error of estimates associated with these formulae are so low; in all instances less than 3 cm compared with > 3 cm of error for Trotter and Gleser formulae (1970). Effectively the procedure has relied on recursive regressions. As a baseline, to reduce the false accuracy, the formulae should only be used for the original derivation: male femur, tibia and radius lengths (all of these are maximum lengths) on the right side and, furthermore, estimates should probably be given with three standard errors to increase the likelihood that the real stature falls within that range.

Currently, however, these are the only formulae specifically derived for populations in near and remote Oceania. There is, however, a need for distinct formulae given that (based on skeletal samples) Pacific populations have relatively shorter distal leg segments (and hence longer femoral segments) than populations from Asia (Biggs, 2003). If a Trotter and Gleser formulae for Mongoloid populations is going to be applied to Pacific populations then the only one approaching appropriateness will be the one using total leg length (i.e., tibia and fibula) since the single proportion that is similar between the groups is the sitting height ratio (i.e., in reverse the total length of the leg relative to height).

None of these formulae help in relation to populations from Papua New Guinea and its archipelago. Houghton (1996: 47) tentatively suggests that the Polynesian formulae might be applied because Melanesian axial heights tend to be relatively large but there is, at the moment, a lack of adequate evidence to support this.

East Asian populations are the next most likely group to require identification in Australia and New Zealand and do have relevant regression formulae. Stevenson (1929) derived regression formulae for northern Chinese males and females, Shitai (cited in Krogman and Iscan, 1986: 321) for southern Chinese, and Fuji (1960) for Japanese. For populations from South-East Asia, Sangvichien, Srisurin and Watthanayingsakul (1985) has published a regression formula for Thais and Bergmann and The (1955) for Javanese.

The alternative to all such formulae is, where possible, to use the anatomical method of reconstructing height; a method much more likely to be feasible in forensic than archaeological situations. The method, derived by Fully (1956) requires measurement of the talus and calcaneus in anatomical position, total length of the tibia (i.e., excluding the tibial spine), bicondylar (or physiological length of the femur), anterior height of the first sacral segment, maximum height of the corpus of the C2–L5 vertebra measured separately, and basion-bregma height of the cranium. While the initial publication is somewhat unclear on these measurements, a recent review by Raxter et al. (2006) details the specifics. These measurements are then added together with a correction fraction. Raxter et al. (2006) suggest that the Fully correction of 10.5 cm (for those with a height between 153.6–165.4 cm) is rather short and instead propose incorporating an age correction as well so that:

Living stature = $1.009 \times$ skeletal height $- 0.0426 \times$ age $+ 12.1$.

Or living stature = $0.996 \times$ skeletal height $+ 11.7$ (no age correction applied).

The advantage is that the work by Bidmos (2005), King (2004) and Raxter et al. (2006) suggests that there are no systematic biases due to sex or ancestry. This makes it one method that potentially can be applied across the southern hemisphere. It does, however, give rather less hope for those dealing with fragmentary remains. However, it should be noted that for archaeological purposes, while stature is a useful indicative measurement, it is not the measurement that should be used for comparison as that needs to be based on the actual long bone measurements.

In common with the other aspects of human identification, it is apparent that stature estimation is fraught. The least reliable measures are those that assume that all southern hemisphere populations fall somehow into one of the three broad groups for whom standards have been established: Caucasoid, Negroid and Mongoloid. The most accurate appears to be the Fully method, although the technique needs to be applied using the appropriate measurement protocols and in the recognition that, while it appears to be nonspecific in relation to sex and ancestry, it so far has only been tested on Caucasian, South African and American black population clusters (Raxter et al., 2006). After all, living stature itself can be difficult to determine (Krogman & Iscan, 1986) let alone estimating it from the dead.

Conclusions

The startling point of this survey is the need for further research relevant to the populations of the Australia–Pacific region. Despite years of research into human variation in the area, the results of this work have rarely been analysed with an applied end in mind. Larnach's work (Larnach, 1978; Larnach & Freedman, 1964; Larnach & Macintosh, 1967) and the work of Houghton (Houghton et al., 1975; Houghton & De Souza, 1975; Houghton & Kean, 1987) are two of the obvious exceptions. Clearly there are areas where further research is needed and where commonly used standards developed elsewhere do need to be tested for their applicability to the populations encountered in the southern hemisphere.

At the same time, however, the application of methods still relies on the background knowledge of the researcher. While methods may be presented as if in a cookbook, the results require interpretation in the light of knowledge of human variation. All aspects of identification are statements of likelihood and as Donlon's (1998) work on sexing points out, false certainty can be seriously misleading. Similarly, statistical results are also statements requiring interpretation in the light of the applicability of the database used to the questions asked of it. Finally, as pointed out by Ubelaker (1996) and Williams et al. (2005), the way that human biology is partitioned is culturally specific and the terms used (e.g., Polynesian, South-East Asian) are interpreted differently in different cultures and hence in different sets of research. In other words, if human identification is to be undertaken, those doing it need to aware of the theory, methods, and materials that underlie what they are about to do, since, after all, these decisions have real import for the living not just the dead.

Acknowledgments

This work was made possible through a summer studentship provided by the Faculty of Arts, University of Auckland. I wish to thank Anna Biggs, Denise Donlon, Bruce Floyd, Gary Heathcote, Sian Halcrow, Mike Pietresewsky and Nancy Tayles for their constructive comments and generosity in responding to my numerous queries.

References

Abbie, A.V. (1957). Metrical characters of a central Australian tribe. *Oceania, 27,* 221–243.

Abbie, A.V. (1975a). *Dental eruption: Studies in physical anthropology.* Canberra, Australia: Australian Institute of Aboriginal Studies.

Abbie, A.V. (1975b). *Ossification: Studies in physical anthropology.* Canberra, Australia: Australian Institute of Aboriginal Studies.

Barker, B. (1973). An additional aid to sexing Aboriginal skulls by measuring mandibular first molars at the cemento-enamel junction. *Archaeology and Physical Anthropology in Oceania, 8,* 127–133.

Bass, W.M. (1987). *Human osteology: A laboratory and field manual.* Columbia, MO: Missouri Archaeological Society.

Bergmann, R., & The, T.H. (1955). The length of the body and long bones of the Javanese. *Documenta de Medicine Geographia et Tropica, 7,* 197–214.

Bidmos, M. (2005). On the non-equivalence of documented cadaver lengths to living stature estimates based on Fully's method on bones in the Raymond A. Dart Collection. *Journal of Forensic Science, 50,* 1–6.

Biggs, A.K. (2003). *The long and the short of it: Variation in limb segment lengths and proportions among Pacific peoples.* Unpublished master's thesis, University of Auckland, Auckland, New Zealand.

Bogin, B. (1999). *Patterns of human growth* (2nd ed.). Cambridge: Cambridge University Press.

Brace, C.L. (1980). Australian tooth size clines and the death of a stereotype. *Current Anthropology, 21*, 141–164.

Brickley, M. (2004). Guidance on recording age at death in juvenile skeletons. In M. Brickley & J. McKinley (Eds.), *Guidelines to the standards for recording human remains* (pp. 21–23). Southampton, England: BABAO.

Brook, A.H., & Barker, D.K. (1972). Eruption of teeth among the racial groups of eastern New Guinea: a correlation of tooth eruption with calendar age. *Archives of Oral Biology, 17*, 751–759.

Brown, P. (1981). Sex determination of Australian Aboriginal crania from the Murray River Valley: A reassessment of the Larnach Freedman technique. *Archaeology in Oceania, 16*, 53–63.

Brown, T. (1973). *Morphology of the Australian skull studied by multivariate analysis.* Canberra, Australia: Australian Institute of Aboriginal Studies.

Brown, T. (1978). Tooth emergence in Australian Aboriginals. *Annals of Human Biology, 5*, 41–54.

Brown, T. (1979). Skeletal maturation rates in Aboriginal Children. *Occasional Papers in Human Biology, 1*, 71–86.

Brown, T., & Barrett, M.J. (1973). Dental and craniofacial growth studies of Australian Aborigines. In R.L. Kirk (Ed.), *The human biology of Aborigines in Cape York* (pp. 69–79). Canberra, Austarlia: Australian Institute of Aboriginal Studies.

Brown, T., & Grave, K.C. (1976). Skeletal maturation in Australian Aborigines. *Australian Pediatric Journal, 12*, 24–30.

Brown, T., Jenner, J.D., Barrett, M.J., & Lees, G.H. (1979). Exfoliation of deciduous teeth and gingival emergence of permanent teeth in Australian Aborigines. *Occasional Papers in Human Biology, 1*, 47–70.

Buikstra, J.E., & Ubelaker, D.H. (1994). *Standards for data collection from human skeletal remains.* Fayetteville, AR: Arkansas Archeological Survey.

Bulbeck, D. (2005a). *Australian Aboriginal craniometrics as construed through FORDISC.* Retrieved March 9, 2006, from http://arts.anu.edu.au/bullda/oz_craniometrics.html

Bulbeck, D. (2005b). *Roonka and the transition from Australoid to Australian craniometrics.* Retrieved March 9, 2006, from http://arts.anu.edu.au/bullda/roonka.html

Chamberlain, A. (1994). *Interpreting the past: human remains.* Berkeley, CA: University of California Press.

Chiu, A., & Donlon, D. (2000). Anthropological and forensic aspects of odontological variation in two contemporary Australian populations. *Dental Anthropology, 14*, 20–37.

Cline, M.C., Meredith, K.E., Boyer, J.T., & Burrows, B. (1989). Decline of height with age in adults in a general population sample: Estimating maximum height and distinguishing birth cohort effects from actual loss of stature with aging. *Human Biology, 61*, 415–425.

Cox, K., Tayles, N.G., & Buckley, H.R. (2006). Forensic identification of 'race': The issues in New Zealand. *Current Anthropology, 45*, 869–874.

Davivgongs, V. (1963a). The femur of the Australian Aborigine. *American Journal of Physical Anthropology, 21*, 457–468.

Davivgongs, V. (1963b). The pelvic girdle of the Australian Aborigine: Sex differences and sex determination. *American Journal of Physical Anthropology, 21*, 443–456.

Dennison, K.J. (1979). Tooth size and sexual dimorphism in prehistoric New Zealand Polynesian teeth. *Archaeology and Physical Anthropology in Oceania, 14*, 123–128.

Diamanti, J., & Townsend, G.C. (2003). New standards for permanent tooth emergence in Australian children. *Australian Dental Journal, 48*, 39–42.

Donlon, D. (1998). Sex determination. In M. Casey, D. Donlon, J. Hope & S. Welfare (Eds.), *Redefining archaeology: Feminist perspectives* (Australian National University Occasional Papers, pp. 98–103). Canberra, Australia: ANU Press.

Donlon, D. (2003). Diversity revealed: Ten years of anthropological case work based in New South Wales, Australia [Abstract]. *Homo, 54*, 151–152.

Duyar, I., & Pelin, C. (2003). Body height estimation based on tibia length in different stature groups. *American Journal of Physical Anthropology, 122*, 23–27.

Eveleth, P.B., & Tanner, J.M. (1976). *Worldwide variation in human growth*. Cambridge: Cambridge University Press.

Fanning, E.A., & Moorrees. C.F.A. (1969). A comparison of permanent mandibular molar formation in Australian Aborigines and Caucasoids. *Archives of Oral Biology, 14*, 999–1006.

Fenner, F. (1939). The Australian Aboriginal skull: Its non-metrical morphological characters. *Transactions of the Royal Society of South Australia, 63*, 248–301.

Formicola, V. (1993). Stature reconstruction from long bones in ancient population samples: An approach to the problem of its reliability. *American Journal of Physical Anthropology, 90*, 351–358.

Friedlaender, J.S., & Bailit, M.J. (1969). Eruption times of the deciduous and permanent teeth of natives on Bougainville Island, Territory of New Guinea: A study of racial variation. *Human Biology, 41*, 51–65.

Frisancho, A.R., Gilding, N., & Tanner, S. (2001). Growth of leg length is reflected in socio-economic differences. *Acta Medica Auxologica, 33*, 47–50.

Fry, E.I. (1976). Dental development in Cook Island children. In E. Giles & J.S. Friedlaender (Eds.), *The measures of man: Methodologies in biological anthropology* (pp. 164–180). Cambridge, MA: Peabody Museum Press.

Fuji, A. (1960). On the relation of long bone lengths of limb to stature. *Bulletin of the School of Physical Education, Juntendo University, 3*, 49–61.

Fully, G. (1956). Une nouvelle methode de determination de la taille. *Annales Medicale et Legale, 35*, 266–273.

Giles, E. (1976). Cranial variation in Australia and neighbouring areas. In R.L. Kirk & A.G. Thorne (Eds.), *The origin of the Australians* (pp. 161–172). Canberra, Australia: Australian Institute of Aboriginal Studies.

Gill, G.W., & Rhine, S. (Eds.). (1990). *Skeletal attribution of race*. Albuquerque, NM: Maxwell Museum of Anthropology University of New Mexico.

Green, M.K. (1990). *Prehistoric cranial variation in Papua New Guinea*. Unpublished doctoral dissertation, Australian National University, Canberra.

Haavikko, K. (1970). The formation and the alveolar and clinical eruption of the permanent teeth: an orthopantographic study. *Proceedings of the Finnish Dental Society, 66*, 101–170.

Halcrow, S.E., Tayles, N.G., & Buckley, H.R. (in press). Age estimation of children in prehistoric Southeast Asia: Are the dental formation methods utilised appropriate? *Journal of Archaeological Science.*

Hanihara, K. (1994). Craniofacial continuity and discontinuity of far easterners in the late Pleistocene and Holocene. *Journal of Human Evolution, 27*, 417–441.

Harris, E., & Bailit, H.L. (1987). Odontometric comparisons among Solomon Islanders and other Oceanic peoples. In J.S. Friedlaender (Ed.), *The Solomon Islands project: A long-term study of health, human biology, and culture change* (pp. 215–264). Oxford: Clarendon Press.

Harris, E., Turner, C.G.I., & Underwood, J.H. (1975). Dental morphology of living Yap Islanders, Micronesia. *Archaeology and Physical Anthropology in Oceania, 10*, 218–234.

Heathcote, G. (1995). *Forensic Anthropology Case Report, No. 95–01*. Mangilao, GU: University of Guam.

Heathcote, G. (1996). A Protocol for scoring three posterior cranial superstructures which reach remarkable size in Ancient Mariana islanders. *Micronesica, 29*, 281–298.

Hoffding, J., Maeda, M., Yamaguchi, K., Tsuji, H., Kuwabara, S., Nohara, Y. et al. (1984). Emergence of permanent teeth and onset of dental stages in Japanese children. *Community Dental Oral Epidemiology, 12*, 55–58.

Hoppa, R.D. (2000). Population variation in osteological aging criteria: An example from the pubic symphysis. *American Journal of Physical Anthropology, 111*, 185–191.

Hoppa, R.D., & Vaupel, J.W. (2002). The Rostock Manifesto for paleodemography: the way from stage to age. In R.D. Hoppa & J.W. Vaupel (Eds.), *Paleodemography* (pp. 1–8). Cambridge: Cambridge University Press.

Houghton P. (1977). Human skeletal remains from excavations in eastern Coromandel. *Records of the Auckland Institute and Museum. 14*, 45–56.

Houghton, P. (1978). Polynesian mandibles. *Journal of Anatomy*, *127*, 251–260.

Houghton, P. (1980). *The first New Zealanders*. Auckland, New Zealand: Hodder & Stoughton.

Houghton P. (1996). *People of the great ocean: Aspects of human biology of the early Pacific*. Melbourne, Australia: Cambridge University Press.

Houghton, P., & De Souza, P. (1975). Discriminant function sexing of prehistoric New Zealand skeletal material from lengths of long bones. *Journal of the Polynesian Society*, *84*, 225–229.

Houghton, P., Kean, M.R. (1987). The Polynesian head: A biological model for *Homo sapiens*. *Journal of the Polynesian Society*, *96*, 223–242.

Houghton, P., Leach, B.F., & Sutton, D.G. (1975). The estimation of stature of prehistoric Polynesians in New Zealand. *Journal of the Polynesian Society*, *84*, 325–336.

Howells, W.W. (1970). Anthropometric grouping analysis of Pacific peoples. *Archaeology and Physical Anthropology in Oceania*, *5*, 192–217.

Howells, W.W. (1973). *The Pacific Islanders*. Wellington, New Zealand: Reed.

Howells, W.W. (1989). *Skull shapes and the map: Craniometric analyses in the dispersion of modern Homo*. Cambridge, MA: Harvard University.

Howells, W.W. (1995). *Who's who in skulls: Ethnic identification of crania from measurements*. Cambridge, MA: Harvard University.

Iscan, M.Y., & Shihai, D. (1995). Sexual dimorphism in the Chinese femur. *Forensic Science International*, *74*, 79–87.

Iscan, M.Y., Loth, S.R., King, C.A., Shihai, D., & Yoshino, M. (1998). Sexual dimorphism in the humerus: A comparative analysis of Chinese, Japanese, and Thais. *Forensic Science International*, *98*, 17–29.

Iscan, M.Y., Yoshino, M., & Kato, S. (1995). Sexual dimorphism in modern Japanese crania. *American Journal of Human Biology*, *7*, 459–464.

Iscan, M.Y., Yoshino, M., & Susumu, K. (1994). Sex determination from the Tibia: Standards for contemporary Japan. *Journal of Forensic Sciences*, *39*, 785–792.

Kamalanathan, G.S., Hauck, H.M., & Kittiveja, C. (1960). Dental development of children in a Siamese Village, Bang Chan 1953. *Journal of Dental Research*, *39*, 453–461.

Katayama, K. (1985). Human skeletal remains from Makin Atoll of the Gilbert Islands, Micronesia. *Man and Culture in Oceania*, *1*, 81–120.

Katzenberg, M.A., & Saunders, S.R. (Eds.). (2000). *Biological anthropology of the human skeleton*. New York: Wiley-Liss.

Kean, M.R., & Houghton, P. (1990). Polynesian face and dentition: Functional perspectives. *American Journal of Physical Anthropology*, *82*, 361–370.

King, C.A., Iscan, M.Y., & Loth, S.R. (1998). Metric and comparative analysis of sexual dimorphism in the Thai femur. *Journal of Forensic Science*, *43*, 954–958.

King, K. (2004). A test of the Fully anatomical method of stature estimation [abstract]. *American Journal of Physical Anthropology* [suppl.], *38*, 125.

Komar, D. (2003). Lessons from Srebrenica: the contributions and limitations of physical anthropology in identifying victims of war crimes. *Journal of Forensic Sciences*, *48*, 713–716.

Konigsberg, L., & Holman, D. (1999). Estimation of age at death from dental emergence and implications for studies of prehistoric somatic growth. In R.D. Hoppa & C.M. Fitzgerald (Eds.), *Human growth in the past: Studies from bones and teeth* (pp. 264–289). Cambridge: Cambridge University Press.

Konigsberg, L.W., Hens, S.M., Jantz, L.M., & Jungers, W.L. (1998). Stature estimation and calibration: bayesian and maximum likelihood perspectives in physical anthropology. *Yearbook of Physical Anthropology*, *41*, 65–92.

Krailassiri, S., Anuwongnukroh, N., & Dechkunakorn, S. (2002). Relationships between dental calcification stages and skeletal maturity indicators in Thai individuals. *Angle Orthodontist*, *72*, 155–166.

Krogman, W.M., Iscan, M.Y. (1986). *The human skeleton in forensic medicine*. Springfield, IL: C.C. Thomas.

Larnach, S.L. (1978). *Australian Aboriginal craniology*. Sydney, Australia: University of Sydney.

Larnach, S.L., & Freedman, L. (1964). Sex determination of the Aboriginal crania from coastal New South Wales, Australia. *Records of the Australian Museum, 26*, 295–308.

Larnach, S.L., & Macintosh, N.W.G. (1967). The use in forensic medicine of an anthropological method for the determination of sex and race in skeletons. *Archaeology and Physical Anthropology in Oceania, 2*, 156–161.

Larnach, S.L., & Macintosh, N.W.G. (1970). *The craniology of the Aborigines of Queensland* (Oceania Monograph No. 15). Sydney, Australia: University of Sydney.

Larnach, S.L., & Macintosh, N.W.G. (1971). *The mandible in eastern Australian Aborigines* (Oceania Monograph No. 16). Sydney, Australia: University of Sydney.

Li, C., & Ji, G. (1995). Age estimation from the permanent molar in northeast China by the method of average stage of attrition. *Forensic Science International, 75*, 189–196.

Liu, W. (1989). Sex determination of the Chinese femur by discriminant function. *Journal of Forensic Sciences, 34*, 1222–1227.

Logan, W., & Kronfeld, R. (1933). Development of the human jaws and surrounding structures from birth to the age of fifteen years. *Journal of the American Dental Association, 20*, 379–427.

Lorenzo, C., Carretero, J.M., Arsuaga, J.L., Gracia, A., & Martinez, I. (1998). Intrapopulational body size variation and cranial capacity variation in Middle Pleistocene humans: The Sima de los Huesos sample Sierra de los Atapuerca, Spain. *American Journal of Physical Anthropology, 106*, 19–33.

Marshall, D.S., & Snow, C.E. (1956). An evaluation of Polynesian craniology. *American Journal of Physical Anthropology, 14*, 405–427.

Massler, M., Schour, I., & Poncher, H. (1941). Developmental pattern of the child as reflected in the calcification pattern of the teeth. *American Journal of Diseases of Children, 62*, 33–67.

Masters, P. (2006). *Time since death.* Unpublished MA Research Portfolio, University of Auckland, Auckland, New Zealand.

Mays, S., & Cox, M. (2000). Sex determination in skeletal remains. In M. Cox & S. Mays (Eds.), *Human osteology in archaeology and forensic science* (pp. 117–130). London: Greenwich Medical Media.

Moorees, C., Fanning, E., & Hunt, E. (1963). Age variation of formation stages for ten permanent teeth. *Journal of Dental Research, 42*, 1490–1502.

Ousley, S., & Jantz, R. (1996). *FORDISC 2.0: Personal computer forensic discriminant functions.* Knoxville: University of Tennessee.

Phenice, T.W. (1969). A newly developed visual method of sexing the os pubis. *American Journal of Physical Anthropology, 30*, 297–302.

Pietrusewsky, M. (1970). Osteological view of indigenous populations in Oceania. In R.C. Green & M. Kelly (Eds.), *Studies in oceanic culture history* (pp. 1–11). Honolulu, HI: Bernice Pauahi Bishop Museum.

Pietrusewsky, M. (1973). A multivariate analysis of craniometric data from the Territory of Papua New Guinea. *Archaeology and Physical Anthropology in Oceania, 8*, 12–23.

Pietrusewsky, M. (1976). *Prehistoric human skeletal remains from Papua New Guinea and the Marquesas.* Honolulu, HI: Social Sciences & Linguistics Institute University of Hawaii at Manoa.

Pietrusewsky, M. (1979). Craniometric variation in Pleistocene Australian and more recent Australian and New Guinea popluations studied by multivariate procedures. *Occasional Papers in Human Biology, 1*, 83–123.

Pietrusewsky, M. (1983). Multivariate analysis of New Guinea and Melanesian skulls: A review. *Journal of Human Evolution, 12*, 61–76.

Pietrusewsky, M. (1984). Metric and non-metric cranial variation in Australian Aboriginal populations compared with populations from the Pacific and Asia. *Occasional Papers in Human Biology 3.* Canberra, Australia: Australian Institute of Aboriginal Studies.

Pietrusewsky, M. (1989). A study of skeletal and dental remains from Watom Island and comparisons with other Lapita people. *Records of the Australian Museum, 41*, 235–292.

Pietrusewsky, M. (1990a). Craniofacial variation in Australasian and Pacific populations. *American Journal of Physical Anthropology, 82*, 319–340.

Pietrusewsky, M. (1990b). Craniometric variation in Micronesia and the Pacific: A multivariate study. *Micronesica, 2*, 373–402.

Pietrusewsky, M. (1990c). Lapita-associated skeletons from Watom Island, Papua New Guinea, and the origins of the Polynesians. *Asian Perspectives, 28*, 83–89.

Pietrusewsky, M. (1997). Biological origins of Hawaiians: Evidence from skulls. *Man and Culture in Oceania, 13*, 1–37.

Pietrusewsky, M. (2004). Multivariate comparisons of female cranial series from the Ryukyu Islands and Japan. *Anthropological Science, 112*, 199–211.

Pietrusewsky, M., & Ikehara-Quebral, R. (2001). Multivariate comparisons of Rapa Nui Easter Island, Polynesian, and circum-Polynesian crania. In C.M. Stevenson, G. Lee & F.J. Morin, (Eds.), *Pacific 2000. Proceedings of the Fifth International Conference on Easter Island and the Pacific* (pp. 457–494). Los Osos, CA: Easter Island Foundation.

Pretty, G.L., Henneberg, M., Lambert, K.M., & Prokopec, M. (1998). Trends in stature in the South Australian Aboriginal Murraylands. *American Journal of Physical Anthropology, 106*, 505–514.

Rainio, J., Hedman, M., Karkola, K., Lalu, K., Petola, P., Ranta, H. et al. (2001). Forensic osteological investigations in Kosovo. *Forensic Science International, 121*, 166–173.

Raxter, M., Auerbach, B., & Ruff, C. (2006). Revision of the fully technique for estimating statures. *American Journal of Physical Anthropology, 130*, 374–384.

Ray, L.J. (1959). Metrical and non-metrical features of the clavicle of the Australian Aboriginal. *American Journal of Physical Anthropology, 17*, 217–226.

Rhine, S. (1990). Non-metric skull racing. In G.W. Gill & S. Rhine (Eds.), *Skeletal attribution of race* (pp. 9–15). Albuquerque, NM: Maxwell Museum of Anthropology University of New Mexico.

Richards, L.C., & Miller, S.L.J. (1991). Relationships between age and dental attrition in Australian Aboriginals. *American Journal of Physical Anthropology, 84*, 159–164.

Richards, L.C., & Telfer, P.J. (1979). The use of dental characters in the assessment of genetic distance in Australia. *Archaeology and Physical Anthropology in Oceania, 14*, 184–194.

Ross, A., & Kongisberg, L. (2002). New formulae for estimating stature in the Balkans. *Journal of Forensic Science, 47*, 165–167.

Sangvichien, S., Srisurin, V., & Watthanayingsakul, V. (1985). Estimation of stature of Thai and Chinese from the length of the femur, tibia and fibula. *Siriraj Hospital Gazette, 37*, 215–218.

Saunders, S.R. (2000). Subadult skeletons and growth-related studies. In M.A. Katzenberg & S.R. Saunders (Eds.), *Biological anthropology of the human skeleton* (pp. 1–20). New York: Wiley-Liss.

Scheuer, L., & Black, S. (2000). *Developmental juvenile osteology.* San Diego: Academic Press.

Sjovold, T. (1990). Estimation of stature from long bones utilizing the line of organic Correlation. *Human Evolution, 5*, 431–447.

Smith, B.H. (1991). Standards of tooth formation and dental age assessment. In M. Kelley & C.S. Larsen (Eds.), *Advances in dental anthropology* (pp. 143–168). New York: Wiley-Liss.

Smith, B.H. (1992). Life history and the evolution of human maturation. *Evolutionary Anthropology, 1*, 134–142.

Snow, C.E. (1974). *Early Hawaiians.* Lexington, KY: The University Press of Kentucky.

Song, H., Lin, Z.Q., & Jai, J.T. (1992). Sex diagnosis of Chinese skulls using multiple stepwise discriminant function analysis. *Forensic Science International, 54*, 135–140.

Stevenson, P.H. (1929). On racial differences in stature long bone regression formulae, with special reference to stature reconstruction formulae for the Chinese. *Biometrika, 21*, 303–321.

Stewart, T.D. (1979). *Essentials of forensic anthropology, especially as developed in the United States.* Springfield, IL: Thomas.

Sutton, D.G. (1979). The prehistoric people of eastern Palliser Bay. *National Museum Bulletin, 21*, 185–203.

Swindler, D.S. (1991). The cephalofacial complex in the Lakalai of New Britain, Melanesia. In T. Brown & S Molnar (Eds.), *XVII Pacific Science Congress* (pp. 21–26). Adelaide, Australia: University of Adelaide Dental School.

Tanner, J.M., Hayashi, T., Preece, M.A., & Cameron, N. (1982). Increase in length of leg relative to trunk in Japanese children and adults from 1957 to 1977: Comparison with British and with Japanese Americans. *Annals of Human Biology, 9*, 411–424.

Townsend, G.C., & Brown, T. (1979). *Tooth size characteristics of Australian Aborigines: Occasional papers in human biology* (pp. 17–38). Canberra, Australia: Australian Institute of Aboriginal Studies.

Townsend, G.C., Richards, L.C., & Carrol, A. (1982). Sex determination of Australian Aboriginal skulls by discriminant function analysis. *Australian Dental Journal, 27*, 320–326.

Townsend, S. (2002). *Sex determination of juvenile remains using ancient DNA.* Unpublished master's thesis, University of Auckland, Auckland, New Zealand.

Trotter, M. (1970). Estimation of stature from intact long limb bones. In T.D. Stewart (Ed.), *Personal identification in mass disasters* (pp. 71–84). Washington, DC: Smithsonian Institution.

Trotter, M., & Gleser, G.C. (1952). Estimation of stature from long bones of American Whites and Negroes. *American Journal of Physical Anthropology, 10*, 463–514.

Trotter, M., & Gleser, G.C. (1958). A re-evaluation of estimation of stature based on measurements of stature taken during life and of long bones after death. *American Journal of Physical Anthropology, 16*, 79–124.

Trotter, M., & Gleser, G.C. (1977). Corrigenda to 'estimation of stature from long limb bones of American whites and negroes', American Journal of Physical Anthropology 1952. *American Journal of Physical Anthropology, 47*, 355–356.

Turner, C.G. (1989). Teeth and prehistory in Asia. *Scientific American, 260*, 88–96.

Turner, C.G. (1990). Major features of sundadonty and sinodonty, including suggestions about East Asian microevolution, population history, and late Pleistocene relationships with Australian Aboriginals. *American Journal of Physical Anthropology, 82*, 295–317.

Ubelaker, D.H. (1996). Skeletons testify: Anthropology in forensic science AAPA luncheon address: April 12, 1996. *Yearbook of Physical Anthropology, 39*, 229–244.

Ubelaker, D.H. (1999). *Human skeletal remains: Excavation, analysis, interpretation.* Washington, DC: Taraxacum.

Ulijaszek, S. (1996). Age of eruption of deciduous dentition of Anga children, Papua New Guinea. *Annals of Human Biology, 23*, 495–499.

Usher, B. (2002). Reference samples: the first step in linking biology and age in the human skeleton. In R.D. Hoppa & J.W. Vaupel (Eds.), *Paleodemography: Age distributions from skeletal samples* (pp. 29–47). Cambridge: Cambridge University Press.

van Dongen, V.R. (1963). The shoulder girdle of the Australian Aborigine. *American Journal of Physical Anthropology, 21*, 469–488.

Weisler, M.I., & Swindler, D.S. (2002). Rocker jaws from the Marshall Islands: Evidence for interaction between eastern Micronesia and west Polynesia. *People and Culture in Oceania, 18*, 23–33.

White, T.D. (2000). *Human osteology.* (2nd ed.). San Diego: Academic Press.

Williams, F.L., Belcher, R., & Armelagos, G. (2005). Forensic misclassification of ancient Nubian crania: implications for assumptions about human variation. *Current Anthropology, 46*, 340–346.

Wiriyaromp, W. (1984). A prehistoric population from north east Thailand. In D.T. Bayard (Ed.), *Southeast Asian Archaeology at the XV Pacific Science Congress: the Origins of Agriculture, Metallurgy and the State in Mainland Southeast Asia* (pp. 327–335). Dunedin, New Zealand: Department of Anthropology, University of Otago.

Wood, W.B. (1976). Ossification variation in two populations from Papua New Guinea. In R.L. Kirk & A.G. Thorne (Eds.), *The origin of the Australians* (pp. 245–263). Canberra, Australia: Australian Institute of Aboriginal Studies.

Wood, W.B., Briggs, C., & Donlon, D. (2002). Forensic osteology. In I. Freckelton & H. Selby (Eds.), *Expert evidence* (pp. 601–802). Sydney, Australia: Thomson Lawbook Co.

Wood, W.Q. (1920). The tibia of the Australian Aboriginal. *Journal of Anatomy, 54*, 232–257.

Wright, R.V.S. (1992). Correlation between cranial form and geography in *Homo sapiens*: CRANID — A computer program for forensic and other applications. *Archaeology in Oceania, 27*, 128–134.

Yamada, H., Kawamoto, K., Tairea, T., & Rere, T.V. (1999). Early emergence of permanent teeth in children of the Cook Islands. In N. Shibata & K. Katayama (Eds.), *Prehistoric Cook Islands: People, life and language: An Official Report for Kyoto University Cook Islands Scientific Research Programme KUCIP in 1989–1998* (pp. 195–212). Rarotonga, Cook Islands: Cook Islands Library and Museum.

Geographic Origin and Mobility Recorded in the Chemical Composition of Human Tissues

Donald Pate

The chemical composition of human tissues may provide information about recent or long-term residence in various geographic localities. Elemental and isotopic signatures in foods and water from particular geographic regions are recorded in the tissues of human consumers. Tissues with different biochemical turnover rates (e.g., skin, fingernails, hair, teeth, and bones) record residence for different temporal periods of a person's lifetime and thus offer a geographic life history for individuals. Initial analyses of stable sulphur and carbon isotopes in modern human hair from five different countries (Brazil, India, Japan, Canada, and Australia) distinguished individuals from different regions and prompted Katzenberg and Krouse (1989) to argue that chemical analyses of human tissues had the potential to make significant contributions to forensic case studies in relation to identifying geographic origin and human mobility.

In cases where recently deceased individuals cannot be identified on the basis of fingerprints, dental records, personal effects, physical anthropology, facial approximation, DNA profile, or other traditional methods, chemical analyses of tissues provide additional information that can be employed in relation to identification. Potential applications of chemical analyses of human tissues in relation to forensic cases include victim identification (determination of recent and long-term residence of individuals associated with clandestine burials, missing persons cases, mass graves, natural disasters, or terrorist activities), demonstration of recent travel (in association with suspected terrorist activities, people-trafficking, smuggling, or illegal immigration) and repatriation of unprovenanced human remains held in museums and private collections (Beard & Johnson, 2000; Ehleringer, 2003; Fraser, Meier-Augenstein, & Kalin, 2006; Pate, Brody, & Owen, 2002; Pye 2004a, 2004b).

This chapter reviews chemical techniques employed in studies of geographic origin and provides a number of case studies to demonstrate particular applications. Although chemical analyses of human tissues are used widely in physical anthropology and archaeology (Pate, 1994; Katzenberg, 2000; Katzenberg & Harrison, 1997; Schoeninger & Moore, 1992; Schwarcz & Schoeninger, 1991; Sealy, Armstrong & Shrire, 1995), applications to forensic cases have been limited.

Human Tissues and Geographic Provenance

Chemical analyses of skin, hair and fingernails provide information about short-term (days to months) diet and environmental exposure, while teeth and bones record long-term signatures (years to decades). In relation to sample collection from living individuals, skin, hair and nails can be obtained in a noninvasive manner; whereas, teeth and bone require invasive techniques. Tooth enamel and cortical samples from long bones are preferred in relation to buried human remains due to their lower susceptibility to postmortem chemical alterations in the burial environment (Budd Montgomery, Evans, & Barreiro, 2000; Pate & Hutton, 1988; Pate, Huton, & Norrish, 1989).

Hair has a very rapid turnover rate relative to nails. In general, growth rates in scalp hair are approximately 0.25 cm per week, while an entire nail represents about 6 months of growth (or about 0.05 cm per week). Thus, in relation to sampling, hair offers a good chronological resolution along the length of the shaft, and the isotopic composition of hair is more consistent with dietary uptake than are isotopic values in nails (Ayliffe, Cerling, Robinson, West, Sponheimer et al., 2004; Fraser et al., 2006; Harkey, 1993; West, Ayliffe, Cerling, Robinson, Karren et al., 2004). The chemical composition of teeth provides a record of childhood diet and residence (Hillson, 1996, 2000; Smith, 1991), while bone relates to a long-term average of dietary composition and habitat use over decades. Thus, in an adult skeleton, teeth will provide information regarding childhood residence and bone offers data about the last decades of life (Pate, 1994, in press).

Developmental stages in permanent tooth crowns provide three phases (Hillson, 2000: 249; Smith, 1991) that can be employed to examine changes in human residence through time: (a) incisors, canines and first molars are initiated during the first year after birth (or just before birth) and are completed between 3 years and 7 years of age, (b) premolars and second molars start formation during the second and third years after birth and are completed between 4 years and 8 years of age, and (c) third molars are initiated any time between age 7 and 12 years and are completed sometime between 10 years and 18 years of age.

Following completion of development, the chemical constituents of teeth do not change during the remaining lifetime of the individual. In contrast, bone continues to change its chemical composition throughout the lifetime of the individual (Pate 1994: 164–165). Consequently, the chemical analysis of teeth and bones provides an opportunity to address changes in diet and residence from childhood to adulthood. Analyses of different teeth from the same individual allow a refinement of childhood dietary reconstruction and habitat use to three stages of maturation. Finally, a combination of bone and tooth chemistry values allows comparisons between the last several decades of life and various subadult stages (Sealy et al., 1995).

Hair and nails are metabolically inert tissues composed of the protein keratin (Hobson, 1999; Rubenstein & Hobson, 2004). In contrast, bone contains both organic collagen (protein) and inorganic hydroxyapatite (mineral) components (Pate, 1994). Tooth crowns are composed of a hard outer layer of enamel that overlies a softer dentine. The inner parts of tooth roots consist primarily of dentine, while the outer portions are composed of cementum. Inorganic hydroxyapatite is the primary chemical component of enamel, dentine and cementum. Enamel consists of approximately 95% hydroxyapatite, 4% water and 1% organic matter, while dentine is 70% hydroxyapatite, 18% organic matter (mainly collagen) and 12% water (Hillson, 1996; Mann, 2001; Woelfel & Scheid, 2002).

Elemental and Isotopic Applications

Both elemental and isotopic concentrations in human and animal tissues have been employed to demonstrate residence in geographic regions with distinct geochemical signatures. A large number of major and trace elements vary in concentration across landscapes and are incorporated into human tissues in relation to dietary intake and environmental exposure (Price, 1989; Priest & van de Vyver, 1999; Pye, 2004b). These include barium, strontium, lead, copper, zinc, nickel, magnesium, chromium, cadmium, aluminium, and arsenic. Fluoride concentrations in teeth may also be used to distinguish between geographic areas with differences in the fluoride levels in drinking water. Chemical 'fingerprints' for different regions are identified employing an extensive suite of major and trace elements (Pye, 2004b). Distinct elemental values in soils and plants are passed up the food chain to animals, including humans.

Isotopes are variants of the same element with differing numbers of neutrons in their nuclei. In relation to isotopic measurements, more positive isotope values indicate greater concentrations of the heavier isotope versus the lighter isotope relative to a standard, for example, greater amounts of ^{13}C versus ^{12}C in the tissue examined. Relative concentrations of two isotopes of the same element in water, soils, and plants are employed to distinguish geographic regions. Isotopes of strontium ($^{87}Sr/^{86}Sr$), oxygen ($^{18}O/^{16}O$), hydrogen ($^2H/^1H$), carbon ($^{13}C/^{12}C$), and lead ($^{206}Pb/^{204}Pb$, $^{207}Pb/^{206}Pb$, $^{208}Pb/^{206}Pb$) in tooth enamel and isotopes of carbon ($^{13}C/^{12}C$), nitrogen ($^{15}N/^{14}N$), and sulphur ($^{34}S/^{32}S$) in proteins (e.g., bone collagen, hair, and nails) are the most common chemical constituents used in human and animal tissue analyses addressing residence and mobility (Budd, Millard, Chenery, Lucy, & Roberts 2004; Müller, Fricke, Halliday, McCulloch, & Wartho, 2003; Pate, in press; Pye, 2004a, 2004b; Richards, Fuller, Sponheimer, & Robinson, 2003; Rubenstein & Hobson, 2004). Studies employing a combination of two or more isotopic techniques, for example, Sr, O, and Pb, improve the reliability of inferences about residence and mobility.

Isotope ratios in inert tissues such as hair and nails reflect food-web conditions at the time of tissue formation and remain unchanged despite movement to different geographic localities (Rubenstein & Hobson, 2004: 259). Thus, sections of these tissues provide a sequential record of geographic residence.

In general, the carbon, nitrogen, strontium, lead, and sulphur isotopic composition of human tissues are related to isotopic values in ingested foods (Ambrose, 1991; Beard & Johnson, 2000; Gulson, Jameson, & Gillings, 1997; Hobson, 1999; Pate, 1994, in press; Richards, Fuller, & Hedges, 2001, Richards et al., 2003). Foods derived from marine and terrestrial ecosystems show distinct isotopic values (Schoeninger DeNiro, & Tauber, 1983; Schoeninger & DeNiro, 1984). Carbon isotope values are also affected by the photosynthetic pathways of dominant plants in various habitats. For example, C_4 grasses dominate tropical ecosystems and C_3 grasses dominate cooler, temperate regions resulting in a general decrease of the proportion of C_4 to C_3 grasses with increasing latitude (O'Leary, 1988). Nitrogen isotope values are affected by trophic level and climate with more positive values associated with higher levels of the food chain, for example, carnivores, and increasing aridity. Strontium, lead, and sulphur isotope values vary according to geological source materials and differences are passed up marine and terrestrial foodwebs to human consumers. Because seawater Sr is well mixed, the strontium isotope composition is relatively constant throughout the oceans of the world (Pate, 1994: 168). In contrast, terrestrial sediments show distinct strontium isotopic values related to the relative presence of different source materials, such as carbonates versus granites. Lead isotope ratios vary in a systematic manner in various geographic regions as a 'result of radiogenic isotopic evolution and therefore as a function of age, parent isotope abundance, and subsequent remodelling of crustal material' (Montgomery, Budd, & Evans, 2000: 372).

In contrast, oxygen and hydrogen isotope values vary according to the composition of ingested water (local drinking water and water contained in foods) and foods (Fricke, Clyde, & O'Neill, 1998; Longinelli, 1984; Sharp, Atudorei, Panarello, Fernandez, & Douthitt, 2003). When food sources are isotopically related to local meteoric water (e.g., plants and animals derived from the same region), the isotopic composition of human tissues should correlate well with that of the local water. Isotope values of precipitation change systematically with altitude and latitude resulting in distinct oxygen and hydrogen isotope ratios for waters derived from different geographic regions. Maps showing the distinct oxygen and hydrogen isotopic composition of surface waters and groundwater for various global regions are being developed in relation to studies addressing geographic residence and mobility (see Darling & Talbot, 2003; Darling, Bath, & Talbot, 2003).

Short-Term Isotopic Variability in Hair and Nails

In order to examine the utility of isotopic analyses of hair and nails as a means to identify an individual's recent movements, geographic origin, and geographic life history, Fraser et al. (2006) conducted a longitudinal study examining carbon, nitrogen, hydrogen, and oxygen isotopic variability in these tissues. Scalp hair and fingernail samples were collected from 20 British and non-British adult volunteers at Queen's University, Belfast, every 2 weeks for a minimum period of 8 months in order to address isotopic variability in individuals residing in the same habitat. Subjects included in the study had been living in Belfast for at least the past 6 months, but were originally from a range of geographic regions worldwide. In addition, in order to establish isotopic variability on a global scale, samples were collected from individuals from Belgium, France, the Netherlands, India, Norway, Sudan, Syria, Australia, and the United States.

In relation to the longitudinal study, the data show a relatively low degree of natural variation in the nitrogen and carbon isotope values of hair and fingernails. In contrast, greater variations were observed in the hydrogen and oxygen isotope values of the same samples. Both nitrogen and oxygen isotope values in nails were significantly more variable than those in hair from the same individual. The authors argue that the rapid formation rate of hair in comparison to nails makes hair less susceptible to subsequent biochemical processes that could alter original isotopic signatures. Thus, in comparison to nails, hair most likely provides a more reliable short-term indicator of the isotopic composition of ingested foods and local environmental chemistry.

Plots of carbon versus nitrogen and hydrogen versus oxygen isotope values for hair and nails derived from the worldwide isotopic database (Figure 12.1) demonstrated that it was possible to differentiate between the majority of the countries

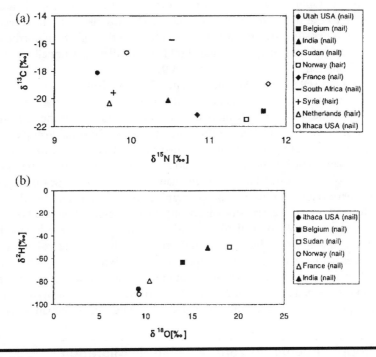

Figure 12.1

Plots of measured isotopic composition of human hair and fingernail samples derived from a global sample (adapted from Fraser et al. 2006: 1114).

located in Europe, Africa, and Asia, and the two regions in North America (cf. Katzenberg & Krouse, 1989). Hydrogen and oxygen isotopes provided better geographic discrimination than did carbon and nitrogen isotopes. Furthermore, the hydrogen isotope values in hair showed a strong correlation with the hydrogen isotopic composition of local water consumed by individuals.

Thus, the determination of hydrogen and oxygen isotope concentrations in stands of hair by mass spectrometry provide a simple, noninvasive method to address short-term changes in residence associated with travel. The reliability of the technique is dependent on the development of hydrogen and oxygen isotopic maps showing variations in local water and food composition for various regions of the world. Both intracontinental and intercontinental variability needs to be established.

The Alpine Iceman: Residence and Mobility

A well-preserved 5200 year-old human mummy, the 'Iceman', was recovered from a glacier along the Italian–Austrian border in 1991 (Bortenschlager & Oeggl, 2000). The excellent preservation of body tissues in this frozen mummy provided a unique opportunity to conduct a range of analytical determinations addressing past lifestyle and behaviours for this Neolithic individual. Mitochondrial DNA extracted from the Iceman closely resembled that of central and northern Europeans, including residents of the alpine region (Handt et al., 1994). Unfortunately, better spatial resolution relating to geographic origin could not be determined on the basis of molecular genetics due to the poor preservation of nuclear DNA. Pollen and moss recovered from the intestines suggested that the Iceman inhabited the vicinity of northern Italy during late adulthood (Dickson, Oeggl, Holden, Handley, O'Connell, & Preston, 1996; Dickson et al, 2000; Oeggl, 1996, 2000).

Müller, Fricke, Halliday, McCulloch and Wartho (2003) used four isotopic tracers (Sr, Pb, O, C) in teeth (enamel and dentine), bone (cortical and trabecular), and intestinal contents to provide more detailed information about the Iceman's residence and mobility from childhood through adulthood. Regional isotopic variability associated with geological substrates and hydrology was employed to demonstrate that the Iceman spent his entire life in an area within 60 km south of the discovery site. Differences in isotope values between enamel and bone suggest that he resided in the northern regions of his lifetime geographic range during adulthood.

The Iceman provides a case study involving a well-preserved human body with a range of tissues available for analysis. Forensic cases involving frozen human bodies from a range of contexts including mountain climbing, hiking, and skiing accidents, plane crashes, and avalanches should benefit from the extensive research associated with the Iceman. The various biochemical and physical anthropological analyses performed on the Iceman offer a model that may contribute to the improvement of procedures employed in victim identification cases involving frozen human remains.

Grasshopper Pueblo, Arizona: Prehistoric Migration

Strontium isotope ratios in the bones and teeth of prehistoric humans from the 14th century archaeological site at Grasshopper Pueblo, Arizona, United States, were compared to differentiate lifelong residents from immigrants (Beard & Johnson, 2000; Ezzo, Johnson, & Price, 1997; Price, Johnson, Ezzo, Ericson, & Burton, 1994). Grasshopper Pueblo was constructed and populated over a period of approximately 150 years. Thus, it was suspected that the local population consisted of a mixture of long-term residents and immigrants who arrived at the site at different periods throughout its occupation. It was hypothesised that strontium isotope values in bone should represent dietary strontium content during the latter stages of life, while tooth enamel values should reflect childhood diet and residence. Bone and tooth isotopic values of relatively sedentary field mice were employed as a measure of the local strontium isotope signature for the site. A number of skeletons had bone-tooth strontium isotope values similar to those of the field mice, indicating long-term residence at the site. In contrast, other individuals had isotopic values that were distinctly different from the local controls (Figure 12.2). These latter individuals were identified as migrants who had spent their childhood in another region.

Population Movements in Ancient Britain

Budd et al. (2004) employ oxygen and strontium isotopes in the tooth enamel of ancient burial populations to examine the movement of individuals away from areas of childhood residence. Tooth samples were taken from 53 individuals excavated from six burial sites in England. Sites date from c. 3500 BC to the 16th century AD. Strontium isotope values at some sites, such as West Heslerton in North Yorkshire,

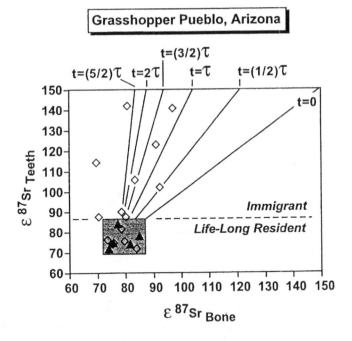

Figure 12.2
Plot of bone strontium isotope values in tooth enamel vs. bone mineral for the 14th century Grasshopper Pueblo, Arizona. Open diamonds represent tooth-bone pairs from the same human skeletons. The gray box indicates isotopic compositions for local Sr where the black triangles show values for field mice (adapted from Beard & Johnson 2000: 1058).

showed local variation that was comparable with that of regional variation. Thus, in these cases it would not be possible to infer migration or long-term local residence on the basis of tooth enamel strontium isotope values. In contrast, oxygen isotope values showed distinct regional variability that could be employed to infer population movements. Rainfall in Great Britain has oxygen isotope values that range from –4.5 ‰ in the extreme west to –8.5 ‰ in inland pockets of the northeast. Thus, tooth enamel oxygen isotope values that fall outside this range suggest a geographic origin somewhere outside of Great Britain.

Isotopic research at the Repton site in Derbyshire focused on skeletal remains associated with a Viking occupation in AD 873–874. On the basis of highly distinctive grave goods and burial mode, three individuals from this period were considered to be of Scandinavian origin. One of these individuals showed a distinctive tooth enamel oxygen isotope ratio of –10.1‰ that equates to a precipitation value of –10.8‰. This value is far too negative for precipitation falling in Great Britain, but is characteristic of rainfall in eastern Sweeden (Figure 12.3). The other two individuals had similar enamel oxygen isotope values that were widely divergent from the first individual (equal to precipitation values of –6.9‰ and –6.7‰). These values fall within the range of precipitation for Great Britain and are similar to those for the western portion of the country. However, they are also similar to values for northern

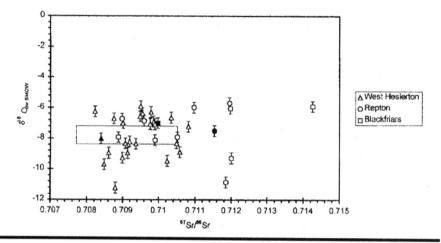

Figure 12.3

Plot showing the relationship between oxygen isotope values of childhood drinking water (recorded in tooth enamel) and tooth enamel strontium isotope values for medieval populations from southern England (adapted from Budd et al. 2004: 133).

France, the Low Countries, and the west coast of Denmark. The use of an additional isotope may improve the ability to distinguish these alternative geographic regions.

Both the United States and British case studies involving archaeological human remains provide models for the employment of oxygen and strontium isotopic analyses of bones and teeth in relation to the determination of childhood versus adulthood residence. As with the other case studies addressed above, applications of isotopic techniques to forensic cases examining residence and mobility will depend on the establishment of controls for environmental isotopic values in local and regional geographic areas of concern.

Repatriation of Indigenous Human Remains

Pate et al. (2002) employed measurements of carbon and nitrogen isotope values in bone collagen as a means to examine the potential geographic origin of unprovenanced Australian Aboriginal skeletons held by the South Australian Museum. The Aboriginal remains had been recovered by members of the general public, collectors and police from late Holocene surface deposits in various regions surrounding the city of Adelaide. However, information regarding the original provenance of the skeletal remains in relation to site of burial and possible area of residence had been lost. Isotopic values for Aboriginal skeletal remains excavated from archaeological sites of known provenance (Figure 12.4) were used to establish isotope signatures for the geographic regions surrounding the ancient burial grounds. These signatures were then employed to assign likely geographic origins for the unprovenanced Aboriginal skeletons (Figure 12.5).

Over 80% of the unprovenanced sample (80/95) could be assigned to a particular geographic zone on the basis of isotopic values, and a further 14% (13/95) were assigned to areas intermediate between two geographic zones. Only two of the 95

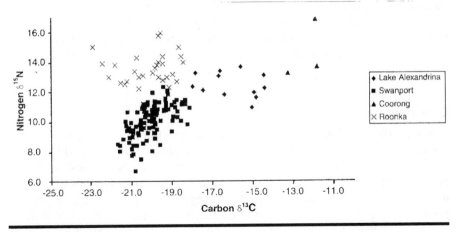

Figure 12.4
Diagram showing stable carbon and nitrogen isotope data points for individual Aboriginal skeletons of know geographic origin from archaeological sites in south-eastern South Australia (adapted from Pate et al. 2002: 3).

individuals possessed anomalous isotopic values in relation to the standard values derived from known geographic localities. In this case, bone collagen stable carbon and nitrogen isotope values allowed the determination of regions of adult residence for a majority of the unprovenanced Aboriginal human remains held by the museum. The use of additional isotope techniques could provide more precise geographic information regarding residence, especially in relation to the two individuals who could not be assigned to a region and those who were assigned to intermediate geographic zones.

In recent times, there have been a significant number of requests for the repatriation of ancient indigenous human remains held in museum and other research

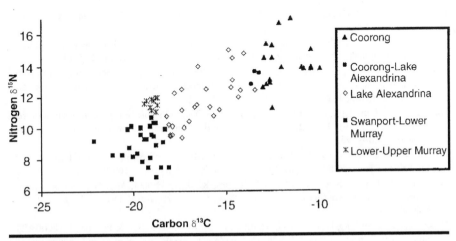

Figure 12.5
Diagram showing stable carbon and nitrogen isotope data points for individual Aboriginal skeletons of unknown provenance that have been assigned to geographic regions in southeastern South Australia (adapted from Pate et al. 2002: 4)

collections. Isotopic analyses of human bones and teeth provide one means to assess or confirm the geographic provenance of skeletal remains held by various institutions. In addition, the identification of long-term sedentary lifeways and associations with particular landscapes via isotopic analyses of skeletal remains has the potential to make significant contributions to indigenous native title cases.

Conclusions

Isotopic analyses of human tissues have the potential to make significant contributions to forensic science in relation to information about short-term and long-term residence in geographic localities with distinct geochemical 'signatures' or 'fingerprints'. The primary limitation to these applications is the requirement for the establishment of isotopic distribution maps for a range of isotopes in a large number of geographic regions worldwide. The employment of these techniques in forensic contexts will depend on detailed data regarding environmental variability in isotopic values across landscapes and further documentation of quantitative relationships between environmental values and the composition of various human tissues. Depending on the nature of each forensic case, some isotopes or human tissues will be more useful than others in providing information about human movements across particular landscapes.

References

Ambrose, S.H. (1991). Effects of diet, climate and physiology on nitrogen isotope abundances in terrestrial foodwebs. *Journal of Archaeological Science, 18*, 293–318.

Ayliffe, L.K., Cerling, T.E., Robinson, T., West, A.G., Sponheimer, M., Passey, B. et al. (2004). Turnover of carbon isotopes in tail hair and breath CO_2 of horses fed an isotopically varied diet. *Oecologia, 139*, 11–22.

Beard, B.L., & Johnson, C.M. (2000). Strontium isotope composition of skeletal material can determine the birth place and geographic mobility of humans and animals. *Journal of Forensic Sciences, 45*, 1049–1061.

Bortenschlager, S., & Oeggl, K., (Eds.). (2000). *The man in the ice. IV. The iceman and his natural environment.* Vienna: Springer.

Budd, P., Millard, A., Chenery, C., Lucy, S., & Roberts, C. (2004). Investigating population movement by stable isotope analysis: A report from Britain. *Antiquity, 78*, 127–142.

Budd, P., Montgomery, J., Evans, J., & Barreiro, B. (2000). Human tooth enamel as a record of the comparative lead exposure of prehistoric and modern people. *The Science of the Total Environment, 263*, 1–10.

Darling, W.G., Bath, A.H., & Talbot, J.C. (2003). The O and H stable isotopic composition of fresh waters in the British Isles. 2. Surface waters and groundwater. *Hydrology and Earth System Sciences, 7*, 183–195.

Darling, W.G., & Talbot, J.C. (2003). The O and H stable isotopic composition of fresh waters in the British Isles. I. Rainfall. *Hydrology and Earth System Sciences, 7*, 163–181.

Dickson, J.H., Bortenschlager, S., Oeggl, K., Porley, R., & McMullen, A. (1996). Mosses and the Tyrolean Iceman's southern provenance. *Proceedings of the Royal Society of London B, 263*, 567–571.

Dickson, J.H., Oeggl, K., Holden, T.G., Handley, L.L., O'Connell, T.C., & Preston, T. (2000). The omnivorous Tyrolean Iceman: Colon contents (meat, cereals, pollen, moss and whipworm) and stable isotope analysis. *Philosophical Transactions of the Royal Society of London B 355*, 1843–1849.

Ehleringer, J. (2003). Forensics and terrorism: Useful stable isotope approaches. In S.A. Phillips, S. Doyle, M. Coleman & L. Philp (Eds.), *Network developing forensic applications of stable isotope ratio mass spectrometry conference 2002* (pp. 10–11). Kent, England: Forensic Explosives Laboratory, Dstl.

Ezzo, J.A., Johnson, C.M., & Price, T.D. (1997). Analytical perspective on prehistoric migration: A case study from east-central Arizona. *Journal of Archaeological Science, 24*, 447–466.

Fraser, I., Meier-Augenstein, W., & Kalin, R.M. (2006). The role of stable isotopes in human identification: A longitudinal study into the variability of isotopic signals in human hair and nails. *Rapid Communications in Mass Spectrometry, 20*, 1109–1116.

Fricke, H.C., Clyde, W.C., & O'Neil. J.R. (1998). Intra-tooth variations in delta O-18 (PO4) of mammalian tooth enamel as a record of seasonal variation in continental climate variables. *Geochimica et Cosmochimica Acta, 62*, 1839–1850.

Gulson, B.L., Jameson, C.W., & Gillings, B.R. (1997). Stable lead isotopes in teeth as indicators of past domicile: A potential new tool in forensic science? *Journal of Forensic Sciences, 42*, 787–791.

Handt, O., Richards, M., Trommsdorff, M., Kliger, C., Simanainen, J., Georgiev, O., et al. (1994). Molecular genetic analyses of the Tyrolean Ice Man. *Science, 264*, 1775–1778.

Harkey, M.R. (1993). Anatomy and physiology of hair. *Forensic Science International, 63*, 9–18.

Hillson, S.W. (1996). *Dental anthropology*. Cambridge: Cambridge University Press.

Hillson, S.W. (2000). Dental pathology. In M.A. Katzenberg & S.R. Saunders (Eds.), *Biological anthropology of the human skeleton* (pp. 249–286). New York: Wiley.

Hobson, K.A. (1999). Tracing origins and migration of wildlife using stable isotopes: A review. *Oecologia 120*, 314–326.

Katzenberg, M.A. (2000). Stable isotope analysis: A tool for studying past diet, demography and life history. In M.A. Katzenberg & S.R. Saunders (Eds.), *Biological anthropology of the human skeleton* (pp. 305–327). New York: Wiley.

Katzenberg, M.A., & Harrison, R.G. (1997). What's in a bone? Recent advances in archaeological bone chemistry. *Journal of Archaeological Research, 5*, 265–293.

Katzenberg, M.A., & Krouse, H.R. (1989). Application of stable isotope variation in human tissues to problems in identification. *Canadian Society of Forensic Science Journal, 22*, 7–19.

Longinelli, A. (1984). Oxygen isotopes in mammal bone phosphate: A new tool for paleohydrological and paleoclimatological research? *Geochimica et Cosmochimica Acta, 48*, 385–390.

Mann, S. (2001). *Biomineralisation: Principles and concepts in bioinorganic materials chemistry*. Oxford: Oxford University Press.

Montgomery, J., Budd, P., & Evans, J. (2000). Reconstructing the lifetime movements of ancient people: A Neolithic case study from southern England. *European Journal of Archaeology, 3*, 370–385.

Müller, W., Fricke, H., Halliday, A.N., McCulloch, M.T., & Wartho, J-A. (2003). Origin and migration of the alpine Iceman. *Science, 302*, 862–865.

Oeggl, K. (1996). Pollen analysis of the Iceman's colon content. *Program and Abstracts of the Ninth International Palynological Congress* (pp. 118–119). Houston, TX.

Oeggl, K. (2000). The diet of the Iceman. In S. Bortenschlager & K. Oeggl (Eds.), *The man in the ice. IV. The iceman and his natural environment* (pp. 89–116). Vienna: Springer.

O'Leary, M.H. (1988). Carbon isotopes in photosynthesis. *BioScience, 38*, 328–336.

Pate, F.D. (1994). Bone chemistry and paleodiet. *Journal of Archaeological Method and Theory, 1*, 161–209.

Pate, F.D. (in press). The use of human skeletal remains in landscape archaeology. In B. David & J. Thomas (Eds.), *Handbook of landscape archaeology*. World Archaeological Congress Research Handbook Series . Tucson, AZ: Left Coast Press and University of Arizona Press.

Pate, F.D., Brodie, R., & Owen, T.D. (2002). Determination of geographic origin of unprovenanced Aboriginal skeletal remains in South Australia employing stable isotope analysis. *Australian Archaeology, 55*, 1–7.

Pate, F.D., & Hutton, J.T. (1988). The use of soil chemistry data to address post-mortem diagenesis in bone mineral. *Journal of Archaeological Science, 15*, 729–739.

Pate, F.D., Hutton, J.T., & Norrish, K. (1989). Ionic exchange between soil solution and bone: toward a predictive model. *Applied Geochemistry, 4,* 303–316.

Price, T.D. (Ed.). (1989). *Chemistry of prehistoric human bone.* Cambridge: Cambridge University Press.

Price, T.D., Johnson, C.M., Ezzo, J.A., Ericson, J., & Burton, J. (1994). Residential mobility in the prehistoric southwest United States: A preliminary study using strontium isotope analysis. *Journal of Archaeological Science, 21,* 315–330.

Priest, N.D., & van de Vyver, F. (Eds.). (1999). *Trace metals and fluoride in bones and teeth.* Boca Raton, FL: CRC Press.

Pye, K. (2004a). Isotope and trace element analysis of human teeth and bone for forensic purposes. In K. Pye & D.J. Croft (Eds.), *Forensic geoscience: Principles, techniques and applications* (pp. 215–236). Bath, England: Geological Society Publishing House.

Pye, K. (2004b, April). *Isotopic and trace element characterization of human teeth and bones for identification and provenance purposes.* Paper presented at the NITECRIME Workshop, Wellington, New Zealand.

Richards, M.P., Fuller, B.T., & Hedges, R. (2001). Sulphur isotopic variation in ancient bone collagen from Europe: Implications for human palaeodiet, residence mobility, and modern pollutant studies. *Earth and Planetary Science Letters, 191,* 185–190.

Richards, M.P., Fuller, B.T., Sponheimer, M., Robinson, T., & Ayliffe, L. (2003). Sulphur isotopes in palaeodietary studies: A review and results from a controlled feeding experiment. *International Journal of Osteoarchaeology, 13,* 37–45.

Rubenstein, D.R., & Hobson, K.A. (2004). From birds to butterflies: Animal movement patterns and stable isotopes. *Trends in Ecology and Evolution, 19,* 256–263.

Schoeninger, M.J., & DeNiro, M.J. (1984). Nitrogen and carbon isotopic composition of bone collagen from marine and terrestrial animals. *Geochimica et Cosmochimica Acta, 48,* 625–639.

Schoeninger, M.J., DeNiro, M.J., & Tauber, H. (1983). Stable nitrogen isotope ratios of bone collagen reflect marine and terrestrial components of prehistoric human diet. *Science, 220,* 1381–1383.

Schoeninger, M.J., & Moore, K.M. (1992). Bone stable isotope studies in archaeology. *Journal of World Prehistory, 6,* 247–296.

Schwarcz, H.P., & Schoeninger, M.J. (1991). Stable isotope analyses in human nutritional ecology. *Yearbook of Physical Anthropology, 34,* 283–321.

Sealy, J.C., Armstrong, R., & Shrire, C. (1995). Beyond life-time averages: Tracing life histories through isotopic analysis of different calcified tissues from archaeological human skeletons. *Antiquity, 69,* 290–300.

Sharp, Z.D., Atudorei, V., Panarello, H.O., Fernandez, J., & Douthitt, C. (2003). Hydrogen isotope systematics of hair: Archaeological and forensic applications. *Journal of Archaeological Science, 30,* 1709–1716.

Smith, H.B. (1991). Standards of human tooth formation and dental age assessment. In M.A. Kelley & C.S. Larsen (Eds.), *Advances in dental anthropology* (pp. 143–168). New York: Wiley-Liss.

West, A.G., Ayliffe, L.K., Cerling, T.E., Robinson, T.F., Karren, B., Dearing, M.D., et al. (2004). Short-term diet changes revealed using stable carbon isotopes in horse tail-hair. *Functional Ecology, 18,* 616–624.

Woelfel, J.B., & Scheid, R.C. (2002). *Dental anatomy: Its relevance to dentistry* (6th ed.). Philadelphia: Lippincott Williams and Wilkins.

3

Determining Time, Manner, and Cause of Death

The Role of the Coroner

David Ranson

Systems for the investigation of deaths are to be found in most societies. They sit alongside and interact with criminal investigations and trials, civil law processes dealing with insurance contracts, the distribution of a deceased person's estate, and administrative procedures regarding registrations of births, deaths and marriages.

Death investigation systems almost always involve a combination of medical, legal and administrative structures. The differences found among the various jurisdictions around the world arise from a variety of interrelated factors including social, religious, historical, political and legal influences, as well as the development of the medical profession and its specialties.

Broadly, the noncoronial continental systems for death investigation, as well as a number of medical examiner systems, are focused on whether criminal behaviour has brought about a death. By contrast, coroners' death investigations today often take a broader and more public health-based approach, with the coroner inquiring as to whether the conduct that gave rise to a death could or should have been different and whether alternative processes might in the future avoid such deaths. Put another way, coronial investigation is about both accuracy in the public record about deaths and prophylaxis: learning from deaths so as to minimise the risks of recurrence, where possible. This means in practice that the purview of the coroner extends into noncriminal matters such as natural disasters, workplace-related accidents and adverse medical treatment events, to identify just a few examples.

The jurisdiction of the coroner is unlike any other aspect of the legal systems in which it is found (see Henneberg, Chapter 20, for an overview of the Australian legal system). The office is an inquisitorial oasis in the broader adversarial legal landscape, with the coroner functioning as both an investigator assembling the evidence he or she needs, and as a decision-maker, working without the constraints of the rules of evidence and formal procedure. However, coroners are not Royal Commissioners. They do not have an open mandate to investigate at large. A question that is regularly posed in inquests is where the lines need to be drawn, beyond which coroners' investigations, findings and recommendations should not trespass? Essentially, the endpoint of a coroner's investigation is the delivery of a finding or verdict that provides key information regarding who the deceased person was, when and where they died, the cause of the death and how they died.

In practice, remarkably few deaths are referred to the coroner. Instead the vast majority of deaths are investigated by the medical practitioner who was responsible for the care of the individual while alive and this investigation is effectively limited to the medical practitioner providing a death certificate, the contents of which are based on their knowledge of the patient's medical history and any recent medical examination they have undergone. The percentage of total deaths investigated by the coroner varies from jurisdiction to jurisdiction and is usually between 10% and 20%. This is the result of coroner's death investigation systems becoming focused on specific types of deaths, being those deaths that the community has decided should be scrutinised by an independent death investigation system. Common belief is that the coroner only investigates suspicious deaths, and many people are surprised to discover that the coroner's role in death investigation is far wider. Again, while the community often perceives the coroner as the legal official who determines 'cause of death', this is only one of the functions of a coroner. Deaths reportable to the coroner will be discussed further below; however, a critical component of the work of the coroner is the declaration of a deceased person's identity. As a result the discovery of body remains or unknown deceased persons results in the matter being specifically referred to the coroner regardless of whether the cause of death is known.

Death and Society

The death of a person is an event that causes distress for family and friends and has the potential in some situations to lead to concern in the wider community. Although death is a completely natural event, it is one that often upsets the living, who, while grieving for a lost loved one, are confronted with their own mortality (Dickenson, Johnson, & Katz, 2000; Fitzgerald, 1994; Kellehear, 2000; Kubler-Ross, 1997a, 1997b; Parkes, 2004; Raphael, 1984). For the wider community, death challenges the notion of a safe and healthy environment, particularly when the death occurs as a result of a mass disaster, trauma or infectious disease. While the deaths of elderly people (Abrams, 1999) who have been unwell for some time are understandable and explicable, deaths of young people are particularly confronting (Hayford, 2003; Rosoff, 1997).

Death today is a more remote phenomenon than in previous ages. In times gone by the dead person would remain in the community, often in the family home, from the time of death until burial. This would allow the family and friends of the deceased to spend time with each other as they mourned. Today there are many in our community who will never have seen a corpse. In particular, children are often shielded from knowledge about death and contact with the dead. This is in an environment where material and human resources to support and enhance safe and therapeutic contact between the living and the dead as part of the grieving process have never been better.

Deaths associated with a mass disaster, or with a person who has been missing for some time, have their own particular problems for the community, including family and friends. The absence of information regarding what has happened to their loved ones causes not only acute distress but ongoing grief that may remain unresolved for years. While a family and the community may understand that there is a high probability that persons missing following a mass disaster are dead, the lack of formal recovery and identification of the bodies allows for lingering doubt and futile hope that can delay and damage bereavement.

Bereavement is a natural process that affects us all at some stage in our lives. While institutions such as coroners' offices are managing a legal process, it is essential from a broader perspective that they do so in a manner that supports the members of the community who are bereaved as a result of a death subject to a medico–legal investigation. Such support needs to be undertaken in a culturally sensitive way (Parkes, Laugnani, & Young, 1997). The failure to carry out death investigations in a way that keeps to a minimum its counter-therapeutic elements can lead to significant psychopathology that, apart from other considerations, in due course may go on to interfere with the death investigation process through loss or distortion of evidence. False visual identification of deceased persons by bereaved family members is well recognised. It is a particular risk in a mass fatality scenario or where the individual has been missing for some time. The emotional need for closure regarding the missing person results in family members being prepared to visually identify human remains where professional death investigators would class the remains as a visually unidentifiable.

While families and the general community have become increasingly isolated from death, the number of officials and government and public agencies that may become administratively involved with a death has increased. The following are just some of these individuals and groups: the Registrar of Births, Deaths and Marriages; the coroner; cemeteries; crematoria; funeral directors; police; doctors, nurses and other health professionals; hospital and health care agencies; solicitors; probate agencies and courts; bereavement counsellors; religious advisers; accountants; government taxation departments; insurance and life assurance companies; banks and investment institutions; welfare agencies; employers; occupational health and safety officials; government statistics agencies; government health departments and related agencies; licensing agencies (vehicle, professional registration, firearm, fishing, and so on); pension providers, and superannuation companies.

For the family, navigating their way through the bureaucracy associated with winding up the affairs of a deceased relative can sometimes be just as traumatic as coping with their own personal grief.

Coroners have a significant part to play in the community's management of death. Coroners have a duty to investigate certain classes and types of death and to arrive at a 'verdict' or 'findings' concerning the death. The results of the coroner's inquiry find their way to a wide range of organisations where they can influence many other administrative, governmental and nongovernmental agencies. The public media are often keenly interested in the results of inquests and there is widespread reporting of some coroners' findings. As a result, the determination of which types of deaths should be reported to a coroner and how they should be investigated is an important consideration for governments and the community.

The monitoring of deaths in the community is a necessary function of modern government. Legislation requiring and authorising administrative and investigative processes surrounding deaths exists in all jurisdictions, although the structure of the administrative processes are far from uniform, when scrutinised from an international perspective. Put simply, the person legally established as the principal investigator of death in most jurisdictions is generally the medical practitioner who was previously responsible for the medical care of the deceased person. It is this medical practitioner who, acting alone, provides the death certificate and, in some cases, in conjunction with other medical colleagues, the cremation certificate.

The statutory administrative processes for the issuing of a certificate and the registration of the death are usually prescribed by legislation; typically some form of Births, Deaths and Marriages Registration Act. The majority of these registration processes do not involve an independent external investigation process. The administrative official responsible, often the Registrar of Births, Deaths and Marriages, simply registers the cause of death provided by the medical practitioner. This is not to say that, if there is some defect or error on a death certificate, the matter will not be followed up by the registrar and the registry staff. However, the staff of the registry does not usually have, and would not be expected to exercise, the specialist medical or legal investigatory skills that could be found in a coroner's or medical examiner's office or among treating medical practitioners.

With respect to especially complex death investigations, other investigative machinery is brought into play. This small category of death investigations involves a range of specialist doctors, scientists, and others, separate and distinct from the medical practitioners who cared for the patient. Such investigative processes might include a coroner's investigation, or a review by a statutory or ministerial consultative council or health care review committee. In addition, individual health care service agencies such as public hospitals or specialist sections within health departments often have their own investigative processes to review certain classes of deaths occurring within their operational area. The Clinical Excellence Commission in New South Wales in Australia manages two such specialist investigative committees operating in the health service field. These are the Special Committee Investigating Deaths Under Anaesthesia (SCIDUA) and the Special Committee Investigating Deaths Associated with Surgery (SCIDAWS). In the United Kingdom the Confidential Enquiry into Maternal and Child Health (CEMACH) is an example of a self-governing review body composed of representatives of several of the medical royal colleges and funded by the National Institute for Health and Clinical Excellence. These investigative bodies and procedures have diverse powers and obligations. Some take place in a public forum (e.g., the coroner's inquest hearing) whereas others, such as ministerial consultative committees, or hospital morbidity and mortality committees, convene in a setting of anonymity or statutorily protected confidentiality.

Death and the Coroners' Jurisdiction

Before instituting an inquest, a coroner must be persuaded that a dead body is within the jurisdiction or that a person died an unnatural death within the jurisdiction. The definition of 'death' is relatively wide and in some jurisdictions a coroner's investigation can be commenced in relation to a suspected death where no body has been found. Establishing that a death has occurred by reference to remains is sometimes not altogether straightforward. The presence of disembodied parts of a human body may not be determinative. A severed arm or leg has been held not to constitute conclusive evidence that the body from which it comes is dead. Thus, it was held in *Ex parte Brady; Re Oram* (1935) 52 WN (NSW) 109 that the finding of a tattooed arm, severed from a human trunk by a sharp knife, was not sufficient to constitute a body for the purpose of giving the coroner jurisdiction to hold an inquest, since an arm may be removed from a body without loss of life (Clark, 1936). However, it is recorded in *Jervis on the Office and Duties of Coroners* (Matthews & Forman, 1993: 57–58) that in an English case:

> … portions of human lung were found in the sea at the point at which an aircraft had crashed, without any trace of the pilot being found. [T]he person from whom the lung material had come was shown to have had the same blood group as the missing pilot. The coroner held that the lung material constituted a body and accordingly he had jurisdiction because of its presence in his area. Similarly, in another case the coroner held that he had jurisdiction to hold an inquest where the lower half only of a girl's body was found in the street, and the rest was not recovered.

> The question, then, is whether the separate parts of the body that have been located are necessarily inconsistent with the person whose potential death is being investigated still being alive. (Farrell, 2000)

Indeed, coroners often investigate the finding of suspected human remains, which permits a coroner to control the scene and order specialist investigators to attend and carry out their work. In the case of skeletal remains it may well be that these are subsequently identified as those of an animal. At this point the jurisdiction of the coroner ceases and there is no basis for further coronial involvement in the incident. Essentially the role of the coroner in investigating the suspected death at this stage is an administrative one consequent on the coroner's legal jurisdiction. The traditional purview of the coroner was restricted to circumstances where there was a body that could be viewed within the jurisdiction, but it has been held on many occasions that it is quite appropriate for inquests to be held despite the absence of a body.[1]

A local coroner may investigate the deaths of persons ordinarily resident within the jurisdiction that have occurred overseas as a result of a man-made or natural disaster. Today, international travel is far more common than when much coronial legislation was formulated. As a result the need to investigate the sudden and unexpected death of a traveller overseas is not an uncommon requirement of the modern coroner's jurisdiction.

In addition to the presence of a body, a coroner must be satisfied that the body is dead. In terms of coronial practice, obtaining proof of death is usually not a problem. Coroners have tended to take the view that a person is dead if an appropriately qualified medical practitioner has stated that he or she is dead. Traditionally, death was regarded by the law in a similar fashion, with Lord Kilbrandon stating in 1968:

> You will never get an answer to what is death in legislation, because that is a technical professional medical matter. It is entrusted to medical men to say when a man is dead and nobody but a doctor can decide that. (Kilbrandon, 1968: 213)

With the development of organ transplantation, the need for vital body organs to be available for transplantation posed practical, legal and ethical dilemmas for the community (Saul, McPhee, & Kerridge, 2006). The traditional medical view that death could be diagnosed when the circulation of blood and breathing had stopped was clearly inadequate. The advent of intensive care techniques whereby breathing and the circulation of blood could be artificially sustained directly contradicted old attitudes regarding the medical determination of death. With the growth of the medical field of organ transplantation, community concerns that organs would be harvested from people who were not in fact dead emerged. It became clear that traditional medico–legal approaches to the definition of death would need to be reviewed and that new definitions of death and new death diagnosis standards were required. By 1981 the Court of Appeal acknowledged that:

> [M]odern techniques have undoubtedly resulted in the
> blurring of many of the conventional and traditional
> concepts of death . There is, it seems, a body of opinion
> in the medical profession that there is only one true test
> of death and that is the irreversible death of the brain
> stem, which controls the basic functions of the body
> such as breathing. When that occurs it is said that the
> body has died, even though by mechanical means the
> lungs are being caused to operate and some circulation
> of blood is taking place.[2]

However, as a matter of practice, coroners' inquests do not take place while a body is hooked up to life support systems, even though a persistent vegetative state may have commenced and a person may be wholly brain dead. This does not mean that the coronial jurisdiction into a reportable death has not been initiated. The death of a person who has been properly declared brain dead and whose death is reportable to a coroner should be reported to a coroner even if his or her somatic organ systems are being medically supported and maintained. Such a death comes under the coroner's jurisdiction and in principle the coroner has legal control of the body. It could be said that the clinical medical staff managing the brain dead patient are acting under an implied authority of the coroner.

The older notion that the person is dead because a medical practitioner has said that he or she is dead has been clearly superseded by legal definitions as to what constitutes death as a matter of law. Ironically these legal definitions effectively still require a medical practitioner to determine the fact of death by identifying the medical evidence that proves, for example, that either irreversible cessation of all function of the brain or irreversible cessation of circulation of blood in the person's body has occurred. It could be said, therefore, that it is still the case that a person is legally dead if medical practitioners say he or she is dead, although the medical practitioners must now have carried out an agreed set of tests and procedures and followed a formal protocol that is accepted by the medical and legal professions.

The question as to which deaths must be investigated by a coroner is answered by reference to the legislation in the given jurisdiction. A distinction exists between the holding of an inquiry or an investigation, and the holding of an inquest. Today, in Australian states and in New Zealand, as well as in other countries, the legislation varies as to when a coroner is obliged to conduct an inquiry and when an inquest must be held. In general, where there is reasonable cause arising out of an inquiry or investigation for the coroner to suspect that a person has died a violent or unnatural[3] death, or died in circumstances that are unclear, or in a prescribed facility such as a prison, police cell, juvenile facility, or psychiatric hospital, an inquest must be held.[4]

In Victoria, a coroner has jurisdiction to investigate a death if it appears to the coroner that the death is or may be a 'reportable death'. Such a death is defined as a death:

(a) that is connected with Victoria in that the body is in Victoria, the death occurred in Victoria, the cause of death occurred within Victoria, or the deceased ordinarily resided within Victoria at the time of death;

(b) and that:

    (i)   appears to have been unexpected, unnatural, or violent, or to have resulted directly or indirectly from accident or injury;

    (ii) occurred during an anaesthetic, or occurred as a result of an anaesthetic and is not due to natural causes;

    (iii) occurred in circumstances prescribed by regulations under the Act;[5]

    (iv) is the death of a person who, immediately before death, was a person under the control, care or custody of the Secretary to the Department of Community Services, the Secretary to the Department of Justice, or a member of the police force; was a patient in an assessment or treatment centre under the *Alcoholics and Drug-dependent Persons Act 1968* (Vic.), or a was a patient (other than a voluntary patient) under the *Mental Health Act 1986* (Vic.);

    (v) is the death of a person whose identity is unknown; or

    (vi) in the case of a death occurring in Victoria, is a death in respect of which a death certificate pursuant to s 37(1) of the *Births, Deaths and Marriages Registration Act 1996* (Vic.) has not been signed, or in the case of a death outside Victoria, is a death the cause of which is not certified by a person who, under the law in force at that place, is authorised to certify that death.[6]

A coroner with jurisdiction to investigate a death must hold an inquest if the body is in Victoria or if it appears to the coroner that the death, or the cause of death, occurred in Victoria or that the deceased ordinarily resided in Victoria at the time of death and:

(a) the coroner suspects homicide, or

(b) the deceased was immediately before death a person held in care, or

(c) the identity of the deceased is not known, or

(d) the death occurred in prescribed circumstances, or

(e) the Attorney-General directs, or

(f) the State Coroner directs.[7]

A coroner who has jurisdiction to investigate a death may hold an inquest if the coroner believes it is 'desirable'.[8] This is not defined. However, the decision as to whether or not to hold an inquest has been held to be largely a matter of common sense.[9]

The endpoint of a coroner's investigation, whether or not an inquest is held, involves the setting out of a finding and or the delivery of a verdict. The transition from a coroner's verdict to that of a discursive, structured set of findings is a particular feature of the modern development of the coronial jurisdiction as it has moved away from its English origins in Australia, New Zealand, and Canada. Traditionally coroners have to determine who the deceased was, when and where they died, the cause of death and how they died. The identification of individuals who have contributed to a death may also form part of a coroners finding. Indeed, in some jurisdictions the coroner has the power to refer individuals to the Director of Public Prosecutions where the coroner believes a criminal action may have been involved. Historically, coroners and/or their juries were able to add riders to their verdicts in which they could comment on broader matters surrounding the death, including steps that might be taken to prevent such deaths occurring in the future. Modern legislation often permits coroners to make specific recommendations in matters affecting public health and safety and the administration of justice. Indeed, the modern focus on making recommendations and suggestions in the interest of public health and safety is a key factor that distinguishes inquests as they are evolving in Australia, New Zealand, and Canada from those in England and Wales. The power to make a recommendation as part of a finding is not unfettered. There should be a clear nexus between the comments or recommendations made and the circumstances surrounding the death into which the coroner enquires. In the context of an inquest into the deaths of prisoners in a jail fire in Victoria, Nathan J. noted the power to make comments and recommendations but held unequivocally that the 'power to comment is incidental and subordinate to the mandatory power to make findings related to how the deaths occurred, their causes and the identity of any contributory persons'.[10] Although the finding as to how a death occurred or what were the circumstances of death associated with recommendations regarding death prevention is perhaps the most important outcome of a death investigation and inquest, the key administrative outcomes of an inquest, including the determination of the particular items of information required to register the death, remain an important part of the coroner's function. This information is essential in order for the public record to be made complete and if necessary 'set straight'.

The History of the Coronial System of Death Investigation

Why has the office of coroner survived for so long? Sheriffs, reeves, hundreds, eyres, outlawry, deodands, amercements and a myriad of other historically significant institutions have either gone or become ceremonial in character, but the coroner and the coroner's inquest are still with us in many countries. Perhaps it is the successes and attributes of the publicly conducted inquest that has allowed the jurisdiction to survive in many of the countries that inherited their legal system from England. History suggests that the power of the coroner and inquests to achieve social change should not be underestimated. When coroners' findings and recommendations are publicised in the media, they can influence policy-makers and provide the catalyst for significant industrial, medical, hygiene and other reforms.

The true origin of coroners remains obscure. There is evidence of the existence of a coroner, at least in name, as early as the reign of King Alfred (871–910; Knapman & Powers, 1985: 1). In Saxon times the council and court took place within a circular enclosure, often a stone circle. The public official whose task it was to maintain order was the 'coronator' or controller of the 'corona' or circle of audience. In AD 925 too King Aethelstan (924–940) granted the office of 'keeper of the pleas of the Crown' (the *custos placitorum coronae*) to John of Beverly (West, 2005).

It seems most accurate, though, to date the true origins of the institution of 'coroner', as we recognise it, to the Council of Eyre in 1194, During the reign of Richard I (1157–1199) the Chief Justiciar, Hubert Walter, Archbishop of Canterbury, had to address the impoverished state of King Richard's Exchequer, in part due to the funding of the crusades and the need to meet the ransom demand of Leopold of Austria. Recognising that sheriffs were often corrupt, inefficient and overburdened by their multifarious administrative responsibilities Hubert Walter created a new local Crown official to provide a check and balance against the excesses of the sheriffs.

An instruction in the Articles of Eyre of 1194 stated that the justices of Eyre were to ensure the election in every county of three knights and a clerk to be 'keepers of the pleas of the Crown' (*custodes placitorum coronae*). Election was limited to those with certain landed qualifications. To this extent the coroner was a political appointee, albeit with a level of independence. The Latin title was in time shortened to 'coronarius' or 'coronator', anglicised to 'crowner' and then to 'coroner'.

The principal obligation of the coroner was to protect the Crown's investment in its subjects. This incorporated a wide range of duties, but one of which was the investigation of unnatural or suspicious death, particularly those deaths associated with the possibility of a fine being levied on the local community. Following the Norman conquest of England, if a person was found dead it would be presumed that he or she was a Norman. This had the consequence that the local community or 'hundred' would be subject to a significant fine, unless the killer was delivered up to justice within five days. However, the presumption of Normanry was rebuttable: if the local community could prove to the coroner that the deceased person was not a Norman through 'presentment of Englishry'(or in Wales 'Welshry') the fine would not apply. In addition, the coroner had a number of other financial regulatory roles; for instance, he bore responsibility for assessing the value of estates and ensuring that land passed back to the Crown on the conclusion of tenancies. The principal duties of the mediaeval coroner, therefore, were essentially those of a tax gatherer, protecting the pecuniary interests of the Crown, in particular those arising from the administration of the criminal law (Holdsworth, 1964: 84–85) by ensuring the safekeeping of fines, deodands, recognisances, and shipwrecks. A coroner's investigation would often result in the imposition of financial hardship when the coroner pursued monies due to the King as the result of a death or an accident. The ability of the King's coroner to fine the local community and to audit the work of the sheriffs, making them account for all fines collected for the King, would have been a source of considerable irritation and often feelings of resentment.

The role of the coroner in the period between the 15th and 18th centuries is less clear. As the judicial system changed, the importance of the medieval coroner as the King's local representative was dissipated. The work of the coroner became onerous and financially perilous, with coroners having to fund inquests out of their own pockets. A number of these administrative problems were remedied in 1487 when the coroner was permitted to charge a mark per inquest into a homicide, plus fourpence from the goods and chattels of the guilty man. In 1751 legislation was passed to increase the remuneration of coroners for conducting inquests. The fees were paid from county taxes on authorisation by justices of the peace sitting at

Quarter Sessions. The role of justices of the peace as holders of the coroners' purse-strings led to considerable friction between the two offices.

The *Births and Deaths Registration Act 1836* attempted to provide for the registration of every death taking place in England and Wales. It formalised an obligation for coroners to inform local registrars of deaths. If an inquest took place, the coroner's obligation was to provide the registrar with any registrable particulars within eight days. Burial of a body was permissible on receipt of a registrar's certificate, or, if there was an inquest, on a coroner's burial order. However, burial prior to the issue of either document was lawful as long as the person undertaking the burial provided a certificate within 7 days of the interment. This death legislation recognised that the jurisdiction of the coroner was far wider than just the investigation of violent deaths. Integral to the need of the community for statistical information about deaths was the availability of an efficient mechanism for investigation of particular classes of death being those deaths that might have significance for public policy.

The birth of the modern coroner is often tracked back to 1860, when a British parliamentary select committee on coroners[11] recommended abandonment of the role of the coroner as a protector of the financial interests of the Crown. The recommendations were implemented in the *Coroners Act 1887,*[12] which conceptualised the role of the coroner as that of providing a means of investigating the circumstances and causes of deaths, where it was in the public interest that there be an investigation. The role of the coroner was not restricted to deaths involving criminal violence, but held to extend also to deaths that were sudden or unnatural or where the causes were unclear, as well as where deaths occurred in prison 'or in such place or under such circumstances as to require an inquest in pursuance of any Act'.

The Operation of the Modern Office of the Coroner

The organisation of a modern coroner's office is dependent on the administrative structures that are in place to manage and support the coroner's court. In some jurisdictions such as England and Wales the court's administrative structure is usually provided by local government and lies outside the administrative services of the civil and criminal courts. In other jurisdictions it is the police who provide most of the support services for the coroner. Regardless of the exact structure of the organisation of a coroner's office, the tasks that are carried out within the office are remarkably similar from jurisdiction to jurisdiction. In some small offices, one person may carry out many roles, while in larger organisations each role may be taken by an individually trained member of the coroner's staff, seconded government administrative staff, external medical staff, or independent contractors.

The operation of the modern office of coroner is perhaps best explained by consideration of the roles undertaken by the key players.

Coroners

While for the most part the roles of coroners within the jurisdiction are similar and include the general responsibility to investigate reported deaths, hold hearings or inquests into the deaths, and to deliver findings or verdicts, the development of centralised state- or territory-based coroners offices has led to some role changes. The effect of recent coronial legislation has been to create the role of State Coroner (or

Chief Coroner or Territory Coroner, as the case may be) with Deputy Coroners to assist him or her. Generally, legislation provides in reasonably short form for the role of the State Coroner. Section 71 of the *Coroners Act 2003* (Qld) is an example:

> The State Coroner's functions are:
>
> (a) to oversee and co-ordinate the coronial system, and
>
> (b) to ensure the coronial system is administered and operated efficiently, and
>
> (c) to ensure deaths reported to coroners that are reportable deaths are investigated to an appropriate extent, and
>
> (d) to ensure an inquest is held if
>
>> (i) the inquest is required to be held under this Act, or
>>
>> (ii) it is desirable for the inquest to be held, and
>
> (e) to be responsible, together with the Deputy State Coroner, for all investigations into deaths in custody, and
>
> (f) to issue directions and guidelines about the investigation of deaths under this Act; and
>
> (g) any other function given to the State Coroner or a coroner under this Act.[13]

Inherent in such legislation is recognition that coroners and especially State Coroners have several separate and discrete responsibilities that include investigative, administrative, and adjudicative (judicial) functions. It is this combination of judicial and nonjudicial roles that renders the State or Chief Coroner a unique judicial officer.

Clerical Staff

A coroner's clerk[14] is the coroner's main legal and administrative assistant. Coroners' clerks have diverse educational and employment backgrounds but they often have experience in government administration, police administration, court administration, or medical administration. In some jurisdictions, where the coroner's clerk is also a legally trained court clerk, they may have some of the coroner's administrative responsibilities delegated to them, though they are not usually given the power to hold an inquest. The clerk is often an appointed administrative officer within the public service and is therefore bound by public service guidelines as to conduct.

The primary role of the coroner's clerk is to manage the day-to-day case work within a coroner's office and to ensure, through liaison with the coroner, that an appropriate level of investigation has been carried out. The coroner's clerk must ensure that the investigation of the death is sufficient to meet the needs of the coroner in dealing with an inquest or arriving at an appropriate chamber finding or verdict. It is usually the coroner's clerk who will receive the information about a reportable death from the police, a medical practitioner or a member of the public. The clerk will evaluate the case and after discussion with the coroner, or by applying general coronial guidelines, organise the administrative matters resulting in the performance of an autopsy by an appropriately qualified pathologist.

As the first point of call for the community, the coroner's clerk will communicate with members of the family of the deceased about the status of an investigation and deal with inquiries made by parties with an interest in the death. In larger jurisdictions the coroner's clerks will be directly available 24 hours a day, and by applying coroner's guidelines, will decide whether a case reported to the coroner should be accepted by the coroner's office for investigation. It is the coroner's clerk who decides on the initial death investigation procedures that are to be carried out, organises the transportation of the body to an appropriate mortuary, and makes the arrangements for the autopsy ordered by the coroner. In small jurisdictions some of these clerical functions may be carried out by a court clerk or administrative officer attached to the magistrate's court or other local court, whose job includes a special responsibility to assist the coroner.

Where an inquest is to be held, the coroner's clerk has a similar duty to that of court clerks in organising the listing of hearings and ensuring that all interested parties are informed of the proceedings. The court clerk manages the administration of the hearing, including the liaison with legal representatives. At the completion of the inquest, the clerk ensures that the finding or verdict is appropriately recorded and that the death is formally registered with the registrar of births, deaths and marriages. The clerk will ensure that records of the inquest are kept and cross-referenced with any other material relating to the death, including any criminal justice processes that may also be under way in other courts.

In some respects, therefore, it appears that the role of a coroner's clerk is similar to that of any other court clerk: they manage courts, and they deal with legal practitioners and members of the public. However, the role of the coroner's court clerk also involves dealing directly with people who are bereaved, and who may be distressed and temporarily unable to represent their own interests adequately. Addressing this situation takes considerable training and experience; these skills are not necessarily gained through working as a clerk in civil or criminal courts. It may well be that there are some court staff who find this side of coroner's work personally distressing; therefore, it is especially important for personnel support services to be in place within the coroner's jurisdiction.

Police

As mentioned above, in some jurisdictions police officers seconded from other duties may perform some of the court clerical duties. Often they act in a combined liaison/operational role between the coroner and operational police units, including general duty police and detectives. This is a very efficient arrangement in many coroners' investigations. However, where a death involves police operations, such as a death in custody, there is the potential for allegations of conflict of interest. In such cases the coronial service needs to have special procedures in place for the appointment of other investigators, legal counsel, or independent supervisors who can oversee the police investigation. Such cases are a minority within coronial practice; for the most part, the advantages of the close working relationship between coroners and the police outweigh the disadvantages.

In larger coroners' offices the role of the police can be more focused on the inquest, with police personnel assisting the coroner in the hearing by calling witnesses and presenting the evidence contained in the brief to the court. In some cases a police officer attached to the coroner's office will directly act as the leading police investigator. This situation arises when the death is one that demands a level of knowledge in a particular field that the general duty police do not have. Police on general duties have a limited involvement in death investigations, whereas coroners' police assistants deal with the issues on a daily basis. Indeed, coroners' police assistants help in the investigation of many more deaths than a specialist police homicide investigation unit. The investigation of deaths occurring in the setting of mass disasters, medical care as well as transport-related deaths involving aircraft, marine craft and trains is often supervised and managed by coroners' police assistants.

Bereavement Services

In recent years there has been increasing recognition of the need for bereavement services to be available from within the coroner's jurisdiction. As noted above, the clients of a coroner's court who have closest involvement with the staff most commonly are the deceased person's family, who are experiencing a particularly stressful period in their lives. It is ironic that it is at this time that they have to make decisions about such matters as whether to object to an autopsy or donate tissues for transplantation, as well as deal with the logistical issues of arranging a funeral and assisting other members of their family and the deceased's friends. This places a great burden on any family. It may take some time and considerable patience to meet their needs adequately. Any contact with a family in this situation has a direct therapeutic context. Mistakes, insensitivities and poor assumptions made by staff may have serious ramifications for the health of members of the family and for the overall scope and quality of the investigation. It is clearly not possible for court clerks without formal training in bereavement counselling and support to manage their contact with relatives of the deceased on a regular basis. The work involved is time-consuming and would seriously impede the efficiency of the coroner's investigation process.

The introduction of a counselling service based at a coroner's court has the capacity to greatly enhance the services for clients and also to improve the efficiency of the coroner's process. The counselling services are not usually designed to provide long-term bereavement care. They are usually fashioned around acute intervention services to provide initial support, counselling and information in an environment that maximises the autonomy of the family. Inevitably many families will require far longer periods of support and counselling. To enable this, the counselling services at coroners' courts usually have close working relationships with other community support services and health services to which the families can be referred.

Medical Services

The most common external medical investigation service used by a coroner is the autopsy service provided by forensic pathologists. Death investigation systems, such as those operated by a coroner, usually have the power to order that an autopsy be carried out to assist in the determination of the manner, circumstances and cause of death. It is significant that the autopsy and medical aspects of the death scene investigation are carried out very early on in the coroner's investigation process. In many jurisdictions the medical death scene investigation and autopsy are completed within 1 or 2 days of the death. It is the results of these initial medical investigations that often shape the nature of subsequent investigations on behalf of the coroner. As a consequence, the professional relationship between pathologists and coroners' staff is usually close.

Although pathologists are the group of medical practitioners most closely involved in the work of coroners, increasingly a range of other medical specialists are being used by coroners in death investigation. Deaths occurring in the setting of medical treatment may require investigations to be carried out by nonpathology medical specialists. Experts in anaesthetics, intensive care, and accident and emergency services, as well as specialist physicians and surgeons, may have an important role to play in the evaluation of such deaths. Today, the advent of the use of alternative death investigation processes, in addition to or as a replacement for the autopsy, demonstrates the need for a wider range of medical specialists to be engaged by a coroner. Medical investigations incorporating therapeutic management review or postmortem radiology will clearly be enhanced by the involvement of the appropriate clinical specialist or radiologist, rather than expecting a forensic pathologist to try to cover these medical specialist areas in addition to the pathology work.

Where human identification is a specific focus of the coroner's death investigation it is usual for other medical science specialists to become involved. Forensic anthropologists and forensic dentists together with molecular biologists have a major role to play in assisting in the scientific investigation of human identification.

Coordination of Initial Investigations

The quality of the initial investigation that takes place within the first 48 hours after a death sets the scene for all subsequent investigations and is crucial in ensuring that a thorough overall investigation takes place. Errors and omissions in the initial processes of investigation often cannot be corrected later. The coordination of the initial investigation process is therefore a task that is essential.

In the case of most routine death investigations carried out by the coroner, the coordination of the investigation revolves around ensuring that the regular systems and protocols that are in place are followed and documented. In many smaller coroners' offices, much of this coordination is carried out by police officers from the district in which the person died. Court clerical officers and the coroner's legal or police assistants may take over the coordination of the death investigation in larger coroners' offices. Where the death investigation involves a specialist technical area or is particularly complicated, other individuals, including medical specialists such as forensic pathologists or specialist police groups, may assist in the coordination of the investigation.

The involvement of the coroner in this coordination process is variable. In some jurisdictions the coroner will leave the initial coordination of the investigation to police and clerical staff. In other jurisdictions the coroner may insist on being informed of each and every death regardless of the time of day. In jurisdictions with centralised coroner services the coroner may set out protocols that determine which cases he or she should be directly informed about, so that he or she can attend the scene and coordinate the initial death investigation. Scenarios where the coroner may wish to step in and direct the investigation include deaths in custody or during a police response, incidents involving mass loss of life, work-related fatalities, and aviation or marine fatalities.

Exhumations

There are a number of situations that require specialist investigation by the coroner's staff. In the case of a death reported to a coroner after the body has been disposed of by burial, it may be necessary for the coroner to order an exhumation of the body. Such a situation has the potential to be extremely distressing for family members, who may have been unaware that there was any issue in relation to the medical and legal procedures that followed the death. Exhumations may be required particularly where allegations are made, some time after a death, that it was due to an unnatural process such as negligent injury, incompetent medical treatment, or most particularly, homicide. Homicide allegations are sometimes undertaken many years after a death because new information has come to light as a result of other criminal investigations.

When a death that occurred some time before is reported and the body of the person is known to be buried in a cemetery, there needs to be an initial investigation into the alleged circumstances of the death, including the current location of the body with reference to cemetery plot numbers and other funeral records. Although not necessarily a legal requirement, the coroner will usually contact the family of the deceased and consult them regarding the proposed procedures for exhumation and subsequent reinterment of the remains.

The coroner will usually seek the advice of a forensic pathologist regarding the feasibility of conducting the exhumation and the relative likelihood that a post-mortem examination of the exhumed remains will reveal information addressing the issues raised by the allegations that made the death reportable. In order to provide the coroner with this information about the potential for the autopsy to materially assist in the death investigation, the pathologist needs detailed information about the time interval since death and the funeral procedures and processes, including the nature of any embalming procedures performed and the type of encoffining of the body. Information about the depth of burial, the soil composition and the drainage of the cemetery may also be required in order to assess whether the examination of the exhumed remains is likely to lead to new evidence.

Occasionally the nature of the allegation will be such that an examination of the body years later will not reveal information that will resolve the issues. However, as with any autopsy procedure it is difficult to be sure that an autopsy will not assist in the death investigation without actually examining the body. Clearly, if soft tissue injuries or disease processes affecting soft parenchymal organs form the basis of the request for exhumation and there is a high probability that the body is now skeletonised, the coroner may conclude that exhumation is not warranted. On the other hand, suppose it is alleged that a person was strangled rather than dying of natural causes. Even if the body is now skeletonised, examination of the bony remains may be able to demonstrate that the structures forming the laryngeal skeleton in the voicebox at the top of the airway, such as the hyoid bone or the horns of an ossified thyroid cartilage, are damaged in such a way as to suggest that neck compression may have been applied.

If the coroner concludes that an autopsy may provide useful information, he or she will inform the cemetery authorities (and, depending on the circumstances, the family of the deceased) that an exhumation is to be performed. Usually a funeral director and the staff of the cemetery will work with coroner's investigators, including the police and the forensic pathologist and anthropologist, to determine an appropriate time for the exhumation. Frequently exhumations are performed early in the morning, prior to the arrival of members of public at a cemetery, in order to minimise the impact on the local community. The exhumation of a body needs to be carried out with considerable care so as not to disturb other nearby graves. Occasionally, where a plot contains more than one body or where plot markings are unclear, an exhumation may result in the uncovering of other bodies, in which case the issue of identity needs to be very carefully addressed. In such situations it may be necessary to bring more than one body to the mortuary for detailed identification processes as well as pathological examination.

The exhumation of a body from a grave can easily result in damage to the remains if special precautions are not taken. Although mechanical diggers may be used to expose the upper levels of a grave, their use close to the coffin may result in damage to it and/or to the body inside. For this reason a degree of manual digging is usually required towards the end of the mechanical exhumation process. Some coffins are prone to disintegration, particularly those made of veneered chipboard, and in such cases of removal additional support of the coffin may be required during the lifting process, through the use of a stretcher-type device. Where the coffin has completely collapsed or disintegrated, the fabric or plastic lining of the coffin containing the body may be removed directly from the grave, as it can act as a body bag. If this too has been destroyed, a more archaeological approach to the removal of individual portions of human remains from the grave may need to be considered.

The process of exhumation needs to be clearly documented with photographs that include images of the plot site prior to exhumation, any identification markers present on the plot, the exposure of the coffin, the state of the coffin, and any identification markers on the coffin itself. During the removal of the coffin and the body from the grave it may be necessary to take samples or specimens from the region of the grave site. These may include samples of soil from above and below the coffin or from the substance of the coffin itself. Drugs and toxins that were present in the body at the time of death may be identified in the soil adjacent to the coffin rather than in the bodily remains. In some exhumations there will be a visible body fluid drainage area present in the soil adjacent to the coffin. Samples from this region may prove valuable for toxicological analysis. Control samples of soil from some distance away from the grave site must also be taken to ensure that the soil in the cemetery is not generally contaminated with some suspicious chemical substance.

With the completion of the medical examination of exhumed remains and the collection of samples for forensic scientific testing, the body is usually returned to the cemetery within a few days and buried in the same grave plot. It may be necessary for the coroner to assist the family by arranging a further funeral service at the time of reinterment.

The Coroner and Human Identification

In many ways the manner in which a society deals with its dead reflects its attitude to the rights of the individual. The coroner's jurisdiction has as one of its major functions the identification of deceased persons. Even if a death has occurred from natural causes, the fact that the identity of a body is unknown is sufficient grounds for requiring a coroner's investigation. As Victoria's first State Coroner, Hal Hallenstein, observed: '[I]t is a hallmark of our civilisation that we regard it as an affront, an indignity, an abrogation of our responsibilities, that a person could live among us, die and be buried without a name' (Cordner, 1998: vii).

Ultimately it is the coroner who must determine identity on a legal basis. To do so, he or she relies on statements of identification provided by witnesses and on the results of specialist medical and scientific investigations.

The weight that the coroner places on the different types of information uncovered in relation to identity is a critical factor in accurate human identification. The circumstances of a death may suggest the probable identity of the deceased, but this information is rarely sufficient on its own for a coroner to make a formal legal determination of identity. Occasionally, however, this may be the only information available; for example, when a person is washed overboard in an accident at sea and the body is never recovered. All forms of identification have a risk of error, and the size of that risk and the need for certainty are matters that a coroner should take into account when deciding to rely on particular forms of identification in respect of a death under investigation.

The identification of the dead is essential for the lives of others to return to normal. From an emotional standpoint, the uncertainty and anguish suffered by families who have a missing loved one who they fear may be dead can be tremendous. From a practical standpoint, if the identification of the deceased is problematic or proves to be impossible, the consequence can be that many others suffer real hardship. For example, the family may not be able to wind up the financial affairs of the deceased, and disbursement of property according to the deceased's wishes may be significantly delayed.

In the majority of deaths reported to a coroner the identity of the deceased is usually suspected by virtue of the surrounding circumstances. Information on suspected identity allows that person's next of kin or friends to be contacted in order for one of them to view the body and provide a formal and legal statement of identification. Confirmation of identity by the coroner in these cases is simply a matter of ensuring that the legal formalities of visual identification have been carried out and adopting the identity stated, rather than organising specialist medical or scientific procedures.

Interestingly, family and friends called to identify a deceased person are not usually asked to grade the certainty of their identification are on a '10-point scale' or a 'percentage basis'; therefore coroners have no real idea of the level of certainty of the visual identification that they rely on. Similarly there is no detailed information on the validity of the visual identification of the dead[15] performed generally for coroners. By contrast, many of the medical and scientific methods for human identification (e.g., dental examination, fingerprint comparison and molecular biological comparison of DNA) have been subject to specific scientific validation and have been accepted by the legal system as being able to provide an acceptable level of certainty (Reeder, 1999).

Fortunately there are several of these validated independent scientific identification methods, including: fingerprint identification, serological identification, molecular biology (DNA identification), dental identification, cranio-facial reconstruction, medical identification, and radiological identification.

Identification Techniques

Where visual identification is problematic or not possible, autopsy procedures will need to be varied in order to accommodate the additional scientific and medical procedures that may have to be undertaken in order to establish identity. One or more of the procedures listed above will be chosen on the basis of the state of the body, the presumed manner of the person's death, and whether there are criminal issues surrounding the death that require a higher level of proof of identity.

Recording the establishment of identity is also an important issue for the coroner. Proof of identity may have civil and criminal legal implications requiring that it be admitted in evidence in legal proceedings. The results of scientific or medical tests need to be clearly documented and retained in a format that permits them to be adduced in evidence. While it is easy to record and document the results of serological or molecular biology tests in a text-based report, fingerprints, dental examinations, autopsy examinations and radiographs may require forms of visual recording as documentation. On rare occasions, in order to record the establishment of identity or to prove the characteristics of a particular injury, the pathologist may wish to retain all or some of the remains until the case is brought to court. This may conflict with the wishes of the family to bury or cremate the remains of their loved one as soon as possible.

Visual Identification

The identification of someone who was a friend or a relative is almost invariably a very stressful ordeal for the witness. Even in the best of circumstances, where the body is fresh, intact, clean and unmutilated and where it is displayed in a clean, bright, nonthreatening environment such as a modern mortuary, with the support of an enlightened and sensitive staff, the family of the deceased may still find it difficult to identify the body. Inevitably mistakes will be made, occasionally frauds will be perpetrated, and in some cases bodies will be unrecognised and remain visually unidentifiable. There are a variety of reasons why this may be so. The most obvious (and overstated) is 'denial' on the part of the relatives, who just cannot accept that it is a member of their family who has died. However, a dead body may bear much less similarity to the person in life than might be anticipated. In life there is a rich but subtle exchange of signals by means of expressions or gestures between people that mutually reinforce recognition.

Some bodies are completely unrecognisable by any conventional visual criteria. Decomposition processes usually involve a degree of bloating of the body, blackening of the skin and loss of tissues such as eyes, skin, hair, and nails (see Tibbett, Chapter 3, and Forbes, Chapter 15). These changes interfere markedly with the likelihood of successful visual identification. The victim of a fatal fire often has no clothing or documents remaining on the body and items such as jewellery may have completely melted so as to be unrecognisable. Much of the skin, hair, and facial features may be absent with partial incineration and the body may appear almost skeletonised, with just a few internal organs remaining. In fire deaths the extremities can be largely burnt away. It is useless to expect the family to attempt to identify a body that has been so badly damaged. Unfortunately, families do sometimes view and identify bodies that are grossly decomposed, badly burnt or grossly disrupted. Visual identification given in such circumstances must be treated with a high degree of suspicion.

Where complete viewing of the body is not possible, or the body is so distorted that general visual identification is impossible, specific regions of the body may be shown to family or friends to enable them to confirm the suspected identify. Characteristic tattoos, scars, naevi (moles or spots) and congenital abnormalities may be recognised by a family member shown only a small part of the body surface. This approach of using limited viewing of the body must be treated with extreme caution, as it is possible for individuals to have identical tattoos or similar scars; with body distortion and stretching of the skin, the similarities can lead to confusion and possible misidentification.

Fingerprinting

The taking of fingerprints from a deceased person is well established as a technique for confirming identity. It is one of the mainstays of the identification procedures in mass disasters, in part because a record of fingerprints can be stored as a paper record, as an electronic image, and as a coded database entry. In addition, where a fingerprint record is not available for a deceased person, latent prints can be lifted from objects that are likely to have been handled by that person. This ability to use latent fingerprints from a person's normal environment greatly enhances the utility of fingerprints for the identification of deceased persons. Most people whose deaths are investigated by a coroner do not have a criminal record and therefore are unlikely to have their fingerprints recorded on a police database. However, where the identity of the deceased person is suspected and fingerprints can be collected from the body, a comparison can be made between those fingerprints and latent prints lifted from various objects and surfaces at the person's home and place of work.

Molecular Biology

The advent of DNA profiling and related technologies has revolutionised human identification in the last few decades. The cells of the human body contain two main types of DNA: nuclear DNA and mitochondrial DNA. While nuclear DNA is inherited from both parents, mitochondrial DNA in both sexes is derived from the maternal cytoplasm only. This limits its specificity for identification purposes, as individuals from the same maternal line cannot be distinguished. Mitochondrial DNA is present in greater amounts within human cells, enabling extraction of DNA for analysis from much smaller samples, a feature that has more relevance for crime scene collection of biological material than for autopsy sampling. While probing DNA for sequences of base pairs has important implications for identification in criminal investigations and civil matters such as determination of paternity, where a one-to-one match is being sought, such techniques are not necessarily as useful where the requirement is for mass human identification in situations where the identification of those missing is unknown. However, the role of DNA analysis for human identification by the coroner is still relevant. Where DNA analysis is required in coroners' investigations, it is usually applied in quite different circumstances from criminal case work.

For the most part, identification of deceased persons subject to a coroner's investigation does not require the use of DNA technology. Indeed, molecular biological techniques are usually employed only where other methods of identification have failed. The only exception is in the case of a mass disaster, where the use of multiple individual means of identification for each and every body as well as body fragments may be required.

Odontology

The application of forensic odontology to human identification involves two main methods of comparison. The first relates to the anatomical structures of the teeth, the jaws and associated facial regions. Genetic and developmental factors influence the structure and relationship of teeth to various oral structures; as a result there is enormous variation among individuals in relation to their dental anatomy. The second method of comparison relates to the identification and documentation of dental treatment, including the effects of restorative dentistry and other forms of dental treatment. With the improvement in oral hygiene in recent years, many young people show no evidence of having received restorative dentistry. However, the advent of modern radiographic techniques to assess dental structures in the living for the purpose of orthodontics has provided a means of comparison with postmortem forensic odontological radiological examination.

Radiological techniques can reveal not only the presence of dental disease and anatomical configuration of the visible portion of teeth, but also the shape of roots and root sockets, together with the fine structure of bone trabeculae around teeth. These bone features can vary over time and with periodontal disease, but over short time intervals they can be as individual as fingerprints. The use of modern materials for dental fillings and the capacity to match a filling's colour with that of the surrounding tooth may result in the restoration being invisible on simple visual inspection of the mouth, and radiological and surface probing may be required in order to detect it.

In order for a forensic dentist to assist in identifying a deceased person, a detailed orofacial examination of the body is necessary, including the taking of radiographs and in some cases dental impressions of the upper and lower jaws. This can usually be performed as part of the autopsy in collaboration with the forensic pathologist. Occasionally, however, it may be necessary for there to be a resection of the upper and lower jaws and removal of them from the body for specialist dental examination. There is normally no technical difficulty in returning the jaws to the body at the completion of the dental examination to permit appropriate facial reconstruction. Where this is not possible, reconstruction of the lower and middle portions of the facial skeleton is undertaken with the use of prosthetic devices and materials. Access to reference photographs of the person in life may be required in order for this reconstructive work to be carried out accurately.

For forensic dentistry to be able to assist with identification, antemortem dental records of the person suspected to be the deceased need to be available for comparison purposes. This may mean that the coroner will have to issue a warrant to seize the dental records of several dentists. It may well be that some of these records turn out to belong to patients who are not the deceased and are still alive. The privacy that would normally attach to such medical records in a clinical setting should be uppermost in the minds of the dental investigators and the coroner's staff. Where there is no indication as to who the deceased might be, comparison matching cannot be carried out. In this situation, where the remains of the deceased display evidence of particularly characteristic dental work, a postmortem dental chart with radiographs and photographs can be prepared. With the approval of the coroner these may be circulated locally, nationally or internationally within the dental profession. Some aspects of dental reconstructive treatment may be highly individualistic and certain national characteristics of dental work such as crowns and bridgework may be recognisable by dentists from a particular area of practice. Often a dentist will be able to recognise the appearance of a dental reconstruction as being her or his own work; this can significantly narrow the search for the identity of the deceased.

In order for an accurate comparison to be made between the postmortem examination and an antemortem dental record, the recording or documentation processes used need to be standardised and/or translatable between the different notation systems. It is partly for this reason that radiographic films and oral impressions are so useful for comparison purposes, as they are free of the idiosyncrasies of the different forms of dental notation. Dental record systems around the world use different dental charts or odontograms. These charts record the position of each of the teeth that are present in the mouth of a patient. The charts record disease such as caries and note its degree as well as its position in the tooth. The location, shape and nature of restoration of all fillings are also noted, together with the presence of any prosthetic devices such as bridges, crowns, and dentures. Where odontograms are used, the drawing of the characteristics of the tooth provides very useful comparison data. However, numerical data regarding the charting of teeth may be difficult to interpret because of the various numbering systems used throughout the world. For this reason it is essential to have antemortem dental charts evaluated and translated into the local form of dental numbering by a specialist dental practitioner prior to being used for comparison purposes in human identification.

In any jurisdiction there is likely to be a register of missing persons who have been reported to police. While most such persons are found safe and well within 6 months of the report, a small percentage of those reported remain missing despite initial police investigations. The dental records of people who have been missing for some time should be compared with those of human bodies that have been reported to the coroner as unknown deceased persons. In order for this comparison to be performed efficiently it may be necessary to develop a database of the antemortem records of missing persons, which includes their recent dental records, as well as other useful comparison data such as medical records and perhaps in some cases biological material from parents or siblings. From a coroner's perspective, people who have been missing for a long time may constitute suspected deaths; this brings them within the coroner's jurisdiction and empowers the coroner to use coercive powers to seek the appropriate antemortem records

Forensic odontologists are considered by most coroners to be among the most useful medical specialists for ascertaining the identity of deceased persons. Forensic odontological examination is a highly successful investigation method, with a very low risk of error in human identification. Not only can it be used for positive identifications, but it can also easily exclude people who have been suggested to be the deceased person by investigators. Despite the availability today of modern molecular biology techniques to identify people, forensic odontology is an accurate and rapid identification method that can be integrated effectively into the autopsy process.

Pathology

The autopsy provides a wide range of information that can be useful for the purpose of medical identification. However, information relating to disease and anatomical characteristics or anomalies may not have a high degree of specificity with respect to identification. This is because many people in the community may show one or more of these features. For example, many people in the community will have had surgery to remove their appendix or gall bladder, so that the absence of these structures at autopsy is usually of low identification value. However, if other identification systems have reduced the possible identities of a body to a few individuals, one of whom has had significant surgery, then autopsy evidence of the surgical procedure may have a high discrimination value. Despite this, particular patterns of clusters of disease and anatomical characteristics may be highly individual.

Medical information about the presence of disease, together with the description of the general characteristics of a body, can form important information about identity. As part of the routine process of autopsy, the external characteristics of a body are described. These include hair and eye colour, the presence of tattoos, scars relating to surgery or previous injury, and 'birthmarks' or skin lesions. External characteristics on the body can provide useful information that can assist with at least a general classification or group into which the deceased can be placed. In the case of mass disasters where there are many dead, information about previous surgery such as an appendectomy can be highly useful when added to other data. In individual case identification, information about scars from prior surgery may narrow the field of possible missing persons who could be the deceased. The presence of tattoos may also be of use. In the past, tattoos were found commonly in particular groups within society such as military personnel, some drug users, bikers or members of bikie groups, and merchant seamen. Today, however, tattoos are common among young people. This has the result of increasing the pool of persons for whom tattoos may be a useful identifying feature. Even so, many tattoos are very similar, such as butterflies, roses, dragons, snakes, Chinese inscriptions, and particular geometric patterns on particular parts of the body such as the back of the shoulders, the skin over the sacrum, or the buttocks. This reduces their discriminatory utility.

Internal examination of the body can reveal evidence not only of current disease but of previous disease processes. This information can prove useful when compared with antemortem records that include notes of prior medical history. The effects and alterations of anatomy caused by previous surgery can also be identified at autopsy and be important for identification.

In some cases prosthetic devices may be left in the body; for example, in orthopaedic surgery where replacement joint surfaces or internal fixator devices are used. Some of these devices will have serial numbers or batch numbers and it may be possible for the manufacturer's records to be used to identify where the prosthetic device was dispatched. Review and assessment of such devices by an orthopaedic surgeon may be helpful. In the case of evidence of other types of surgery it may be appropriate to obtain the advice of a surgeon from that field of practice, as styles of surgery and techniques employed may differ over time and between different schools of surgical practice. The information that the deceased perhaps underwent a surgical procedure more than 20 years ago in Europe may be a useful discriminator in the process of human identification.

Anthropology

Although a pathologist records details of anatomy during the course of autopsy, the involvement of a specialist anatomist or anatomical anthropologist may provide far more information regarding the possible identity of an individual. Such specialists are regularly involved in examination of skeletal remains. However, they can provide very useful assistance in the case of exhumations and in examination of the decomposed and disrupted remains. In the case of persons who have been involved in explosions, there may be considerable fragmentation of the body, resulting in the need to identify grossly distorted body parts among commingled remains.

Anthropologists are key players in the identification of the deceased. They can help to provide information on race, gender, height, and age from skeletal remains, including the skull (see Littleton, Chapter 11). Examination of the skeleton may also provide information about lifestyle and previous injury (see Buckley & Whittle, Chapter 9).

When unidentified human skeletal remains are recovered from remote locations and/or rural areas, it is frequently the case that animal bones or teeth are included with the human remains. These nonhuman elements have to be identified so that they can be excluded from the investigation process (see Oxenham & Barwick, Chapter 6). Anatomical anthropologists are usually skilled in comparative skeletal anatomy and are ideally suited to carry out this task. In routine investigations conducted for coroners, it is not uncommon for animal remains to be referred to the coroner on the basis that they may represent human remains. In straightforward cases a forensic pathologist is able to distinguish between human and nonhuman bones. However, with some skeletal structures from some animal species this is more difficult and a specialist anatomist may be required to carry out the task.

Many of the tasks carried out by anatomists in human identification rely on reference tables of measurements of bones within the human skeleton. Great care must be taken in ensuring that the reference values used are appropriate to the community from which the deceased is likely to have come. Racial and regional variations in skeletal features related to human size and ageing can pose particular problems. Many of the reference tables available in the literature have come from established anatomical collections of skeletal material that are far from recent. The features that these old collections show may not be representative of the modern community from different cultural and racial groups. It follows that these data sets need to be expanded and continuously updated in order to be of use worldwide in human identification.

Radiology

The use of radiology in human identification has been mentioned above as it is a useful adjunct to the work of many medical and scientific professionals engaged in the task of human identification. Radiographs taken of people in life may be compared with postmortem radiographs taken at the time of autopsy. Even if there has been subsequent severe bone damage at the time of death, reconstruction of bone fragments and subsequent radiology may still provide enough information to enable a direct comparison to be made. Where the skeleton is widely fragmented, it may be possible to match up the characteristic micro-architecture of a bone fragment with a small region of a radiograph taken in life.

A number of areas of the human skeleton show very individual characteristics. The skull is a good example. The pattern of the air sinuses, particularly the frontal sinuses of the skull, may provide enough information to confirm identity. As discussed above, this is usually carried out through the use of two-dimensional x-rays of a skull specimen that is positioned to match the orientation of the original ante-mortem x-ray. The use of three-dimensional computerised tomography scans of the skull can assist with this: a virtual two-dimensional slice can be made of the three-dimensional data set in any plane or position, so as to allow computerised manipulation of the image to match the orientation of the two-dimensional radiograph taken in life.

One of the advantages of radiology in assessing the human skeleton is that it can provide a record of the skeletal structures of the remains, which can be retained even following disposal of the body. Because the specimen is close to the x-ray film when postmortem radiographs are taken, measurements of the bone can be taken from the radiograph directly. Such measurements can be used by anthropologists and radiologists in estimating the deceased's height or measuring key features that can be used to suggest the gender or racial origin of the individual. Computed tomography (CT) scanning of the body provides an ideal three-dimensional record of the remains that allows for detailed measurements of the morphology of individual skeletal structures.

In addition to bone shape and size, radiographs of skeletal structures can also identify the existence of current or previous disease. This is not limited to disease of the bone but can include information about other systemic disease markers that can be seen in bone changes. People who have been subject to debilitating diseases in early life may show lines of maturation arrest: irregularities of bone formation that occurred during childhood bone development.

In skeletal remains of young persons, radiological assessment can assist in determining the probable age of persons at the time of their death from a variety of factors, including the appearance and closure pattern of epiphyses. In older people, radiological assessment of age-related changes and wear patterns may again assist in determining the person's probable age at the time of death, although this is likely to be less precise than the age estimation that can be calculated for younger individuals.

Disaster Victim Identification

Incidents involving mass loss of life, although rare, present real challenges to the community. Events such as natural disasters, acts of terrorism, transportation accidents, building accidents, and warfare often result in multiple deaths. These deaths pose particular problems for coroners. Coroners are responsible for the identification of deceased persons whose deaths are reported to them. In addition, they are responsible for determining the cause of death and in some jurisdictions are required to delve more deeply into the circumstances surrounding the death and to identify the issues involved. With the increase in the movement of people around the world, mass disasters often involve individuals from many different countries and jurisdictions. This can pose problems for international law and raise communication issues in relation to discovering personal information about those who may have died. In cases of mass death in warfare or as a result of acts of terrorism, state security and intelligence issues may also complicate the picture. Both natural and human-made disasters involve similar death investigation processes in respect of the identification of victims; however, the scope of the surrounding investigation may be very different.

Among the major death investigation and death scene management processes involved in a mass casualty scenario, the identification of deceased persons is often the foremost consideration for the community. Coroners have overall responsibility for this function, in addition to their broad death investigation role. While in some mass casualty events visual identification of the victims will be possible, where fire or explosion is involved the bodies may not be identifiable without recourse to special scientific and medical techniques. It is essential that the process put in place to investigate the cause of a major disaster causing multiple loss of life does not interfere with the process of identification of the victims. Identification and incident investigation should go hand in hand; indeed each relies on the other for information. For example, in the case of a bomb blast, identification of the most fragmented body can assist in determining the location of the bomb and perhaps the identity of the 'bomber'. For a coroner who has ultimate legal responsibility for both incident investigation and human identification, the coordination of all phases of a mass disaster investigation is an important responsibility. In most cases a coroner delegates individual tasks to various specialists, and the coordination of the identification of victims is often handled for the coroner by a senior police officer (see Robertson, Chapter 17). This officer is often referred to as the DVI ('Disaster Victim Identification') commander. The DVI commander's functions are to be in operational command of all phases of the DVI process:

- to liaise with the coroner, other police investigators, and emergency service providers
- to maintain a list of all personnel involved in the DVI process for occupational health and safety management
- to ensure that all phases of the process are adequately resourced
- to report to the coroner on the identity of all victims.

When the circumstantial, scientific, medical, and dental information that establishes the identity of a victim has been collected to the police officer's satisfaction, this information is presented to the coroner during the process of reconciliation. The identity of the individual is not confirmed until the coroner is satisfied with the information provided.

The key personnel involved in disaster victim identification include:

- the coroner
- the clerical and administrative staff of the coroner's office
- general duty police
- crime scene investigators
- scene photographers
- fingerprints experts
- missing persons police
- forensic pathologists
- forensic odontologists
- forensic anthropologists
- mortuary technical staff
- forensic radiologists
- forensic biologists (including molecular biologists)
- grief counsellors
- media liaison staff.

In addition to these professionals, many disasters will involve other specialist investigators who, although not directly involved in victim identification, need to work closely and in collaboration with the above personnel. For example, specialist accident investigators such as air safety investigators and maritime investigators may have a role in the investigation of transport accidents involving mass loss of life. In the case of terrorist incidents or warfare, military personnel may also be involved.

Standard disaster response and disaster victim identification procedures have become established internationally over the last few decades. The expansion in international travel, combined with the increase in the number of passengers that a single vehicle such as an airliner can accommodate, has meant that responding to mass disasters is an international enterprise requiring the resources of many different nations. Interpol has a standing committee for disaster victim identification, which has co-ordinated international efforts to standardise the procedures and record systems involved in human identification.

The process of disaster victim identification has been subject to considerable analysis and planning on an international basis. According to current protocols, the process of disaster victim identification can be divided into five phases:

- Phase 1 involves the investigation of the scene of the disaster, including all of the locations where bodies or body parts lie.
- Phase 2 involves the examination of the bodies at the mortuary.
- Phase 3 involves the collection of antemortem information from the community in relation to potential victims of the disaster.
- Phase 4 involves a process of reconciliation where the antemortem and postmortem information is matched to identify each victim.
- Phase 5 involves the process of debriefing all personnel involved in the disaster victim identification procedures, including critical incident stress debriefing and operational effectiveness debriefing.

Each of the phases has its own coordinator who reports directly to the DVI commander. Documentation of victim identification information in all phases uses the international standard Interpol DVI forms. This permits the exchange of standardised information between investigators from different countries and representatives of victims.

The size of a mass disaster has important implications for the success of any response. In a situation such as a civil airliner crash, management of the investigation and identification of hundreds of dead is well within the resources of most countries with established specialist forensic services. When such deaths occur in places with less well-developed services, specialists may need to be brought in from other jurisdictions. However, in places that are dangerous or hazardous as a result of geography, meteorological events, or armed conflict, the investigation of even a relatively small number of deaths may be extremely problematic.

From the perspective of disaster victim identification and the coroner, internal civil conflict and international military conflict pose particular problems. The civilian investigation of military action is often subject to specific legal restrictions in the interests of national security. As a result the jurisdiction of the coroner may be significantly curtailed.

The ability of a military service adequately to resource the identification of deceased military personnel and civilians is often limited, as in many jurisdictions the majority of the specialist investigators required are employed in civilian organisations. Where the need to identify military individuals is considerable, specialist military units are often established. These units, however, often deal with discovered remains of individuals who were reported missing in action many years earlier. The United States military operates the United States Army Central Identification Laboratory in Hawaii, where a large number of anthropologists are involved in the identification of recovered remains of military personnel who went missing in the Pacific region during World War II.

The nature of military activities is considerably more varied today than was perhaps conceived of in the past. Classical warfare activities are rarely a significant part of active military service today. Instead, the military often finds itself dealing with civil disturbance, acts of terrorism, and protective security issues. These events, however, may still involve significant loss of life among both civilians and military personnel. Peacekeeping activities will also involve deaths associated with accidents rather than direct conflict. The nature and sophistication of military activities inevitably entails major transportation and industrial operations, all of which may be associated with traumatic death.

The involvement of civilian agencies such as the coroner in the investigation of such deaths has the potential to lead to conflict. Theoretically it would be easy for a military agency to claim that any death related to its activities represents a security issue that should not be discussed or investigated by a civilian agency. However, the capacity of the military to undertake a complex industrial death investigation may be limited, and increasingly the community expects deaths that do not have a military security issue involved to be thoroughly investigated to the same standard as would occur in civilian activities.

Specialist forensic investigators and coroners' staff who are engaged in the process of human identification following a mass disaster are at particular risk of developing a range of physical and psychological health problems as a result of their experiences. Posttraumatic stress disorder (PTSD) can involve a constellation of symptoms, and the condition has been estimated to occur in approximately 9% of the population during their lifetime (McFarlane, 1993). PTSD is an anxiety disorder that can arise when a person has experienced an event outside the range of usual human experience that would be markedly distressing to almost anyone. Victims of the disorder may experience recurrent dreams or intrusive recollections of the event as well as psychological distress during linked life events such as the anniversary of the original experience. Victims may suffer from psychogenic amnesia, social withdrawal and detachment, restricted emotional responses, sleep disturbance, irritability and difficulties in concentration, among other symptoms.

Given the extraordinary nature of the work associated with responding to mass disasters and the potentially distressing nature of the experiences, critical incident stress debriefing was developed as a technique to potentially reduce the risk of people developing PTSD. The debriefing process was originally designed for emergency service personnel exposed to distressing events while engaged in their professional work. More recently, the critical incident stress debriefing has been made available to bystanders, families, survivors and whole communities affected by the distressing event. It is clear that critical incident stress debriefing provided to whole communities does not prevent the onset of PTSD for everyone. In part this is due to the fact that in any community there will be people with particular vulnerabilities to PTSD as a result of their previous mental health status and experiences. The general process of critical incident stress debriefing applied to large or small groups may not be sufficiently tailored to the needs of particular individuals (Solomon, Gerrity, & Muff, 1993). Individually tailored psychological debriefing is likely to be more effective; while this can be provided specifically to disaster response staff who have been identified as being at risk or who have developed symptoms of a stress-related illness during the disaster response, it is unlikely that such a service can be made available to all people affected by a disaster.

Despite these concerns, critical incident stress debriefing applied to small groups has become a universal part of managing the health of people involved in disaster response. The approach has been largely educational, with groups informed about the nature of common stress reactions and provided with information about stress management techniques and when to seek specialist professional help. The very act of taking part in such group educational sessions may also help people to come to terms with their experiences and to reduce the severity of symptoms that may otherwise have affected them.

Coroners and death investigators have a key role to play in the response to mass disasters involving major loss of life. The increased international mobility of our community throughout the 20th century as a result of overseas work and recreation has given modern disaster response a multinational dimension. Few countries today have the resources to respond to all possible disasters to which their citizens might be subject. In the case of large-scale natural disasters, terrorist acts and military conflicts, political, environmental and social factors play a major role in defining the disaster response process. Internationally it is accepted that the family of a missing person has the right to know whether the person has died and how he or she died. Although this right probably imposes a duty on governments, in coronial jurisdictions it is the coroner who is ultimately responsible for ensuring that disaster investigation leading to disaster victim identification is efficiently performed.

The Inquest

An inquest is an investigative process concerned, among other things, 'to set the public mind at rest where there are unanswered questions about a reportable death'. The process of inquiry is principally inquisitorial but has been described as containing both inquisitorial and adversarial elements, differing from a fundamentally investigatory process such as a Royal Commission. An important aspect of the inquest is that coroners exercise judicial power, notwithstanding the executive nature of their functions, and the fact that proceedings in coroners' courts involve the administration of justice. The rules of evidence do not strictly apply, and there is considerable flexibility of procedure. The role of the coroner is fundamental to the inquest process and is more significant to the outcome of hearings than the role of the judge is in standard civil and criminal hearings. This is because inquests are coroner-driven: the coroner is principal investigator in the sense of generating the search for evidence to be taken into account in the decision-making phase of the inquest. The responsibilities of the coroner were described in some detail by the Master of the Rolls in *R v Coroner for North Humberside, ex parte Jamieson [1995] QB* 1; (1994) 3 All ER 972:

> It is the duty of the coroner as the public official for the conduct of inquests, whether he is sitting with a jury or without, to ensure that the relevant facts are fully, fairly and fearlessly investigated. He is bound to recognize the acute public concern rightly aroused where deaths occur in custody, He must ensure that the relevant facts are exposed to public scrutiny particularly if there is evidence of foul play, abuse or inhumanity. He fails in his duty if his investigation is superficial, slipshod or perfunctory. But the responsibility is his. He must set the bounds of the inquiry. He must rule on the procedures to be followed.

The burden of proof applied in the coroner's inquest is not the same as that required in either criminal or civil jurisdictions. Coroners can only make findings on the basis of proof of the relevant facts on the balance of probabilities in Australian and New Zealand coronial inquests. However, where the matters that are the subject of the coroner's findings are very serious or approximate criminal conduct, the finding will be on the upper end of the balance of probabilities, in accordance with the scale postulated in *Briginshaw v Briginshaw (1938)* 60 CLR 336, 343–344.

As Latham CJ put it:

> There is no mathematical scale according to which degrees of certainty of intellectual conviction can be computed or valued. But there are differences in degree of certainty, which are real, and which can be intelligently stated, although it is impossible to draw precise lines, as on a diagram, and to assign each case to a particular subdivision of certainty. No court should act on mere suspicion, surmise or guesswork in any case. In a civil case, fair inference may justify a finding on the basis of preponderance of probability. The standard of proof required by a cautious and responsible tribunal will naturally vary in accordance with the seriousness or importance of the issue.

Where a coroner has the power to commit trial within their jurisdiction as a result of inquest findings it is of course critical that the inquest burden of proof approximates that to the burden that would apply in a criminal committal hearing. This is a sliding scale of burden of proof can present coroners with real difficulties at an inquest.

During an inquest coroners are routinely assisted by police officers seconded to the coroner's officer for that purpose (Bills, 1998). Where matters are particularly complex, coroners are assisted by solicitors or members of counsel. The role of police officers who assist the coroner during the inquest hearing can be complex. In addition to calling the coroner's witnesses and establishing the basis of the witnesses' evidence by asking them questions, the police officer may also have been directly involved in the management of the overall coroner's investigation prior to the inquest. This places them in a quite different role from that of the legal representatives of those permitted standing at an inquest. Where those given leave to appear at an inquest are not legally represented, the coroner may instruct the police officer assisting to act as their spokesperson and allow them to ask questions of witnesses through the police officer assisting the court. The most common situation in which this occurs is where the family of a deceased person does not have legal representation.

Procedures differ from jurisdiction to jurisdiction in relation to the examination of witnesses at an inquest. While in the United Kingdom it is standard for the coroner to be the first to examine witnesses, in Australia and New Zealand the statement of the witness will be tendered after it has been adopted as true and correct by the witness. The coroner's assistant or counsel assisting may ask supplementary questions before other legal representatives are permitted to ask questions. Questioning takes place in the order permitted by the coroner and on such subjects as are of assistance to the coroner. Practices differ as to whether the person making allegations (often the family of the deceased) should be the first to question; this is often regarded as a sensible sequence. Coroners ask such questions as they deem necessary at any time and should permit the opportunity to ask further questions arising out of the answers given to coroners' questions.

Questioning of witnesses by legal representatives should be directed toward testing assertions made. Questioning must be relevant to the issues before the coroner. It is improper for a coroner unduly to restrict it; legal representatives are entitled to test opinions expressed by experts, to suggest they are of insufficient foundation, and in plain terms, that the witness's views are wrong (see also Henneberg, Chapter 20). Questioning may be forceful, even adversarial; ensuring that witnesses are not harassed or intimidated is a component of the coroner's obligation to ensure fairness of proceedings.

Coroners are not bound to observe the rules of procedure and evidence that apply in other courts of record. This means that objections as to admissibility based on the common law or statutory rules of evidence are not particularly helpful at inquests. The freedom from the constraints of the rules of evidence is an inquisitorial aspect of the coroner's jurisdiction and has been described as one of its advantages. Despite this freedom coroners' courts have a duty to comply with the rules of natural justice and coroners are obliged to act judicially. This means, among other things, that coroners are bound to provide a fair hearing to persons who may be adversely affected by their findings or recommendations.

Conclusions

As we have seen, the office of coroner in its various forms has existed for over a millennium. The endurance of the coroner's inquisitorial jurisdiction within an adversarial system of law is an anomaly that is hard to explain. Its persistence may be explained in part by the fact that the coroner's jurisdiction has operated separately from, but parallel to, the more traditional English legal system. This has provided it with a level of immunity that has allowed it to survive the many developments and changes in direction that have transformed the English legal system and those systems that are derived from it. Despite the long establishment of the office of coroner the jurisdiction has not stagnated. With British colonisation, the coroner's jurisdiction migrated and became established in much of the new English-speaking world. In its new colonial soil many hybrid death investigation systems that have incorporated elements of the traditional office of the coroner have evolved to meet the needs of these rapidly growing new communities. Despite these developments and reforms criticisms of coroners and their courts have begun to emerge. The deference shown in previous times to the complex and diverse roles of coroners has dissipated and fundamental questions have been asked about whether coroners have become an anachronism worth retaining (Sholl, 1940). Bodies such as the lobby group INQUEST have proclaimed that 'the current inquest system is failing. This is heightened by deaths that involve questions of state or corporate accountability' (INQUEST, 2002).[16]

Despite these concerns there have been some real gains in the operation of coroner's death investigation services, in particular the increase in professionalisation of the coroners themselves. There is increasing recognition of the specialised nature of the coronial role. In some Australian jurisdictions, for instance, the practice has developed of appointing only magistrates with particular skills or knowledge as full-time coroners. As a result, fewer 'general duty' magistrates are being shuttled through the jurisdiction for a few weeks of experience of coronial practice and then being expected to act as part-time coroners.

Training programs for coroners are now being developed through coroners' societies and judicial training organisations. It is starting to be recognised that skills beyond competency in law and decision-making are required for the modern coroner. There are some parallels with the skill-set required of Royal Commissioners.

However, there is still little recognition that appointment as a coroner requires significant levels of skill as a manager of death investigations, over and above the possession of those skills in investigation as are found among judicial officers generally. Given that the coroner has an increasingly complex administrative role in supervising and directing the death investigation process, this lack of specialist expertise is emerging as an issue of concern. In addition, although coroners in many jurisdictions have the power to make recommendations regarding public health and safety, knowledge of risk-management theory and practice among coroners is extremely variable. In practice, the phenomenon of the temporary or part-time coroner still remains in many jurisdictions and is perhaps the greatest impediment to the development of the coroner as a death investigation specialist.

The modern jurisdiction of the coroner has a far broader role than could have been imagined 100 years ago. These broader functions include:

- determining the medical cause of death, including social and psychological factors
- advancing medical knowledge, including facilitating accurate statistical information on causes of death
- investigating deaths to allay rumours or suspicion, and thereby to ensure that no foul play or wrongdoing slips through the net
- making recommendations to avoid future fatalities
- checking on the death registration system
- enabling family and friends to find out how the deceased died, assisting in personal and community grieving processes
- providing an independent review and investigation of the deaths of individuals in the care or custody of state agencies
- providing families with medical information that may have direct relevance to the maintenance of their health and wellbeing.

The focus on the role of the coroner in preventing injury and death has become a prominent characteristic in the evolution of coronial law in Australia and Canada, particularly since the mid 1980s. There has been increased recognition that the value of death investigation goes beyond the resolving of legal issues and the simple identification of the facts surrounding the death (Johnstone, 1992). Although even today coroners' inquests are largely directed toward ascertaining direct causes of death, such as accidents or a deficit in provision of care, natural disease deaths (that comprise the majority of coroners' death investigations) are acknowledged as having significant public health implications. Recent developments in the field of human genetics have identified hitherto unknown genetic variations and defects that predispose to, or directly cause, disease and sudden unexpected death. The Long QT syndrome is a good example of such a genetic disease. Although this cardiac conduction abnormality leading to sudden cardiac death from arrhythmia has been recognised for some time, the exact genetic base of the disorder is now being uncovered and diagnostic tests have begun to appear. The identification of such defects has important ramifications for other members of the family of a deceased person. Addressing these issues from a prophylactic perspective has the potential to result in a reduction in morbidity and mortality within the community. As risk management, occupational health and safety and preventive medicine have grown into important vocations, together with integrated systems for coroners' inquiry, the application of these disciplines as part of a coroner's death investigation has assumed a greater importance.

The office of coroner has been remarkable for its ability to evolve from a collector of revenues to an institution focusing on avoidance of preventable death. It has been able to adapt to changing community needs, culture and beliefs regarding death and death investigation. Analysis of the strengths, weaknesses, and future potential of the institution of coroner, uninhibited by the details of its current legislative base, may enable it to be further modified so as to build on its past and facilitate its role as an effective part of society's investigation and response to deaths.

Recommended Reading

Alsop, C. (1992). *Coroner's court inquests: A basic handbook*. Melbourne, Australia: Leo Cussen Institute.

Dorries, C. (2004). *Coroner's courts: A guide to law and practice* (2nd ed.). Oxford: Oxford University Press.

Freckleton, I., & Ranson, D. (2006). *Death investigation and the coroner's inquest*. Melbourne, Australia: Oxford University Press.

Hand, D., & Fife-Yeomans, J. (2004). *The coroner: Investigating sudden death*. Sydney, Australia: ABC Books.

Knapman, P., Powers, M., & Thurston, G. (1985). *The law and practice on coroners: Thurston's coronership* (3rd ed.). Chichester, England: Barry Rose.

Levine, M. & Pyke, J. (1999). *Levine on coroners' courts*. London: Sweet & Maxwell.

Matthews, P. (2002). *Jervis on the office and duties of coroners* (12th ed.). London: Sweet & Maxwell.

Northern Territory, Royal Commission of Inquiry into Chamberlain Convictions, *Report of the Commissioner The Hon Mr Justice T R Morling* (1987).

Selby, H, (Ed.). (1992). *The aftermath of death*. Sydney, Australia: Federation Press.

Selby, H., (Ed.). (1997). *The inquest handbook*. Sydney, Australia: Federation Press

Waller, K. (1994). *Coronial law and practice in New South Wales* (3rd ed.). Sydney, Australia: Butterworths.

Worden, J.W. (1991). *Grief counselling and grief therapy : A handbook for the mental health practitioner*. London: Routledge.

References

Abrams, R. (1999). When parents die: Learning to live with the loss of a parent. (2nd ed.). London: Routledge.

Bills, S. (1998). The police role in coronial investigation. In H. Selby (Ed.), *The inquest handbook* (pp. 22–27). Sydney, Australia: Federation Press.

Clark, H.R. (1936). The law and the coroner. *Medical Journal of Australia, 2*, 565.

Cordner, S. (1998). Foreword. In J.G. Clement & D.L. Ranson (Eds.), *Craniofacial identification in forensic medicine.* London: Edward Arnold.

Dickenson, D., Johnson, M., & Katz, J.S. (2000). Death, dying and bereavement. London: Open University and Sage Publications.

Farrell, B. (2000). *Coroners: Practice and procedure.* Dublin: Round Hall Ltd.

Fitzgerald, H. (1994). *The mourning handbook.* New York: Simon & Schuster.

Hayford, J.W. (2003). *I'll hold you in heaven.* London: Regal Books.

Holdsworth, W. (1964). *A history of English law.* (7th ed.). London: Methuen & Co.

Johnstone, G. (1992). An avenue for death and injury prevention. In H. Selby (Ed.), *The aftermath of death* (pp. 140–184). Sydney, Australia: Federation Press.

Kellehear, A. (2000). *Death and dying in Australia.* Melbourne, Australia: Oxford University Press.

Kilbrandon, Lord (1968). Chairman's closing remarks. In G. Wolstenholme & M. O'Connor (Eds.), *Law and ethics of transplantation* (pp. 212–215). London: Churchill.

Knapman, P., & Powers, M. J. (1985). *The law and practice on coroners.* Chichester, England: Barry Rose Publishers Ltd.

Kubler-Ross, E. (1997a). *Living with death and dying.* London: Simon & Schuster.

Kubler-Ross, E. (1997b). *On death and dying.* London: Prentice Hall.

Matthews, P., & Foreman, J.C. (1993). *Jervis on the office and duties of coroners.* (10th ed.). London: Sweet & Maxwell.

McFarlane, A. (1993). Post-traumatic stress. In I. Freckelton & H. Selby (Eds.), *Expert evidence.* Sydney, Australia: Law Book Company.

Parkes, C. (2004). *Bereavement: Studies of grief in adult life.* London: Penguin.

Parkes, C.M., Laugnani, P., & Young, B. (1997). *Death and bereavement across cultures.* Hove, England: Brunner-Routledge.

Raphael, B. (1984). *The anatomy of bereavement.* London: Routledge.

Reeder, D.J. (1999). Impact of DNA typing on standards and practice in the forensic community. *Archives of Pathology and Laboratory Medicine, 123*, 1063.

Rosoff, B. (1997). *The worst loss.* New York: Henig Holt & Co.

Saul, P., McPhee, J., & Kerridge, I. (2006). Organ donation and transplantation in Australia. In I. Freckelton & K. Petersen (Eds.), *Disputes and dilemmas in health law* (pp. 343–362). Sydney, Australia: Federation Press.

Sholl, R., The Hon Sir. (1940). Coroners' inquests. *Proceedings of the Medico-Legal Society of Victoria, IV*, 173.

Solomon, S.D., Gerrity, E.T., & Muff, A.M. (1993). Efficacy of treatments for post-traumatic stress disorder: An empirical review. *Journal of the American Medical Association, 268*, 633.

West, C. (2005). Kane County Coroner, Kane County, Illinois. *Coroner: An historical perspective.* Retrieved March 1, 2008, from http://www.co.kane.il.us/coroner/history.htm.

Endnotes

1   *R v Secretary of State for the Home Department, ex parte Weatherhead* (1996) 160 JP 627.

2   *R v Malcherek* [1981] 1 WLR 690 [[1981] 2 All ER 422; 73 Cr App R 173; [1981] Crim LR 401] (CA), per the Court at 694.

3   For examples of 'natural deaths', see Matthews P., & Foreman J.C. (1986). Jervis on the office and duties of coroners. (10th ed.). London: Sweet & Maxwell. p.: 118ff.

4   *Coroners Act 1997* (ACT), s 13(1)(k); *Coroners Act 1980* (NSW), s 14B; *Coroners Act 1993* (NT), s 12; *Coroners Act 2003* (Qld), s 12(2); *Coroners Act 2003 (SA)*, s 21; *Coroners Act 1995* (Tas), s 24; Coroners Act 1985 (Vic), s 17; *Coroners Act 1996* (WA), s 22.

5   *Coroners Regulations 1996* (Vic) do not currently prescribe any circumstances.

6   *Coroners Act 1985* (Vic), s 3.

7   *Coroners Act 1985* (Vic), s 17(1). See Clancy v West [1996] 2 VR 647 (CA).

8   *Coroners Act 1985* (Vic), s 17(2).

9   See *Clancy v West* [1996] 2 VR 647 (CA).

10   *Harmsworth v State Coroner* [1989] VR 989, 996, per Nathan J.

11   House of Commons Reports from Committees, 1860, vol 16.

12   *Coroners Act 1887*, 50 & 51 Vict, c71.

13   *Coroners Act 1997* (ACT), s 7 (Chief Coroner); *Coroners Act 1980* (NSW), s 4D; *Coroners Act 1993* (NT), s 4A (Territory Coroner); *Coroners Act 2003* (SA), s 7; *Coroners Act 1995* (Tas), s 7 (re Chief Magistrate in respect of coronial functions); *Coroners Act 1985* (Vic.), s 7; *Coroners Act 1996* (WA), s 8.

14   In the United Kingdom such individuals are often referred to as coroner's officers.

15   This is in contrast to assessment of eyewitness identifications of the living, where, although the knowledge of the individual recognised is often only fleeting, identifications have been relied on only to be later proved erroneous. See Australian Law Reform Commission, Criminal Investigation, Report No. 2 (1975) para 118; Thomson D. (1993). Eyewitness identification. In I. Freckelton & H Selby (Eds), *Expert evidence*, 6-volume loose-leaf service. Sydney: Law Book Company.

16   INQUEST, How the Inquest System Fails Bereaved People: INQUEST's Response to the Fundamental Review of Coroner Services, INQUEST, London, 2002, p 1.

The Use of Insects and Associated Arthropods in Legal Cases: A Historical and Practical Perspective

Ian R. Dadour

Michelle L. Harvey

Forensic entomology has generally been recognised among law enforcement and the wider community as a science employed in the estimation of time since death. The utility of this science in contributing to the provision of time frames resulting in the focusing of valuable investigative resources has certainly been of the greatest importance. However, arthropods have been exploited extensively for their ability to provide information in a multitude of other situations, including cases of neglect, the food industry, and information relating to the cause and manner of death. This chapter will discuss the realm of information obtainable from insects and related groups in the forensic context, including and beyond the recognised time since death applications. Two areas of current research, molecular forensic entomology and entomotoxicology, will be discussed for their potential impact in the field.

Background

Forensic entomology is a wide field encompassing all interactions of insects and other arthropods with the law. The first documented case took place in 13th century China. In *The Washing Away of Wrongs* (as translated by McKnight, 1981, cited in Hall, 1990), Chinese criminalist Sung Tz'u reported a case in which insects were used to identify a murderer. A murder was committed by slashing, and all villagers were ordered to bring their sickles to a single location. All sickles were laid before their owners on the ground, and flies were attracted to a specific sickle, presumably responding to traces of tissue and blood. The owner of the sickle, when faced with this situation, was connected to the crime and he confessed. From this early beginning, exploiting the attraction of flies to decaying matter, forensic entomology has grown to recognise the innate interaction of arthropods and humankind.

Insects and arthropods in general are enormously successful organisms, exploiting a wide variety of niches and therefore making them an omnipresent taxon. The ability to recognise these invertebrates and predict their behaviour makes them a useful source of information in a forensic context.

A wide variety of arthropods are found in association with humankind, however, in a forensic context it is generally the insect groups Coleoptera (beetles) and Diptera (flies) that are used to provide information. The basic premise of forensic entomology, in terms of death investigations, is that insects are attracted to the nutrient rich yet ephemeral carrion. The arrival of insects occurs in a predictable yet locality specific succession, with each taxon arriving when conditions on the substrate are most suited to their needs. This therefore means that knowledge of the behaviour of local insect taxa in relation to carrion facilitates inferences about the stage of decomposition, given an assemblage of particular taxa present at a point in time.

The Calliphoridae, or blowflies, are the most studied decomposition insects, and are considered the most useful insects as they are the first to arrive following death and therefore initiate the arthropod succession. Following death, female flies are attracted to the body, depositing eggs or live larvae around orifices and wounds. Larvae are responsible for the secretion of enzymes and spread of bacteria that result in the decomposition of tissues, and they feed on the byproducts of this process, resulting in the removal of the soft tissues. Following cessation of feeding, they leave the body to pupate under nearby objects or in surrounding material, and after a period of metamorphosis emerge as adult flies. Knowledge of the timing of these stages and the effect of numerous variables on development allows the specific estimation of age of calliphorid individuals, based on taxon specific developmental data for known conditions.

The ability to employ the predictability of insect behaviour in conjunction with specific estimates of insect age allows the provision of time frames in a variety of situations. This may provide investigators with defined temporal periods for investigation and therefore focusing of valuable resources. However, forensic entomology may also provide large amounts of other information. Applications of this science have generally been categorised as urban, stored-product or medicolegal in nature (Lord & Stevenson, 1986, cited in Hall, 1990), and it is these three categories that will form the basis of discussion in this chapter.

Urban Applications

The urban aspect of forensic entomology involves the interaction of insects with humans and their environment. The implications of such cases may therefore be health and safety related. They may include the breeding of flies in livestock and similar facilities (Hall, 2001), and the infestation of buildings by termites, cockroaches and other nuisance insects (Hall, 1990).

Agricultural facilities such as feedlots and commercial animal-related facilities such as abattoirs and poultry facilities may provide ideal environments for the breeding of pest insects, particularly flies. The production of flies in the hospitable conditions provided in many such facilities holds significant nuisance value for the community at large, with the potential for litigation against responsible bodies where negligence can be shown.

Termites (Isoptera) are pest insects with the potential to inflict serious structural damage in the urban environment. The issues of termite extermination and damage are important facets of urban forensic entomology (Hall, 2001), with huge financial implications for the real estate industry. Other structural insect pests include the

Coleoptera, whose often concealed activity may have enormous impact in the timber and furniture industries. The prevention of insect damage under this category of forensic entomology is highly reliant on the employment of highly trained and experienced personnel in detecting the presence of subversive insect taxa.

The urban aspect of forensic entomology may also involve the infestation of wounds and body orifices in humans, generally in the very young and the elderly (Benecke & Lessig, 2001; Benecke, Josephi, & Zweihoff, 2004; Goff, Brown, Hewadikaram, & Omori, 1991; Lord, 1990). The presence of fly larvae in wounds and orifices may result in allegations of neglect and mistreatment against carers and/or guardians, and determination of the circumstances surrounding the infestation relies heavily on the forensic entomologist. The application of size measurements of larvae to developmental data may result in estimation of the age of larvae. In the case of infestation of hospital patients, the age of larvae may provide a time frame that may either clear or incriminate the hospital carers. In cases of neglect, the age of larvae may provide a useful indication of the duration of the period of neglect (Amendt Krettek, & Zehner, 2004; Benecke, 1998; Benecke & Lessig, 2001), a very useful piece of information in subsequent cases of litigation.

Benecke and Lessig (2001) used fly larvae in conjunction with successional information and developmental data to estimate both the period of antemortem neglect and postmortem interval (PMI) in a single case. The presence of *Muscina stabulans*, often attracted to decaying organic matter, with a preference for human faeces over corpses, along with *Fannia canicularis*, a common species on urine and faeces, allowed estimation of the antemortem neglect period, and the primary carrion coloniser *Calliphora vomitoria* was used to estimate the PMI. In this way, it was shown there was a high likelihood that the child had been neglected prior to death.

Stored-Product Applications

Under the stored-product aspect of forensic entomology, stored commodities may be infested by arthropods in what may be a health and/or economic issue. Infestations may include the harvesting and storage of crops and subsequent invasion by an insect pest, or the invasion of foodstuffs in the domestic kitchen by insect pests.

The stored-product aspect also encompasses the infestation of food sold by retailers to the public (Hall, 2001), which may result in prosecution and substantial fines. In such situations, the size/developmental stage of insects, together with ambient conditions may be used to estimate the age of insects and therefore minimum time since infestation. Time frames provided may be used to determine whether infestations are the fault of the retailer, or are the result of storage issues or even deliberate contamination by a consumer. The identification of arthropod parts or fragments may also aid in tracing the origin of the pest contaminant.

Medico–Legal Applications

The most widely recognised facet of forensic entomology is the medico–legal aspect, promoted widely in recent film and fiction. The wide-ranging applications of this aspect may apply to cases of neglect, myiasis (infestation of the body by insect larvae), violent crime and ultimately, death.

The main applications include (a) determination of time and location of human death (Hall, 1990), (b) determination of circumstances surrounding death (Hall, 1990; Roeterdink, Dadour, & Watling, 2004), (c) evidence of postmortem corpse relocation (Benecke, 1998), and (d) association of a suspect with a death scene.

The estimation of PMI relies on the knowledge of the predictable succession expected in any given locality to estimate the minimum period elapsed before arrival of a particular taxon, and the temporal significance of the concurrent inhabitation of any given assemblage of taxa. In addition, in the early stages of decomposition, developmental data may aid in the provision of a more defined PMI estimate, given the ability to use data for the highly researched blowfly taxa.

Insects may provide a useful insight into the manner and cause of death of an individual. In the latter stages of decomposition, the absence of soft tissues may prevent visualisation of wounds. The collection of fly larvae around particular areas may be a good indication of some kind of open wound where a specific gunshot or stab wound may not be visible. Roeterdink et al. (2004) developed a technique for the extraction of gunshot residues from the alimentary canal of fly larvae, a useful technique for the identification of the incidence of gunshots where the advanced decomposition of a body may prevent other inference. Other methods of entomotoxicology enable the identification of the presence of drugs and their metabolites from the insects found on the deceased.

A specific locality generally has a characteristic assemblage of insects that may separate the area from any other. The occurrence of a particular taxon in this area may be a unique finding, and therefore when a body is found in locality A with an insect taxon known only to occur in locality B, investigators are provided with an indication that a body may have been shifted following death. By the same token, the presence of a particular insect on the body of a suspect, in their belongings or in association with a vehicle may provide a useful clue as to the movements of an individual, and perhaps even tie a suspect to a victim on the basis of that taxon.

The estimation of PMI is based not only on knowledge of insect behaviour and development, but an understanding of the numerous variables that may affect insect colonisation, succession and decomposition. Burial, wrapping, temperature, season, sun/shade ratio, clothing, vegetation, indoor/outdoor location and rainfall are just some of the factors that may affect decomposition, and therefore the estimation of PMI. An awareness of the possible implication of any of these factors in a particular case, and their potential effect on the decomposition process is vital. Such knowledge relies on thorough research of these factors and their possible impact, and decomposition studies consequently feature prominently in the forensic entomology literature. There are a variety of other areas of research in the field that are currently extending the utility of insects in relation to legal cases, and two areas, the molecular and entomotoxicological facets, will be discussed further for their potential impact in the field.

Future Applications

As scientific technologies evolve to provide more accurate and insightful information, these technologies are being applied in a forensic context to elucidate the circumstances surrounding legal cases. In forensic entomology, cutting-edge technologies are being adapted to the analysis of arthropod evidence to develop new ways that insects and their related taxa can contribute to investigations.

Molecular Techniques

The proliferation of DNA-based techniques being applied to forensic casework in general has extended to forensic entomology since the early 1990s. The polymerase chain reaction (PCR) and its ability to exponentially amplify small amounts of DNA collected from a crime scene have made it possible to study both entire arthropods and their fragmentary remains long after their departure from a scene.

The estimation of PMI using insects relies fundamentally on the accurate identification of insects collected from a corpse, most frequently immature stages of the Calliphoridae (blowflies). The high interspecific morphological similarity of these immature stages makes identification challenging, and may result in the application of inappropriate developmental data in PMI estimation and, therefore, an erroneous estimate. Rearing of immature stages has been used to allow identification from the adult stages, but this is time consuming and plagued by numerous complications. In recent years, molecular techniques have been applied to address the identification problem, most commonly utilising PCR of the mitochondrial DNA (mtDNA), followed by sequencing and phylogenetics analysis for clustering of conspecific individuals (e.g., Harvey, Dadour, & Gaudieri, 2003a; Harvey, Mansell, Villet, & Dadour 2003b; Wallman & Donnellan, 2001; Wallman, Leys, & Hogendoorn, 2005). These techniques have the ability to identify individuals with greater accuracy and efficiency than the previous morphological and rearing approaches to identification. The development of rapid diagnostic assays negating the need for sequencing will further accelerate the process of identification. In addition, potential exists that with further molecular study, individuals may be able to be traced to a specific geographical provenance, and therefore incidences of postmortem relocation of remains detected and primary crime scenes located, significantly narrowing and directing investigative resources to appropriate locations.

A further application of molecular techniques in the field of forensic entomology has been the extraction of ingested host DNA from the alimentary canal of larval calliphorids. The ability to estimate PMI relies on the assumption that larvae used in calculations have completed their entire development on the host (carrion) in question. The importance of confirming the host on which an individual has developed becomes vital in a number of situations, including (a) where a body has been deposited in a place where garbage or other suitable food source is also located, (b) where multiple bodies are present in the same area and it is unclear which body larvae may have fed on, providing problems in the use of larvae in PMI estimation, and (c) where animal or other carcasses may be present nearby.

Carvalho, Dadour, Groth and Harvey (2005) established the potential to extract ingested DNA from the alimentary canal of *Calliphora dubia* in their second day of the pupal stage. A variety of other studies have further confirmed the ability to isolate and detect host DNA from larval calliphorids (Campobasso, Linville, Wells, & Introna, 2005; Linville & Wells, 2002; Wells, Introna, Di Vella, Campobasso, Hayes, & Sperling, 2001). While DNA may be detected and identified to a species level, it appears unlikely, given the degradation of the template under the action of digestive enzyme in the insect alimentary canal, that an individual human may be profiled based on ingested DNA from calliphorid immatures. The ability to confirm the species affinity of the food source remains, however, a useful confirmation in assuring the basic assumptions in PMI estimation.

Entomotoxicology

Insects feeding on host tissues may potentially ingest a variety of substances present in the host body. These substances and their metabolites may be detected through analytical techniques applied to the insects themselves following collection from the host, and used as indicators of manner and cause of death. In some situations decomposition may be considerably advanced, and arthropods form useful specimens for toxicological analysis where traditional tissues and fluids are not available (Gagliano-Candela & Aventaggiato, 2001; Introna, Campobasso, & Goff, 2001). Arthropods feeding on the tissue ingest drugs and toxins introduced into the host while still alive, and therefore form a useful record. While blowfly larvae form a useful source for analysis, predatory beetles, such as Staphylinidae that feed on the larvae, may secondarily accumulate toxins and be important indicators (Introna et al., 2001).

The extraction of drugs from blowfly larvae has been a well-researched area in the forensic entomology literature. Analysis is generally performed using thin layer chromatography (TLC), gas chromatography or high pressure liquid chromatography coupled to mass spectrometry (GC/MS, HPLC/MS). A variety of drugs and substances have been isolated from larvae, including barbiturates, benzodiazepines, antidepressants, phenothiazine, and opiates/opioids (Bourel, 2001; Carvalho, Linhares, & Trigo, 2001; Goff, Omori, & Goodbrod, 1989; Goff et al., 1991; Hedouin et al., 1999; Sadler, Fuke, Court, & Pounder, 1995; Tracqui, Keyser-Tracqui, Kintz, & Ludes, 2004).

Also important in entomotoxicology is study of the effect of various drugs and toxins on insect development (Introna et al., 2001). Many substances have been shown to affect the rate of growth of larvae (Goff & Lord, 1994), including diazepam (Carvalho et al., 2001) and morphine (Bourel et al., 1999; Zhao, Hu, Zhang, Feng, & Wang, 2005). The effect of such substances on insect development is of critical importance in the estimation of PMI, as incidence of accelerated or retarded growth may result in significant error in subsequent calculations when not considered.

Tracqui et al. (2004) declare entomotoxicology to be a useful field for qualitative analysis, but caution against placing too much emphasis on the results of such analyses. While a positive result confirms the presence of a substance, a negative result does not mean the substance is not present in the host, but that it was not ingested. In addition, they found quantitative inference to be useless, as a multitude of factors may affect drug concentration in the insects. According to Introna et al. (2001), very little is known about the exact mechanisms behind larval accumulation and elimination of drugs and toxins and therefore their potential to record meaningful quantitative values.

A new interest in entomotoxicology has been the extraction of gunshot residues from blowfly larvae. Of considerable importance in any death investigation is the cause of death; however, in cases of advanced decomposition, larval feeding activity and the decomposition of soft tissues may distort wounds and leave little tissue in a suitable state for toxicological analysis. Roeterdink et al. (2004) optimised a technique based on inductively coupled plasma-mass spectrometry (ICP-MS) to extract and detect the gunshot-related elements lead (Pb), barium (Ba) and antimony (Sb) from larvae feeding on a shot substrate. Preliminary indications are that the elements are held within the crop and eliminated from the insect's system, and not incorporated into the

230

tissues of the larvae, meaning that detection at pupal level is unlikely given the purging of the alimentary canal prior to pupation. The authors acknowledge the need for establishing background levels of these elements from nonshot substrate (in the case of a homicide, a piece of intact tissue with no gunshot); however, this new application represents a useful foray for forensic entomology into providing inference relating to cause of death.

Conclusions

A multitude of applications exist for the use of arthropods in relation to legal matters. The diversity of biology present across the arthropods enables them to exploit an enormous variety of habitats, making them an important source of information in a wide variety of situations. Traditionally recognised applications under the urban, stored-product and medico–legal facets are increasingly being complemented by the adaptation of new techniques that extend the range and nature of information obtainable from insects and related taxa. The domain of arthropod fauna in forensic entomology is no longer simply in the estimation of time since death, but as the source of an endless array of applications to contribute to the investigation of legal issues in the wider community.

References

Amendt, J., Krettek, R., & Zehner, R. (2004). *Forensic entomology. Naturwissenschaften, 91,* 51–65.

Benecke, M. (1998). Six forensic entomology cases: Description and commentary. *Journal of Forensic Sciences, 43,* 797–805.

Benecke, M., Josephi, E., & Zweihoff, R. (2004). Neglect of the elderly: Forensic entomology cases and considerations. *Forensic Science International 146* (suppl. S), S195–S199.

Benecke, M., & Lessig, R. (2001). Child neglect and forensic entomology. *Forensic Science International, 120,* 155–159.

Bourel, B., Fleurisse, L., Hedouin, V., Cailliez, J-C, Creusy, C., Gosset, D., & Goff, M.L. (2001). Immunohistochemical contribution to the study of morphine metabolism in Calliphoridae larvae and implications in forensic entomotoxicology. *Journal of Forensic Sciences, 46,* 596–599.

Bourel, B., Hedouin, V., Martin-Bouyer, L., Becart, A., Tournel, G., Deveaux, M. et al. (1999). Effects of morphine in decomposing bodies on the development of *Lucilia sericata* (Diptera: Calliphoridae). *Journal of Forensic* Sciences, *44,* 354–358.

Campobasso, C.P., Linville, J.G., Wells, J.D., & Introna, F. (2005). Forensic genetic analysis of insect gut contents. *American Journal of Forensic Medicine and Pathology, 46,* 161–165.

Carvalho, F., Dadour, I., Groth, D., & Harvey, M. (2005). Isolation and detection of ingested DNA from the immature stages of *Calliphora dubia* (Diptera: Calliphoridae). *Forensic Science, Medicine and Pathology, 1,* 261–265.

Carvalho, L.M.L., Linhares, A.X., & Trigo, J.R. (2001). Determination of drug levels and the effect of diazepam on the growth of necrophagous flies of forensic importance in southeastern Brazil. *Forensic Science International, 120,* 140–144.

Gagliano-Candela, R., & Aventaggiato, L. (2001). The detection of toxic substances in entomological specimens. *International Journal of Legal* Medicine, *114,* 197–203.

Goff, M.L., Brown, W.A., Hewadikaram, K.A., & Omori, A.I. (1991). Effects of heroin in decomposing tissues on the development rate of *Boettcherisca peregrina* (Diptera: Sarcophagidae) and implications of this effect on estimation of post-mortem intervals using arthropod development patterns. *Journal of Forensic Sciences, 36,* 537–542.

Goff, M.L., & Lord, W.D. (1994). Entomotoxicology: A new area for forensic investigation. *American Journal of Forensic Medicine and* Pathology, *15,* 51–57.

Goff, M.L., Omori, A.I., & Goodbrod, J.R. (1989). Effect of cocaine in tissues on the rate of development of *Boettcherisca peregrina* (Diptera: Sarcophagidae). *Journal of Medical Entomology, 26*, 91–93.

Hall, R.D. (1990). Medicocriminal entomology. In E.P. Catts & N.H. Haskell (Eds.), *Entomology and death: A procedural guide* (pp. 1–8). Clemson, SC: Joyce's Print Shop.

Hall, R.D. (2001). Perceptions and status of forensic entomology. In J.H. Byrd & J.L. Castner (Eds.), *Forensic entomology: The utility of arthropods in legal investigations* (pp. 1–15). Boca Raton, FL: CRC.

Harvey, M., Dadour, I., & Gaudieri, S. (2003a). Mitochondrial DNA cytochrome oxidase I gene: Potential for distinction between immature stages of some forensically important fly species (Diptera) in Western Australia. *Forensic Science International, 131*, 134–139.

Harvey, M., Mansell, M., Villet, M., & Dadour, I. (2003b). Molecular identification of some forensically important Calliphoridae (Diptera) of southern Africa and Australia. *Medical and Veterinary Entomology, 17*, 363–369.

Hedouin, V., Bourel, B., Martin-Bouyer, L., Becart, A., Tournel, G., Deveaux M. et al. (1999). Determination of drug levels in larvae of *Lucilia sericata* (Diptera: Calliphoridae) reared on rabbit carcasses containing morphine. *Journal of Forensic* Sciences, 44, 351–353.

Introna, F., Campobasso, C.P., & Goff, M.L. (2001). Entomotoxicology. *Forensic Science International, 120*, 42–47.

Linville, J.G., & Wells, J.D. (2002). Surface sterilization of a maggot using bleach does not interfere with mitochondrial DNA analysis of crop contents. *Journal of Forensic Sciences, 47*, 1055–1059.

Lord, W.D. (1990). Case histories of the use of insects in investigations. In E.P. Catts & N.H. Haskell (Eds.), *Entomology and death: A procedural guide* (pp. 9–37). Clemson, SC: Joyce's Print Shop.

Roeterdink, E.M., Dadour, I.R., & Watling, R.J. (2004). Extraction of gunshot residues from the larvae of the forensically important blowfly *Calliphora dubia* (Macquart) (Diptera: Calliphoridae). *International Journal of Legal Medicine, 118*, 63–70.

Sadler, D.W., Fuke, C., Court, F., & Pounder, D.J. (1995). Drug accumulation and elimination in *Calliphora vicina* larvae. *Forensic Science International, 71*, 191–197.

Tracqui, A., Keyser-Tracqui, C., Kintz, P., & Ludes, B. (2004). Entomotoxicology for the forensic toxicologist: Much ado about nothing? *International Journal of Legal Medicine, 118*, 194–196.

Wallman, J., & Donnellan, S. (2001). The utility of mitochondrial DNA sequences for the identification of forensically important blowflies (Diptera: Calliphoridae) in southeastern Australia. *Forensic Science International, 120*, 60–67.

Wallman, J., Leys, R., & Hogendoorn, K. (2005). Molecular systematics of Australian carrion-breeding blowflies (Diptera: Calliphoridae) based on mitchondrial DNA. *Invertebrate Systematics, 19*, 1–15.

Wells, J.D., Introna, F., Di Vella, G., Campobasso, C.P., Hayes, J., & Sperling, F.A.H. (2001). Human and insect mitochondrial DNA analysis from maggots. *Journal of Forensic Sciences, 46*, 685–687.

Zhao, W., Hu, S., Zhang, M., Feng, X., & Wang, B. (2005). Effects of morphine on *Lucilia sericata* growth accumulated degree hour and deduction of decedent post-mortem interval. *Shengtaixue Zazhi, 24*, 1361–1364.

Forensic Chemistry: Applications to Decomposition and Preservation

Shari Forbes

Decomposition and preservation are complex processes involving chemical pathways that can be influenced by the many variables present within the surrounding environment (Gill-King, 1997; Vass, Bass, Wolt, Foss, & Ammons, 2002). In order to understand these processes, a multidisciplinary approach is required that encompasses a broad range of scientific disciplines (Tibbett, Carter, Haslam, Major, & Haslam, 2000). To date, considerable focus has centred on the areas of pathology (Clark, Worrell, & Pless, 1997; Corry, 1978; Polson, Gee, & Knight, 1985), entomology (Amendt, Krettek, & Zehner, 2004; Archer, Bassed, Briggs, & Lynch, 2005; Hall & Donovan, 2001; see also Dadour & Harvey, Chapter 14), anthropology (Iscan, 2001; Komar, 2003; Steadman & Haglund, 2005), and more recently archaeology (Haglund, Conner, & Scott, 2001; Menez, 2005; Skinner, Alempijevic, & Djuric-Srejic, 2003; Spennemann & Franke, 1995), in order to gain a better understanding of these complicated processes and the factors that influence them.

Depending on the investigating discipline, the process of decomposition can be defined by a number of different stages (see also Tibbett, Chapter 3). In forensic pathology, the changes associated with the early postmortem period and the ability of select phenomena to assist in the estimation of postmortem interval is particularly important (Dix & Graham, 2000). Specifically, pathological changes including rigor, livor, and algor mortis are useful in approximating the time of death (Di Maio & Di Maio, 2001). As these phenomena pass, the stages of decomposition are often described by autolysis, putrefaction, liquefaction, and skeletonisation (Clark et al., 1997; Janaway, 1996; Janssen, 1984; Polson et al., 1985).

In forensic entomology, the stages are more generally defined by the physical condition of the carcass and the associated arthropods (Payne & King, 1968). The description may vary slightly, but stages usually include fresh, bloat, active decay, advanced decay, and dry remains (Rodriguez & Bass, 1983; VanLaerhoven & Anderson, 1999). Similar to forensic pathology, forensic entomology is primarily used to determine postmortem interval of decomposed remains. However, the use of entomology spans a larger timeframe than pathology and can be used for remains that are days, weeks, months or years postmortem (Goff, 2000).

Since anthropologists are predominantly called on to analyse skeletal remains in a forensic investigation (Iscan & Loth, 1997), the decomposition stages described in forensic anthropology tend to focus towards the later postmortem period. Comparable to those listed for entomology, the five major categories include fresh, early decomposition, advanced decomposition, skeletonisation, and extreme decomposition (that refers to the decomposition of skeletal material; Galloway, 1997). As forensic archaeologists work closely with forensic anthropologists (Dirkmaat & Adovasio, 1997; Skinner et al., 2003; Ubelaker, 1997), these stages often overlap between the two disciplines. One of the main roles of the forensic archaeologist is to locate and recover decomposed or skeletal remains in order to assist the anthropologist in establishing the identity of the deceased, and in some instances determining the events surrounding the death (Iscan, 2001; Roberts, 1996).

In referring to the various stages of decomposition, it is evident that a multidisciplinary approach is necessary to understand the many transitions that occur as decomposition proceeds. Although the above stages traverse the early, intermediate and late phases of decomposition, there are additional important processes that occur during these periods that have not been investigated as extensively. Of particular importance is the chemical degradation processes that commence immediately following death (Evans, 1963) and represent the basis for many of the observed phenomena associated with decomposed remains. Additionally, the processes associated with soft tissue preservation also warrant examination. Investigation of these processes has the potential to provide additional evidence that may assist investigations involving death, disaster and abuse. Hence, this chapter will focus on decomposition and preservation chemistry and its role in forensic science.

Chemistry of Decomposition

The process of decomposition commences within minutes following death (Vass et al., 2002) and involves a myriad of complex chemical changes that will usually lead to skeletonisation (Clark et al., 1997). The processes of rigor, livor and algor mortis often represent the first observable chemical changes to occur postmortem. Rigor mortis is the result of a chemical reaction that occurs when glycogen, normally used to provide energy for the contraction of muscles, is depleted causing the muscles in the body to stiffen. The change occurs within hours following death but is 'reversible' and will pass after approximately 24 to 36 hours (Wright, 2005).

Livor mortis results from the gravitational settling of the blood in the lowest points of the body (Dix & Graham, 2000). The change is initially observed as a red discolouration of the skin but the colour will change to purple as the oxygen in the haemoglobin begins to dissociate (Clark et al., 1997). Livor mortis can be observed as early as 1 hour after death (Wright, 2005) and will become 'fixed' approximately 10 hours after death as the fat in the dermis solidifies, causing the blood-filled capillaries to close (Dix & Graham, 2000).

Algor mortis refers to the normal cooling of the body following death. The process will continue until the body temperature equilibrates with the surrounding environmental temperature. The change occurs as a result of the postmortem cessation of the metabolic processes that normally maintain a body temperature of approximately 37 °C (Clark et al., 1997). Due to their importance to forensic pathologists, these chemical processes have received considerable attention in the literature. However, the chemical changes, which often follow these phenomena, have been largely overlooked with regard to the process of decomposition.

The human body consists predominantly of water with the remaining matter being made up of biological macromolecules; namely proteins, lipids, and carbohydrates (Gill-King, 1997; Vass et al., 2002). During the decomposition process, each of these macromolecules will eventually degrade (depending on environmental variables) to their basic components via a number of complex chemical pathways. Both the chemical pathways and the resulting decomposition products are important to an overall understanding of decomposition chemistry.

Protein Degradation

Protein degradation results from the effects of bacterial enzymes that denature the proteins to their constituent amino acids (Gill-King, 1997). The process is often referred to as proteolysis and occurs at low pH levels that are necessary for the formation of the enzymes (Corry, 1978). Certain amino acids that are produced during the decomposition process have been identified as being important tissue biomarkers for estimating postmortem interval. A study involving the decomposition of human remains detected a correlation between specific amino acids (alanine, methionine, serine, histidine, aspartate, leucine, phenylalanine, glutamate, praline, cysteine, and valine), the tissue type, and the postmortem period (Vass et al., 2002). The empirical model proposed as a result of the study has been successfully applied to forensic cases involving postmortem interval estimation.

Amino acids can, depending on environmental conditions, undergo deamination (loss of an amine group) or decarboxylation (loss of a carboxyl group). Loss of an amine group and a hydrogen atom from an amino acid yields ammonia, which is readily used by higher plants and microbes, and will accumulate in the soil or groundwater system (Dent, Forbes, & Stuart, 2004). Accumulation of ammonia will cause a shift in pH to neutrality or alkaline (Janssen, 1984). Ammonia can be readily converted to ammonium that is used by plants. The result of ammonium accumulation is an increase or acceleration of vegetative growth in the area as a result of the added nutrients (Hunter & Martin, 1996). An increase in vegetative growth compared to the surrounding vegetation can provide a useful indicator for locating decomposing remains. Variations in vegetation may also occur as a result of decomposition that can cause changes in flowering or fruiting patterns (Hunter & Martin, 1996), or more importantly, the identification of certain species that are only associated with disturbed locations (i.e., grave sites).

Decarboxylation of amino acids by bacterial enzymes results in a loss of the α-carboxyl group and liberation of carbon dioxide. Amino acid precursors available during decomposition include ornithine, lysine, histidine, tyrosine, tryptophan, and phenylalanine. The biogenic amines that form as a result of the decarboxylation of these amino acids are putrescine, cadaverine, histamine, tyramine, tryptamine, and phenylethylamine, respectively (Nadon, 1998). The production of biogenic amines is dependent on the availability of microorganisms capable of amino acid decarboxylation, and the presence of environmental conditions suitable for bacterial and enzyme production. Bacteria capable of decarboxylating amino acids through the enzymes they produce include *Enterobacteriaceae*, *Clostridium*, and *Lactobacillus* (Shalaby, 1996).

A considerable number of amines have been identified in decomposed soft tissue (Corry, 1978; Vass et al. 2002) and two particular diamines, putrescine and cadaverine, are regularly referred to in a forensic context due to their apparent offensive odour (Gill-King, 1997). It has been suggested that volatile putrescine and cadaverine can be detected by cadaver dogs at low concentrations (Killam, 1990). However, recent studies investigating the volatile organic compounds that evolve from decomposing remains have failed to identify these specific diamines among 80 to 424 volatile substances detected (Statheropoulos et al. 2005; Vass et al., 2004). Another protein degradation byproduct, dimethyl disulfide (DMDS) was, however, identified in high concentrations and is likely a key component, along with other sulphur compounds, of the offensive odour associated with decomposition.

Lipid Degradation

Adipose tissue is comprised of adipose cells, blood vessels, fibroblasts, and nerve fibres (Ruiz-Gutierrez et al., 1992). Human adipose tissue consists predominantly of neutral lipids, the major ones being triacylglycerols. Triacylglycerols (also referred to as triglycerides) are triesters of glycerol with three long-chain fatty acids. Oleic, palmitic, linoleic, stearic, myristic, palmitoleic, and vaccenic acids account for more than 90% of the fatty acid composition of triacylglycerols (Calder, Harvey, Pond & Newsholme, 1992). Following death, the neutral lipids are hydrolysed by intrinsic tissue lipases to yield a mixture of unsaturated and saturated fatty acids (Evans, 1963). As decomposition proceeds, the amount of free fatty acids increases while the neutral lipids decrease.

In an aerobic environment, oxidation of unsaturated fatty acids (i.e., palmitoleic, oleic, linoleic, and vaccenic acid) will yield products of aldehydes and ketones (Janaway, 1996). Conversely in an anaerobic environment, hydrogenation of unsaturated fatty acids will increase the yield of saturated fatty acids during decomposition. Analysis of putrefactive liquid after four years decomposition showed a fatty acid composition of predominantly myristic, palmitic, stearic, and oleic acid (Cabirol, Pommier, Gueux, & Payen, 1998). The same fatty acids are often identified in a solid lipid preservation product known as *adipocere*. The chemical process that yields adipocere will be discussed in a later section.

Of the numerous byproducts that can form during the protein and lipid degradation processes, volatile fatty acids (VFAs) are particularly useful in forensic science. Analysis of soil samples from directly beneath a decomposing body can demonstrate the presence of volatile fatty acids in the soil solution. Specifically, a correlation has been shown between the ratio of propionic, butyric, and valeric acids released into the soil and the decompositional rate of human remains (Vass et al., 1992). Establishing a decompositional rate allows investigators to calculate a maximum time since death estimation. This technique has been successfully applied to forensic cases and, in each case reported, the timeframe generated was within the timeframe when the person went missing.

The analysis of VFAs has also been used in human rights investigations in the former Yugoslavia (Tuller, 1991). Soil samples collected from a mass grave in Croatia were analysed for the presence of VFA, approximately 6 years after burial. The analysis identified the short-chain fatty acids: iso-butyric and iso-valeric, as well as the long-chain fatty acids: capric, lauric, myristic, palmitic, stearic, and oleic. The positive findings of fatty acids in the grave soils confirmed the site as a suspected crime scene many years after the event had occurred. The method may also be used to successfully identify grave sites in the absence of human remains or other physical evidence.

Carbohydrate Degradation

Although carbohydrate degradation has less of an application to forensic science, the process is still important to decomposition chemistry. As with proteins and lipids, decomposition will cause the body's carbohydrates to break down to their individual components, namely glucose (Vass et al., 2002). The action of microorganisms can cause the degradation of complex polysaccharides, such as glycogen, to glucose monomers (Dent et al., 2004). Fungi have the ability to decompose the sugars to a range of organic acids including glucuronic acid, oxalic acid and citric acid (Waksman & Starkey, 1931). Oxalic acid has been detected in liver, kidney, heart, and muscle tissue over a range of postmortem periods and is a critical biomarker in the estimation of postmortem interval of decomposed remains (Vass et al., 2002). The conversion of oxalic acid to glycolic acid has been observed in the liver and kidney and is considered a key feature of the carbohydrate degradation process.

Bacteria will decompose carbohydrates via a number of different pathways that are dependent on the surrounding environmental conditions. In an aerobic environment, glucose monomers will degrade initially to organic acids, including lactic and pyruvic acid, and finally to carbon dioxide and water (Evans, 1963). In an anaerobic environment, butyric and acetic acid will be produced in addition to alcohols such as ethanol and butanol (Gill-King, 1997). The process of bacterial carbohydrate fermentation also yields decomposition gases including methane, hydrogen sulphide, and hydrogen.

Chemistry of Preservation

As with decomposition, the process of natural preservation of soft tissue is entirely dependent on the surrounding environmental conditions. Factors such as temperature, humidity, moisture levels, and the action of microorganisms can all have a major influence on soft tissue preservation in nature (Sledzik & Micozzi, 1997). The most common forms of natural preservation observed in a forensic context are mummification by desiccation and adipocere formation.

Mummification by Desiccation

Mummification results from the desiccation or dehydration of tissue and occurs when the surrounding environment is extremely dry (Clark et al., 1997). Mummification can take place soon after death if the conditions are optimal and the body rapidly loses moisture via evaporation. Desiccation can occur in the entire body or in discrete portions of the body that are exposed to the desiccating environment. Rapid desiccation of soft tissue prevents decomposition by inhibiting the actions of enteric microorganisms and soil bacteria (Sledzik & Micozzi, 1997). Mummification is often associated with macroscopically well-preserved skin that appears dark and leathery.

Although very few studies have focused on the chemical processes of mummification in a forensic context, the analysis of natural mummification in much older remains can provide useful information that can be applied to forensic investigations. As with decomposition, preservation of skin and other tissue occurs via protein and lipid pathways. The main compound classes typical in postmortem skin include triacylglycerols, fatty acids, and proteins (Bereuter, Mikenda, & Reiter, 1997).

Very little gross structural change occurs in skin immediately following death. The outer skin surface is dominated by proteins while the inner surface contains more triacylglycerols. Once the process of mummification commences, the proteins, saturated triacylglycerols, and unsaturated triacylglycerols are released within the tissue. Desiccation will cause changes in protein content along with possible changes in the secondary protein structure (Gniadecka et al., 1999). Disintegration of the epidermis during mummification will lead to a loss of proteins and a predominance of triacylglycerols (Bereuter et al., 1997). Triacylglycerols will eventually decompose to their constituent fatty acids (Mayer, Reiter, & Bereuter, 1997).

Monocarboxylic acids in the carbon range C_{12}–C_{26} have been identified in mummified tissue with the dominant fatty acid being palmitic, stearic or oleic acid (Gulacar, Susini, & Klohn, 1990; Makristathis et al., 2002). The dominant fatty acid has been shown to vary with the position of the body; an investigation of the desiccated tissue of a hanging corpse identified palmitic acid as the main fatty acid, while an investigation of mummified remains found lying in an apartment identified oleic acid as the main fatty acid in the mummified tissue (Bereuter, Lorbeer, Reiter, Saidler, & Unterdorfer, 1996). The difference in fatty acid composition is most likely due to the loss of liquid oleic acid from the hanging corpse as a result of gravitational forces.

Adipocere Formation

Adipocere forms from the adipose tissue of decomposing remains and is often identified as a white solid substance that can vary in consistency from soft and paste-like to hard and brittle (Fiedler & Graw, 2003). Adipocere formation occurs as a result of the actions of aerobic and anaerobic putrefactive bacteria (Vane & Trick, 2005). Depending on the environment in which it forms, adipocere can be observed in as little as 30 to 90 days after death (Dix & Graham, 2000; Fiedler & Graw, 2003). Its formation can lead to the preservation of soft tissue and internal organs. As a result, the body becomes very resistant to decomposition.

Adipocere formation occurs because of the hydrolysis and hydrogenation of the body's lipids into a mixture of fatty acids. Adipocere is predominantly characterised by saturated fatty acids including myristic, palmitic, and stearic acids. The presence of oleic acid has also been reported, along with hydroxy-stearic acid and oxo-stearic acid that form through hydrogenation and dehydrogenisation of the respective unsaturated double bonds (Takatori, 1996). Conjugation of the fatty acids with bivalent metallic ions forms insoluble soaps, such as calcium salts of fatty acids, thus contributing towards its harder consistency (Stuart, Craft, Forbes, & Dent, 2005).

Adipocere formation is also highly dependent on the surrounding environment. Factors including temperature, moisture, oxygen content, soil type, method of burial, and clothing can all contribute towards its formation (Forbes, Stuart, & Dent, 2005a,

2005b, 2005c). Although it is most commonly observed on bodies recovered from water, its formation is not uncommon in soil burials and other anaerobic environments.

In a forensic context, the importance of adipocere lies in its preservation ability. Facial traits of adipocere-preserved remains may still be visible many months or even years after decomposition would normally occur (Kahana et al., 1999). Numerous cases have been reported whereby the preservation of facial features was sufficient to allow for visual identification of the body (Dix & Graham, 2000; Fiedler & Graw, 2003). Preservation of the tissue surrounding wounds may also assist a forensic investigation. For example, adipocere formation around a gunshot wound allowed for its identification after a 12-month burial in damp soil. The actual point of entry in the skin could be recognised and demonstrated that the shooting was carried out at a close contact range (Mant, 1987).

Conclusions

In a taphonomical context, the study of decomposition and preservation processes relies heavily on a multidisciplinary approach encompassing fields such as pathology, entomology, chemistry, anthropology and archaeology. Many of the phenomena associated with death are observed in either the immediate or later stages of the post-mortem period. However, the chemical processes that occur in the transitional period also have an important application to forensic science. Preliminary studies of decomposition chemistry and preservation chemistry have identified important protein and lipid degradation products that can assist in estimating the postmortem period or establishing a burial site. Additional studies in this area have the potential to significantly contribute to international criminal investigations involving death, disaster, and abuse.

References

Amendt, J., Krettek, R., Zehner, R. (2004). Forensic entomology. *Naturwissen*, *91*, 51–65.

Archer, M.S., Bassed, R.B., Briggs, C.A., & Lynch, M.J. (2005). Social isolation and delayed discovery of bodies in houses: The value of forensic pathology, anthropology, odontology, and entomology in the medico-legal investigation. *Forensic Science International*, *151*, 259–265.

Bereuter, T.L., Lorbeer, E., Reiter, C., Saidler, H., & Unterdorfer, H. (1996). Post-mortem alterations of human lipids — part I: Evaluation of adipocere formation and mummification by desiccation. In K. Spindler (Ed.), *Human mummies: A global survey of their status and the techniques of conservation*. (pp. 265–273). New York: Wien.

Bereuter, T.L., Mikenda, W., & Reiter, C. (1997). Iceman's mummification: Implications from infrared spectroscopical and histological studies. *Chemistry — A European Journal*, *3*, 1032–1038.

Cabirol, N., Pommier, M.T., Gueux, M., & Payen, G. (1998). Comparison of lipid composition in two types of human putrefactive liquid. *Forensic Science International*, *94*, 47–54.

Calder, P.C., Harvey, D.J., Pond, C.M., & Newsholme, E.A. (1992). Site-specific differences in the fatty acid composition of human adipose tissue. *Lipids*, *27*, 716–720.

Clark, M.A., Worrell, M.B., & Pless, J.E. (1997). Post-mortem changes in soft tissues. In W.D. Haglund & M.H. Sorg (Eds.), *Forensic taphonomy: The post-mortem fate of human remains* (pp. 151–164). Boca Raton, FL: CRC Press.

Corry, J.E.L. (1978). A review. Possible sources of ethanol ante- and post-mortem: Its relationship to the biochemistry and microbiology of decomposition. *Journal of Applied Bacteriology*, *44*, 1–56.

Dent, B.B., Forbes, S.L., & Stuart, B.H. (2004). Review of human decomposition processes in soil. *Environmental Geology, 45,* 576–585

Di Maio, D.J., & Di Maio, V.J.M. (2001). *Forensic pathology: Practical aspects of criminal and forensic investigation* (2nd ed.). Boca Raton, FL: CRC Press.

Dirkmaat, D.C., & Adovasio, J.M. (1997). The role of archaeology in the recovery and interpretation of human remains from an outdoor forensic setting. In W.D. Haglund & M.H. Sorg (Eds.), *Forensic taphonomy: The post-mortem fate of human remains* (pp. 39–64). Boca Raton, FL: CRC Press.

Dix, J., & Graham, M. (2000). *Time of death, decomposition and identification: An atlas.* Boca Raton, FL: CRC Press.

Evans, W.E.D. (1963). *The chemistry of death.* Springfield, IL: Charles C. Thomas.

Fiedler, S., & Graw, M. (2003). Decomposition of buried corpses, with special reference to the formation of adipocere. *Naturwissen, 90,* 291–300.

Forbes, S.L., Stuart, B.H., & Dent, B.B. (2005a). The effect of the burial environment on adipocere formation. *Forensic Science International, 154,* 24–34.

Forbes, S.L., Stuart, B.H., & Dent, B.B. (2005b.) The effect of soil type on adipocere formation. *Forensic Science International, 154,* 35–43

Forbes, S.L., Stuart, B.H., & Dent, B.B. (2005c). The effect of the method of burial on adipocere formation. *Forensic Science International, 154,* 44–52

Galloway, A. (1997). The process of decomposition: A model from the Arizona-Sonoran desert. In W.D. Haglund & M.H. Sorg (Eds.), *Forensic taphonomy: The post-mortem fate of human remains* (pp. 139–150). Boca Raton, FL: CRC Press.

Gill-King, H. (1997). Chemical and ultrastructural aspects of decomposition. In W.D. Haglund & M.H. Sorg (Eds.), *Forensic taphonomy: The post-mortem fate of human remains* (pp. 93–108). Boca Raton, FL: CRC Press.

Gniadecka, M., Edwards, H.G.M., Hart Hansen, J.P., Nielsen, O.F., Christensen, D.H., Guillen, S.E. et al. (1999). Near-infrared Fourier transform Raman spectroscopy of the mummified skin of the alpine Iceman, Qilakitsoq Greenland mummies and Chiribaya mummies from Peru. *Journal of Raman Spectroscopy, 30,* 147–153.

Goff, M.L. (2000). *A fly for the prosecution: How insect evidence helps solve crimes.* Cambridge, MS: Harvard University Press.

Gulacar, F.O., Susini, A., & Klohn, M. (1990). Preservation and post-mortem transformations of lipids in samples from a 4000-year-old Nubian mummy. *Journal of Archaeological Science, 17,* 691–705.

Haglund, W.D., Connor, M., & Scott, D.D. (2001). The archaeology of mass graves. *Historical Archaeology, 35,* 57–69.

Hall, M., & Donovan, S. (2001). Forensic entomology: What can maggots tells us about murders? *Biologist, 48,* 249–253.

Hunter, J.R., & Martin, A.L. (1996). Locating buried remains. In J. Hunter, C. Roberts, & A. Martin (Eds.), *Studies in Crime: an Introduction to Forensic Archaeology* (pp. 86–100). London: B.T. Batsford.

Iscan, M.Y. (2001). Global forensic anthropology in the 21st century. *Forensic Science International, 117,* 1–6.

Iscan, M.Y., & Loth, S.R. (1997). The scope of forensic anthropology. In W.G. Eckert (Ed.), *Introduction to Forensic Sciences* (pp. 343–369). Boca Raton, FL: CRC Press.

Janaway, R.C. (1996). The decay of buried human remains and their associated materials. In J. Hunter, C. Roberts & A. Martin (Eds.), *Studies in crime: An introduction to forensic archaeology* (pp. 58–85). London: B.T. Batsford.

Janssen, W. (1984). *Forensic histopathology.* New York: Springer.

Kahana, T., Almog, J., Levy, J., Shmeltzer, E., Spier, Y., & Hiss, J. (1999). Marine taphonomy: Adipocere formation in a series of bodies recovered from a single shipwreck. *Journal of Forensic Science, 44,* 897–901.

Killam, E.W. (1990). *The detection of human remains.* Springfield, IL: Charles C Thomas.

Komar, D.A. (2003). Twenty-seven years of forensic anthropology casework in New Mexico. *Journal of Forensic Science, 48*, 521–524.

Makristathis, A., Schwarzmeier, J., Mader, R.M., Varmuza, K., Simonitsch, I., Chavez, J.C. et al. (2002). Fatty acid composition and preservation of the Tyrolean Iceman and other mummies. *Journal of Lipid Research, 43*, 2056–2061.

Mant, A.K. (1987). Knowledge acquired from post-War exhumations. In A. Boddington, A.N. Garland & R.C. Janaway (Eds.), *Death, decay and reconstruction: Approaches to archaeology and forensic science* (pp. 65–78). Manchester, England: University Press.

Mayer, B.X., Reiter, C., & Bereuter, T.L. (1997). Investigation of the triacylglycerols composition of iceman's mummified tissue by high-temperature gas chromatography. *Journal of Chromatography, B 692*, 1–6.

Menez, L.L. (2005). The place of a forensic archaeologist at a crime scene involving a buried body. *Forensic Science International, 152*, 311–315.

Nadon, C.A. (1998). The quantification of biogenic amines in low-temperature stored vacuum-packaged and carbon dioxide modified atmosphere-packaged fresh pork. Unpublished master's thesis, University of Manitoba, Canada.

Payne, J.A., & King, E.W. (1968). Arthropod succession and decomposition of buried pigs. *Nature, 219*, 1180–1181.

Polson, C.J., Gee, D.J., & Knight, B. (1985). *The essentials of forensic medicine* (4th ed.). Oxford: Pergamon Press.

Roberts, C.A. (1996). Forensic anthropology 1: The contribution of biological anthropology to forensic contexts. In J. Hunter, C. Roberts & A. Martin (Eds.), *Studies in crime: An introduction to forensic archaeology* (pp. 101–121). London: Routledge.

Rodriguez, W.C., & Bass, W.M. (1983). Insect activity and its relationship to decay rates of human cadavers in east Tennessee. *Journal of Forensic Science, 28*, 423–432.

Ruiz-Gutierrez, V., Montero, E., & Villar, J. (1992). Determination of fatty acid and triacylglycerol composition of human adipose tissue. *Journal of Chromatography B, Biomedical Applications, 581*, 171–178.

Shalaby, A.R. (1996). Significance of biogenic amines to food safety and human health. *Food Research International, 29*, 675–690.

Skinner, M., Alempijevic, D., & Djuric-Srejic, M. (2003). Guidelines for international forensic bio-archaeology monitors of mass grave exhumations. *Forensic Science International, 134*, 81–92.

Sledzik, P.S., & Micozzi, M.S. (1997). Autopsied, embalmed, and preserved human remains: distinguishing features in forensic and historic contexts. In W.D. Haglund & M.H. Sorg (Eds.), *Forensic taphonomy: The post-mortem fate of human remains* (pp. 483–495). Boca Raton, FL: CRC Press.

Spennemann, D.H.R., & Franke, B. (1995). Archaeological techniques for exhumations: A unique data source for crime scene investigations. *Forensic Science International, 74*, 5–15.

Statheropoulos, M., Spiliopoulou, C., & Agapiou, A. (2005). A study of volatile organic compounds evolved from the decaying human body. *Forensic Science International, 153*, 147–155.

Steadman, D.W., & Haglund, W.D. (2005). The scope of anthropological contributions to human rights investigations. *Journal of Forensic Science, 50*, 23–30.

Stuart, B.H., Craft, L., Forbes, S.L., & Dent, B.B. (2005). Studies of adipocere using attenuated total reflectance infrared spectroscopy. *Forensic Science, Medicine and Pathology, 1*, 197–202.

Takatori, T. (1996). Investigations on the mechanism of adipocere formation and its relation to other biochemical reactions. *Forensic Science International, 80*, 49–61.

Tibbett, M., Carter, D.O., Haslam, T., Major, R., & Haslam, R. (2004). A laboratory incubation method for determining the rate of microbiological degradation of skeletal muscle tissue in soil. *Journal of Forensic Science, 49*, 560–565.

Tuller, H. (1991). *Dirty secrets: blood protein and VFA analysis of soil from execution and grave sites in the former Yugoslavia.* Unpublished master's thesis, Michigan State University, MI.

Ubelaker, D.H. (1997). Taphonomic applications in forensic anthropology. In W.D. Haglund & M.H. Sorg, (Eds.), *Forensic taphonomy: The post-mortem fate of human remains* (pp. 77–90). Boca Raton, FL: CRC Press.

Vane, C.H., & Trick, J.K. (2005). Evidence of adipocere in a burial pit from the foot and mouth epidemic of 1967 using gas chromatography-mass spectrometry. *Journal of Forensic Science, 154,* 19–23.

VanLaerhoven, S.L., & Anderson, G.S. (1999). Insect succession on buried carrion in two biogeo-climatic zones of British Columbia. *Journal of Forensic* Science, *44,* 32–43.

Vass, A.A., Barshick, S.A., Sega, G., Caton, J., Skeen, J.T., Love, J.C., & Synstelien, J.A. (2002). Decomposition chemistry of human remains: A new methodology for determining the post-mortem interval. *Journal of Forensic Science, 47,* 542–553.

Vass, A.A., Bass, W.M., Wolt, J.D., Foss, J.E., & Ammons, J.T. (1992). Time since death determinations of human cadavers using soil solution. *Journal of Forensic Science, 37,* 1236–1253.

Vass, A.A., Smith, R.R., Thompson, C.V., Burnett, M.N., Wolf, D.A., Synstelien, J.A. et al. (2004). Decompositional odor analysis database. *Journal of Forensic Science, 49,* 760–769.

Waksman, S.A., & Starkey, R.L. (1931). *The soil and the microbe.* New York: Wiley.

Wright, R.K. (2005). Investigation of traumatic deaths. In S.H. James & J.J. Nordby (Eds.), *Forensic science: An introduction to scientific and investigative techniques* (2nd ed.; pp. 43–59). Boca Raton, FL: CRC Press.

Forensic Identification in Fatal Crocodile Attacks

Walter B. Wood

Forensic anthropology is the science of identification of unknown individuals by skeletal examination and analysis for medicolegal or coronial purposes. Normally this involves the determination of the age, sex, race, stature and physique, and the pathology, injuries and anomalies affecting the unidentified skeletal remains. An estimate of time since death and any skeletal evidence of the possible cause of death may also be noted.

Because many forensic anthropologists come from a background in physical anthropology and/or archaeology, they may also be involved in the search for, and the location and recovery of human remains from a variety of forensic contexts. Some forensic anthropologists have also developed an interest and considerable expertise in facial reconstruction and a number of sophisticated computer programmes and digital imaging devices have been especially developed for this purpose. Since 1974, there have been a number of publications dealing with crocodile attacks in Australia (Caldicott, Croser, Manolis, Webb, & Britton, 2005; Edwards, 1998; Mekisic & Wardill, 1992; Webb, Yerbury, & Onions, 1978). These have all tended to review and analyse the circumstances that led up to the attacks and the injuries caused by such attacks. Three papers (Burke, 1987; Davidson & Solomon, 1990; Mekisic & Wardill, 1992) have described the injuries caused to the victims of a fatal crocodile attack, but only Burke 1987 deals with the method used to identify the victim of such an attack.

In my role as a forensic consultant in human bone identification in Queensland over a period of 30 years (1971 to 2001), I was approached in 1985 to assist in the identification of bone fragments recovered from the stomach of a captured crocodile following a fatal crocodile attack in northern Queensland. This was followed some years later by my examination of the remains of a second victim that had washed up on a tropical beach 3 days after a fatal attack and other remains that were recovered from the stomach of a 3 m crocodile that was killed nearby 5 days after the attack.

Experience in victim identification in the above two cases, as well as studies by my postgraduate research students into the effects of crocodile digestion on human bone (Ford, 1994; Weldon, 2000) and a continuing interest in the identification techniques used in 16 other fatal attacks across northern Australia since 1974, have stimulated me into writing this chapter.

Australian Crocodiles

Two species of crocodile inhabit Australian waterways: (a) the saltwater Crocodile-*Crocodylus porosus*, and (b) the freshwater crocodile — *Crocodylus johnstoni*. Both species are found extensively across the tropical north of the country from Broome in the west to Rockhampton in the east. They can live for up to 70 years or more in the wild, they can inhabit both fresh and salt water, and they can survive for many months without food.

The Freshwater Crocodile — *C. johnstoni* (Webb & Manoulis, 1989)

The freshwater crocodile (*C. johnstoni*) is restricted to the Australian mainland and tends to inhabit freshwater streams, waterholes, swamps and billabongs further upriver (for some hundreds of kilometres) than their saltwater relative. Their common name belies the fact that they are also quite tolerant of saltwater, and there are limited areas further downstream in the tidal regions of northern rivers where both species may be found to coexist. They rarely attain a length greater than 3 m or a weight more than 100 kg, with the males attaining a greater size and weight than the females. They have long narrow snouts and fine peg-like teeth. They are riverbank feeders consuming mainly insects, crustacea and small fish. Unlike saltwater crocodiles they nest and rarely feed through the northern dry and are more tolerant of other crocodiles in close proximity, especially when they are forced to congregate into small permanent waterholes along the course of otherwise dried up river systems.

The Saltwater (Estuarine) Crocodile — *C. porosus* (Webb & Manoulis, 1989)

The total range of the saltwater crocodile extends from India and Sri Lanka in the west, through South-East Asia, Indonesia, northern Australia, Papua New Guinea and the larger islands of the southwest Pacific in the east. In Australia, their habitat extends from Broome in Western Australia, across the Northern Territory to Rockhampton in Central Queensland, with occasional sightings of isolated animals further south.

Saltwater crocodiles tend to frequent estuarine areas and neighbouring open beaches. However, they can extend up tropical river systems for more than 100 km, especially where the rivers wander through flat coastal flood plains. The flood plains are usually associated with extensive freshwater billabongs, swamps and lagoons where the crocodiles can nest and often take up permanent residence.

The females rarely achieve a length of more than 3 m. The largest authenticated saltwater crocodiles (invariably males) have approximated 6 m or more in length and weighed more than 1000 kg.

Crocodile Behaviour

Saltwater crocodiles are much larger and more aggressive in their behaviour than fresh water crocodiles. They are less tolerant of other crocodiles in their vicinity and cannibalism of juvenile crocodiles by larger animals may play a significant role in the control of total population numbers in the wild.

Saltwater crocodiles are more active at night and over the summer months of November to April (the so-called 'wet season' in the north) when they actively feed, nest and mate. However, being opportunistic feeders if they are hungry they will accept a meal where and whenever the occasion presents. Smaller animals exist on a variety of insects, crustacea, fish, birds, lizards, aquatic reptiles, turtles, and small mammals. Larger animals will attack larger prey in or near the water, including large mammals (marsupials, dogs, feral cats and pigs, cattle, buffalo, horses and humans) and are also known to be attracted to carrion on or near the beaches or river banks.

Saltwater crocodiles have large peg-like teeth and broad robust jaws that are adapted for grasping, holding and crushing their prey. They are furtive hunters, using sight, hearing and smell to silently stalk and approach their prey. They can remain under water for up to 1 hour and can launch themselves with incredible speed half their body length out of the water to seize prey on nearby land, in the air or in low-lying branches of overhanging shrubs or trees.

They first try to subdue their prey by crushing vital parts (e.g., the head, neck, or chest) or by dragging and holding them underwater until they drown. With larger prey that resists being dragged into the water, they will attempt to throw them off balance by grasping a body part and rolling violently.

Once their victim is subdued, they will swallow smaller prey whole, but larger prey must first be butchered before being swallowed. This is achieved by crushing their prey in their jaws, by violently thrashing their heads from side to side, and by rolling their bodies rapidly in the water (the so-called death roll) until parts of the body come adrift. This process usually results in severe mutilation of the carcass, and a quantity of scattered body remains. As crocodiles have relatively small stomachs for their overall body size (Webb & Manoulis, 1989) there are usually leftover remains in the vicinity of a successful crocodile attack on large prey (see Figure 16.1). Body parts may be thrown up onto the nearby bank of a waterhole or stream, caught in the branches of overhanging trees or left in the water to drift away with the flow of the stream or tide. In estuaries and open sea waters, unconsumed remains may attract further soft tissue predation by other common marine scavengers, such as crabs, turtles, fish, sharks, and so on; see Figure 16.1(f) and Figure 16.2(e).

The Saltwater Crocodile Digestive Process

The mechanical and chemical digestive processes of the saltwater crocodile are extremely efficient and can rapidly break down most consumed soft tissues of their prey. Because of the extreme acidity of crocodile gastric juices that can reach pH 1.7 (Ford, 1994), they can also demineralise bones (and teeth) that tend to be retained in their stomachs until completely digested (Ford, 1994; Weldon, 2000; see Figures 16.3 and 16.4). According to Fisher (1981), it is rare to find calcified bones or bone remnants in crocodile scats.

Tissues containing keratin or chitin (e.g., hair, feathers, claws, nails, thick skin, crab shells) are particularly resistant to the crocodile digestive process and often collect into hair balls that can remain in the crocodile's stomach for some time and may be periodically regurgitated (see Figure 16.5). Ingested stones (gastroliths) also are present in the stomachs of many crocodiles larger than 2 m — see Figure 16.5(f). They are thought to be accidentally swallowed by crocodiles when grabbing for prey and are thought to assist with the mechanical breakdown and digestion of food items (Webb & Manoulis, 1989).

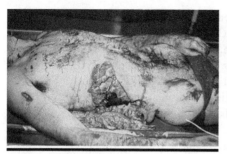

Figure 16.1(a)

A mutilated body recovered within 24 hours of an attack. Note the severe laceration of the right abdominal wall with partial evisceration of gut contents, and scattered superficial lacerations and puncture wounds of the right groin and upper limb.

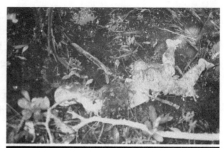

Figure 16.1(b)

The mutilated and rapidly decomposing body of a crocodile attack victim missing both upper limbs. The remains were recovered 2 days after an attack. Facial identification of the victim was not possible. Final identification was achieved by photographic dental superimposition onto an antemortem photograph of the smiling victim.

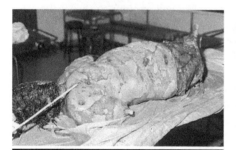

Figure 16.1(c)

The mutilated torso and head of a crocodile attack victim displaying avulsion of all four limbs, recovered 1 day after a fatal attack. The right chest wall and pectoral girdle has been crushed and is overlain by an arcade of skin lacerations and puncture wounds caused by the teeth of a large crocodile. Extensive skin slippage has already occurred due to the rapid onset of decomposition.

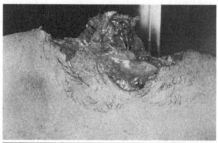

Figure 16.1(d)

Avulsion of the head and neck caused by a fatal crocodile attack. The remains were recovered the same day as the attack. Note the circumferentially orientated abrasions and lacerations of the adjacent skin surrounding the avulsion site due to the violent rolling of the crocodile as it twisted off the head of the victim.

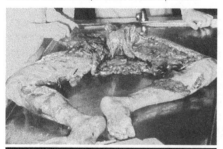

Figure 16.1(e)

The extremely lacerated lower half of a crocodile attack victim recovered on the 3rd day after the attack. The noningested specimen consisted of two separate lower limbs each with an attached hemipelvis which had been transected from the upper torso below the L4 vertebral level. Multiple fractures and dental puncture wounds were present in the bones of both specimens.

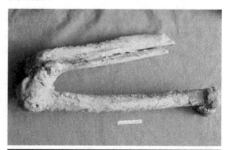

Figure 16.1(f)

The noningested, articulated and defleshed right lower limb specimen (missing the distal leg and foot) of a crocodile attack victim which was washed up on a beach on the third day after an attack. There were multiple dental puncture wounds made by crocodile teeth present on the distal femur and proximal tibia. Numerous superficial cuts and abrasions of the femoral shaft were due to other marine scavengers; see Figure 16.2(e).

Figure 16.1
Unconsumed remains.

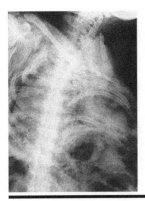

Figure 16.2(a)
X-ray of the crushed chest of a victim. Note the multiple fractured and displaced ribs, and fractures and puncture wounds of the blade of the right scapula; the dislocated right acromioclavicular joint; the dislocation of the cervical spine at C7/T1 vertebral level; and the missing distal-shaft of the left clavicle. The remainder of the left pectoral girdle and upper limb has been avulsed.

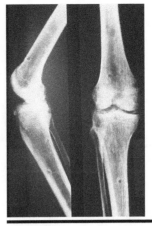

Figure 16.2(b)
Lateral and posterior radiographs of the right knee region of an avulsed R lower limb recovered 3 days after an attack. These display numerous puncture wounds of the distal femur and proximal tibial shaft.

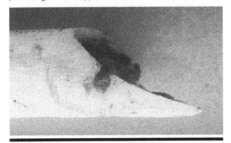

Figure 16.2(c)
A crocodile tooth puncture wound and adjacent cortical bone score marks associated with an oblique fracture of the distal tibial shaft in a defleshed lower limb washed up on a beach 3 days after a fatal attack.

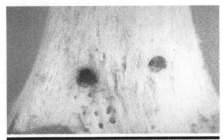

Figure 16.2(d)
Two typical round puncture wounds present in the distal end of a femur caused by crocodile teeth. Note the smaller vascular foramina nearby. Vascular openings and puncture wounds in the cortical bone of ingested specimens allows the penetration of demineralising gastric juices into the underlying cancellous bone and marrow cavity. This precipitates rapid and progressive destruction of the bone ends and the spread of demineralisation along the endosteal surface of the bone shaft.

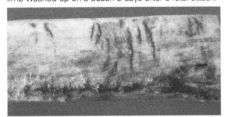

Figure 16.2(e)
Elongated cuts and parallel abrasions of the cortical bone surface, apparent on a femoral shaft washed ashore 3 days after a fatal crocodile attack. The bone had been completely stripped of soft tissue. The marks were caused by noncrocodilian marine predators and scavengers feeding on the soft tissue of the lower limb. The fine parallel striations apparent in the upper centre field have been identified as caused by parrot fish of the family Scuridae.

Figure 16.2
Skeletal trauma in unconsumed remains.

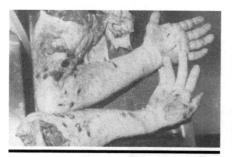

Figure 16.3(a)

Two mutilated, avulsed and ingested upper limb specimens recovered from a crocodile's stomach 4 days after a fatal attack. Segments of degloved palmar and digital skin present among the stomach contents provided readable fingerprints that matched antemortem prints from the victim — see Figures 16.5(a) and 16.5(b).

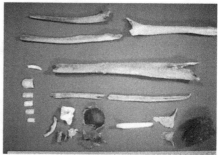

Figure 16.3(c)

Crocodile ingested human remains recovered 25 days after a fatal attack. Clockwise from above left: left radius and ulna, distal portion of left humerus; right tibia (with postmortem saw cut); right fibula (with midshaft fracture); hairball; 2 unidentified flat bone fragments; rib fragment; unidentified cartilage; four decalcified and unidentified bone fragments; set of five fingernails; ? decalcified metacarpal shaft fragment. Note the destruction of the articular ends of the long bones: extensive thinning of all the long bone shafts with softening and curling of the remaining ends of the shafts.

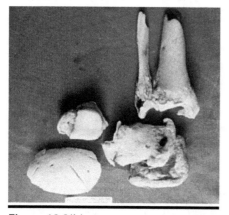

Figure 16.3(b)

Ingested lower ends of an articulated tibia and fibula recovered from a crocodile's stomach 5 days after an attack, together with an isolated talus; a calcaneus and associated undigested skin from the heel; and skin from the sole of the foot. Note the erosion and perforation of cortical bone on the distal ends of the tibia and fibula and lateral surface of the calcaneum; and the plates of undigested articular cartilage peeling away from the articular surfaces of the talar and subtalar joints.

Figure 16.3

Ingested remains.

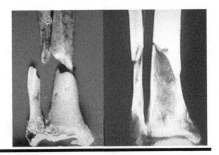

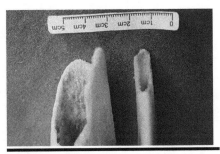

Figure 16.4(a)
A photograph (left) and x-ray (right) of the articulated fragments of a distal tibia and fibula (lower half of image) recovered from a crocodile's stomach 5 days after a fatal attack These are matched with the noningested proximal tibia and fibula (upper half of image) of a defleshed lower limb washed up onto a nearby beach 2 days earlier. Note the matching fracture lines of the ingested and noningested specimens; the extensive demineralisation (radiolucency and thinned cortical bone) and rounded and thinned edges of the fracture sites on the ingested bone fragments compared with the neighbouring noningested bones.

Figure 16.4(b)
The frayed, rounded and thinned fracture sites of a tibia and fibula specimen recovered from a crocodile's stomach (5 days). The cortical bone thickness of each bone shaft was already reduced by approximately 50% compared with that of the bones from the matching noningested specimen recovered from a nearby beach 2 days earlier; see Figure 16.3(b) and Figure 16.4(a).

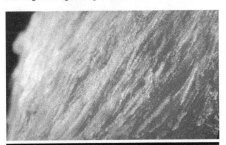

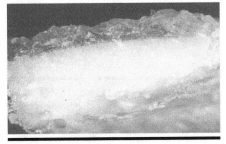

Figure 16.4(c)
A low-powered (× 10) image of the surface of an ingested tibial shaft (5 days). Note the roughened fibrous appearance and surface undulations due to the shedding of large parallel collagen bundles released from the bony matrix by the demineralisation process.

Figure 16.4(d)
A low powered (× 10) cross-sectional view of an ingested tibial shaft (5 days). Note the progression of demineralization from the periosteal surface (transparent zone — above) towards the still mineralised white opaque endosteal surface (below).

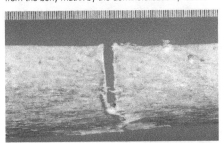

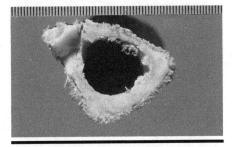

Figure 16.4(e)
Surface appearance of the midshaft of an ingested tibia (25 days) with a postrecovery saw cut. Note the rough fibrous appearance of the periosteal surface and the frayed edges of the saw cut.

Figure 16.4(f)
Cross-sectional appearance of the midshaft of an ingested tibia (25 days). Note the reduced cortical thickness and the frayed and fibrous appearance of the outer cortical bone due to demineralisation and mechanical digestive processes.

Figure 16.4
Effects of crocodile digestion on bone.

Section 3:

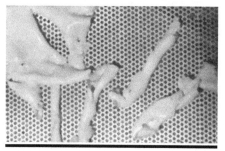

Figure 16.5(a)
Fragments of degloved palmar and digital skin recovered from a crocodile's stomach 4 days after an attack, from which legible finger prints were obtained and used for identification of the victim; see Figure 16.3(a) and Figure 16.5(b).

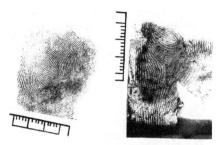

Figure 16.5(b)
The antemortem fingerprint of a crocodile attack victim (left) compared with a postmortem print (right) obtained from degloved digital skin recovered from a crocodile's stomach 4 days after an attack; see Figure 16.3(a) and Figure 16.5(a).

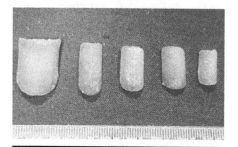

Figure 16.5(c)
A complete set of manicured and undigested finger-nails recovered from a crocodile's stomach (25 days). This demonstrates the relative resistance of keratinised tissues to the digestive process.

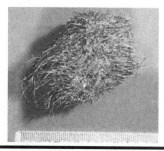

Figure 16.5(d)
A typical hair ball recovered from the stomach of a crocodile 25 days after a fatal crocodile attack. Human head and pubic hair was recovered from its surface and was consistent with hair which matched antemortem samples recovered from the victim's toiletry and bathroom.

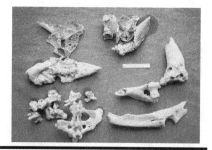

Figure 16.5(e)
The skeletal and skin remnants of an ingested turtle (upper left and lower portions of image) and the carapace and claw remnants of ingested crustacea (upper right) that were included with human remains recovered from a crocodile's stomach.

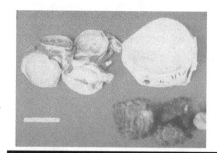

Figure 16.5(f)
Nonbiological remains (soft drink cans, a plastic margarine container, and gastroliths) that were recovered from a crocodile's stomach that also contained human remains.

Figure 16.5
Miscellaneous crocodile stomach contents.

Crocodile Attacks

Both species of crocodile will attack humans and cause nasty soft tissue injuries if humans invade their territory, adventure too close to their nests, or corner them in a threatening situation (Caldicott et al., 2005; Edwards, 1998; Kar & Bustard, 1983; Mekisic & Wardill, 1992; Webb et al., 1978). However, only saltwater crocodiles have been known to attack humans as a food source and to cause fatal injuries.

Well before Europeans ventured into Australia's north in the middle of the 19th century, crocodiles and crocodile attacks were already woven into local Aboriginal folklore and mythology and were well recognised as a permanent risk by resident Aborigines whenever they ventured into or near the water. From the 1850s to World War II, occasional fatal attacks were reported in the newspapers but on the whole they were poorly documented.

For more than 20 years following the World War II there was uncontrolled shooting and trapping of crocodiles in northern Australia, especially for saltwater crocodile skins that were highly prized for their leather-making qualities. Crocodiles were shot by the tens of thousands, and by the mid- to late-1960s their numbers had depleted dramatically and they were placed on the endangered species list.

Since the introduction of crocodile protection legislation (Western Australia, 1969; Northern Territory, 1971; Queensland, 1974) there has been a rapid recovery of animal numbers, resulting in a steady increase in both average animal size and in animals reaching maturity (Webb, 1986). Associated with this recovery has been a steady increase in the numbers of people populating and visiting our tropical north where ecotourism and fishing charters have become major money spinners in the 'Top End'. This has led to the increasing probability that humans and crocodiles will cross paths more frequently and that the incidence of crocodile attacks on humans (with potential fatalities) will also increase.

Fatal Crocodile Attacks Since 1974

Saltwater crocodiles become dangerous to humans and potential human-killers once they attain a length of approximately 3 m and a body weight of more than 150 kg. This means that most fatal attacks are caused by the larger male individuals. From 1974 to 2005 inclusive, 18 fatal crocodile attacks were recorded across northern Australia (Table 1). The attacks were not restricted to, or concentrated in, the 'wet' season but were scattered throughout the various months of the year. A brief summary of the recovered remains and the recovery times is presented in Table 2.

Of the 18 victims, no remains were recovered in two cases (Cases 15 and 16 were both witnessed attacks). No details of the recovery date of the victim's remains were available for two other cases (Cases 3 and 4). Of the remaining 14 cases, unconsumed remains were recovered in 13 cases, with four cases (Cases 1, 7, 10 and 12) including both types of remains (unconsumed and ingested). There was only one case (Case 5) in which ingested remains alone were recovered from a crocodile captured 25 days after the attack.

All the unconsumed remains were recovered within 3 days (72 hours) of the reported attack. Seven of these were recovered within the first 24 hours of the attack; three within 24 to 48 hours, and three within 48 to 72 hours. In the five cases involving the recovery of ingested remains, the respective recovery dates were 1, 2, 4, 5 and 25 days after the attack.

Table 1

Fatal Crocodile Attacks 1974–2005

Case no.	Sex	Age	Date	Locality*
Case 1	M	32	25/04/75	Mission River, Weipa, NQ
Case 2	M	28	7/10/79	Gove Peninsula, NT
Case 3	F	—	30/06/80	Cato River, NT
Case 4	M	—	25/11/80	Wyndham, WA
Case 5	F	43	21/12/85	Daintree River, NQ
Case 6	F	31	11/02/86	Staaton River, NQ
Case 7	M	39	11/06/86	McArthur River, NT
Case 8	M	40	17/03/87	East Alligator River, NT
Case 9	F	24	29/03/87	Prince Regent Sound, WA
Case 10	M	37	26/06/87	Bamaga, NQ
Case 11	M	25	30/09/88	Cato River, NT
Case 12	M	43	11/05/90	Groote Eylandt, NT
Case 13	M	44	24/12/93	Jardine River, NQ
Case 14	F	23	22/10/02	Kakadu National Park, NT
Case 15	M	21	21/12/03	Finniss River, NT
Case 16	M	60	16/08/05	Normanby River, NQ
Case 17	M	37	24/09/05	Groote Eylandt, NT
Case 18	M	55	29/09/05	Coburg Peninsula, NT

Note: * NQ, north Queensland; NT, Northern Territory; WA, Western Australia.

Physical Effects of Crocodile Attack (see Figures 16.1, 16.2, and 16.4)

Because crocodiles crush and butcher human prey, it is almost inevitable that any remains will display a wide variety of residual soft and hard tissue injuries. These consist of bite marks, dental puncture wounds and severe lacerations and abrasions of the skin with associated soft tissue crushing and mutilation; avulsion of large chunks of soft tissue including skin, muscle, nerves and fat; fractures, puncture wounds, and/or dislocations of bones and joints; crush injuries of the chest, pelvis and head; avulsion of appendages (head and/or limbs); organ evisceration; and torso transection. The presence of soft tissue bruising associated with any of the above injuries indicates that the victim was still alive at the time the particular injury occurred.

Personal examination of the ingested remains of two of the victims (Case 5 and Case 10) and information obtained from the postmortem reports, coronial inquests, radiographs and photographs of two other victims in which ingested remains were recovered (Case 7 and Case 12) have revealed the effects of the crocodile's digestive tract on human remains recovered up to 25 days after an attack (see Figures 16.3 and 16.4). The ingested remains included whole or partial limbs; a human head; portions of the vertebral column and thoracic cage; various soft tissues including skin, muscle, tendons, nerves, and cartilage; cervical, thoracic and abdominal viscera; fingernails, and human hair. The results of these observations are recorded below.

Ingested Human Remains Recovered 1 Day After Attack: Case 12

The following notes are based on information derived from the postmortem report on the victim. The ingested remains consisted of skin of the foot with associated metatarsal bones and the 2nd to the 5th toes with attached tendons, a number of lower anterior rib fragments, fragments of an incomplete liver, the left and right lungs, the heart, the stomach, and remnants of the small intestine.

Table 2
Summary of Recovered Remains and Recovery Times

Case no.	Recovered remains	Recovery time (after attack)
1	Unconsumed remains: both lower limbs	day 2
	Ingested remains: head, trunk and upper limbs	day 2
2	Unconsumed remains: full body	day 1
3	Unconsumed remains: torso only	nda*
4	Unconsumed remains: full body	nda*
5	Ingested remains only: L upper limb bones; R lower limb bones; rib fragment;	
	a metacarpal shaft; fingernails; hair; unidentified cartilage and decalcified bone fragments	day 25
6	Unconsumed remains: limbless head and torso	day 1
7	Ingested remains: head; both upper limbs; upper half of transected torso to L4 level	day 4
	Unconsumed remains: lower half of transected body below L4 level	day 3
8	Unconsumed remains: headless body	day 1
9	Unconsumed remains: full body missing both upper limbs	day 2
10	Ingested remains: R lower leg and posterior foot	day 5
	Unconsumed remains: R thigh bone (femur) and bones of R upper leg	day 3
11	Unconsumed remains: lower half of transected body below L4 vertebra	day 2
12	Ingested remains: thoracic and abdominal viscera; fragments of ribs and R forefoot	day 1
	Unconsumed remains: transected upper and lower halves of eviscerated body	
	missing R forefoot	day 3
13	Unconsumed remains: full body	day 1
14	Unconsumed remains: full body	day 1
15	No remains recovered	—
16	No remains recovered	—
17	Unconsumed remains: full body multiple fractures, lacerations and puncture wounds	day 1
18	Unconsumed remains: full body skull fractures; bruised and lacerated head, neck	
	and upper trunk	day 1

Note: * nda, no details available.

Observations and Comments

All ingested soft tissues of the foot, the anterior thoracic wall, and the viscera displayed evidence of autolysis and partial digestion. The exposed metatarsal bones and rib fragments were still hard and white in consistency and showed minimal evidence of demineralisation. The remains were associated with some well digested avian bones, feathers and several 2 cm to 5 cm pebbles

Ingested Human Remains Recovered 4 Days After Attack: Case 7

The following notes are based on information derived from the postmortem report and by personal examination of the associated postmortem photographs. The ingested remains consisted of skin and soft tissues from the face and neck including the hyoid-larynx complex, both right and left upper limbs, see Figure 16.3(a); large sheets of skin from the trunk and upper limbs; multiple loose fragments of degloved epidermis from the hands and fingers, see Figure 16.5(a); fragments of bone from the skull vault, base and jaws; a number of loose teeth; sections of the thoracolumbar vertebral column down to L4 with posterior rib fragments still attached; numerous loose rib fragments; scalp and beard hair.

Observations and Comments

Both ingested right and left upper limbs were completely degloved of epidermal tissue and displayed moderate digestion of associated soft tissues. There were multiple loose segments of degloved epidermis from the hands and fingers with dermatoglyphic patterns still clearly visible. Irregular antemortem scarring was apparent on the degloved right 4th and 5th fingers with finger tip loss and nail dystrophy. Dark brown, wavy scalp hair was present and collected into a hairball ring.

All exposed bony surfaces displayed a fibrous appearance. The numerous loose rib fragments were completely decalcified, being rubbery and flexible. Bone fragments from the jaws and skull were partially decalcified. Sections of the thoracolumbar vertebral column (down to L4 vertebra) displayed partially eroded and decalcified vertebral bodies. The teeth displayed extensive demineralisation and enamel loss that destroyed specific identifying features. A postmortem compound fracture of the L humerus displayed marked thinning (digestion) of the exposed ends of the bone.

X-rays of the R upper limb revealed a poorly united antemortem fracture of the distal R ulna with surrounding callus formation. The fourth lumbar vertebra (L4) present in the ingested remains matched with the fifth lumbar vertebra (L5) present on an unconsumed R lower limb and hemipelvis segment recovered separately, thus confirming that they were from the same individual.

Ingested Remains Recovered 5 Days After Attack: Case 10, Figure 16.3(b)

The following notes are based on information derived from personal examination and observation of the remains. The ingested remains consisted of the lower quarter of an articulated right tibia and fibula, an isolated R talus bone, an isolated R calcaneum with associated skin and subcutaneous tissue of the heel and posterior sole of the foot, an isolated segment of thick skin and dense connective tissue from the sole of the foot.

Observations and Comments

The lower portions of the R tibia and R fibula were still held together by the distal tibio-fibular ligaments, but were stripped of other soft tissue except for periosteal remnants and plates of partly dislodged articular cartilage. Considerable decalcification and cortical erosion affected all exposed surfaces of the ingested bones resulting in a superficial fibrous appearance. The edges of the fracture sites on the proximal ends of the tibial and fibular remnants were smooth and rounded by the digestive process. There was irregular cortical destruction and perforation of the cancellous filled distal ends of the tibia and fibula. Similar damage affected the exposed lateral and medial surfaces of the calcaneum and talus bones of the foot.

Thin white plates of undigested articular cartilage were peeling away from the underlying articular surfaces of the distal tibia, the fibula, the talus and the calcaneum. Well preserved thick skin of the heel was still present and attached to the calcaneum by partially digested dense connective tissue. The loose segment of thick skin from the sole of the foot was largely unaffected by digestion and displayed clear dermatoglyphic patterns and superficial antemortem cuts and puncture marks.

Isolated puncture wounds (from a broken crocodile tooth) were obvious as shallow depressed cortical fractures on the anterolateral surface of the distal tibial shaft and the lateral surface of the calcaneum.

X-rays — see Figure 16.4(a) — revealed the extent of the demineralisation in the ingested bones compared to the bones in the unconsumed remains that were recovered 2 days earlier (over 50% reduction in cortical thickness adjacent to the fracture line). They also revealed the close matching of the fracture sites in the tibia and fibula in both the ingested and unconsumed remains that indicated that they were from the same individual.

The ingested human remains were intermixed with partially digested bones and undigested skin and shell of a turtle, crustacean shells, gastroliths, two drink cans, and a plastic margarine container — see Figure 16.5(e) and Figure 16.5(f).

Ingested Remains Recovered 25 Days After Attack: Case 5, Figure 16.3(c)

These descriptions were obtained by personal examination and observation of the remains. The ingested remains consisted of a fractured L humerus (the lower two-thirds of the shaft only), a L radius (shaft only), a L ulna (shaft only), a R tibia (shaft only, sawn in half after recovery); a R fibula (shaft only, fractured into two pieces), a ?metacarpal shaft, two small unidentified flat bone fragments, unidentified plates of articular cartilage, unidentified fragments of demineralised bone, a full set of five manicured fingernails, pubic and head hair (recovered from the surface of a gastric hairball).

Observations and Comments

The ingested long bone remnants were of a light greenish brown colour with their articular ends completely eroded away by the digestive process. However, the distinctive human shape and form of the bone shafts could still be recognised — see Figure 16.3(c). They were extremely thin and light in weight, with a fibrous cortical surface and eroded, softened, frayed and curled bone ends. The fibula was in two parts due to a midshaft fracture that was probably postmortem in nature. There were scattered fenestrations along the shaft of the fibula where erosion of the cortical bone surface had penetrated through into the marrow cavity. The tibial shaft had been partly sawn through then broken in half after recovery by police investigators to fit the remains into a specimen bottle — see Figure 16.4(e).

Radiographs of the recovered long bones displayed marked radiolucency and extreme cortical thinning of the long bone shafts (due to demineralisation) when compared to normal bones of the same type and size.

A hairball of mainly porcine (pig) origin had human pubic and head hair adherent to its surface — see Figure 16.5(d). A small quantity of lead shot was also recovered from the crocodile's stomach.

The lower rib fragment included with the ingested remains was recovered from the river bed near where the crocodile was captured and was of a different colour and consistency from all the other ingested bony remains. It was white and hard to the touch and displayed no evidence of digestion or demineralisation.

Decomposition and Degradation of Remains Following Fatal Crocodile Attacks

The heat and humidity of the northern Australian tropical environment and the often severe mutilation of the remains of a victim of fatal crocodile attack result in any unconsumed remains that are exposed out of water undergoing rapid decomposition. Skin blistering and slippage occurs within 1 day to 2 days and complete skeletonisation may occur within 1 week to 3 weeks.

Immersion of any unconsumed remains in water will hinder and slow down the effects of exogenous necrotising agents (e.g., fly maggot activity), but because of the relatively high water temperature, endogenous bacterial decomposition will still proceed apace — see Figure 16.1(c). This may be aided especially in estuarine and open sea waters by other marine predators scavenging on the remains. In one case (Case 10) an unconsumed lower limb from a victim was reduced to just its skeletal elements within three days of the reported attack — see Figure 16.1(f).

Additional factors need to be known and considered when dealing with ingested remains that are exposed to the extremely destructive chemical and mechanical digestive processes experienced in a crocodile's stomach. Of particular importance is the effect of crocodile digestion on bones and teeth. In other circumstances bones and teeth are the most durable parts of the body and usually play a significant role in the postmortem identification process. It has been shown by consideration of the case material reported above (Cases 7 and 10), and by controlled laboratory and field experiments (Ford, 1994; Weldon, 2000) that within 4 days to 5 days of ingestion, bones and teeth rapidly demineralise and lose many of their characteristic identifying features. Cortical bone progressively loses mineral from any exposed surface (periosteal or endosteal) and develops a rough fibrous appearance on the exposed bony surfaces; see Figures 16.4(e) and 16.4(f). Teeth lose their enamel crowns and cancellous areas of the skeleton (long bone ends, vertebral bodies, ribs and short bones of the hands and feet) start to corrode and disintegrate; see Figure 16.3(b). Case 5, however, demonstrates that even 25 days after ingestion, remnants of ingested human long bones may still be present and their distinctively human size, shape and form may still be identified even though the bones are close to complete disintegration; see Figure 16.3(c).

Cases 7 and 10 also demonstrate that the thick keratinised skin of the fingers and palms and the soles of the feet can survive ingestion for at least 5 days with the preservation of their dermatoglyphic patterns and the possibility of recovering finger, palm, and sole prints from the victim for possible identification; see Figures 16.3(b), 16.5(a) and 16.5(b). Fingernails — see Figure 16.5(c) — and human hair can also survive relatively unaffected for more than 25 days (Case 5) with the hair being potentially useful in identification of the victim; see Figure 16.5 (d).

Victim Identification

Investigation and identification of victims of fatal crocodile attack have followed the standard inquiries and practices applied universally to missing people and to the identification of unknown victim's remains. Specific questions that need to be asked and considered by investigating authorities include:

(a) When was the victim noticed and/or reported to be missing?
(b) When was the victim last seen to be alive?
(c) Was the victim known to be in or near the water at the time they went missing?
(d) Did the victim leave any physical evidence that they had been in the vicinity (e.g., footprints, discarded clothing, cameras, fishing gear, or other cultural artefacts, parked vehicles, water craft that were abandoned, swamped or overturned)?
(e) Was there any knowledge or evidence of crocodile activity near where the victim disappeared?
(f) Did anyone witness a crocodile take the victim?

(g) Were any unconsumed human remains recovered in the vicinity of the reported attack?

(h) Did any recovered remains display evidence consistent with a crocodile attack (e.g., tearing or crushing injuries, tooth marks, avulsion of body parts)?

(i) Was there any evidence of bruising of any associated soft tissues (evidence that the victim was alive at the time of the attack)?

(j) Were any human remains recovered from the stomach of a captured and/or slaughtered crocodile in the area?

(k) What were the postmortem findings on the remains?

(l) How were the remains identified as those of the reported victim?

The normal means of victim identification require the matching of antemortem data of a missing person (the suspected victim) with postmortem data obtained from the human remains being investigated. These include:

(a) facial recognition by a relative, friend, or a person who knew the victim during life

(b) dental records (if available) including written records of missing or absent teeth, dental anomalies, fillings, plates, dental casts and radiographs

(c) photographs that allow the possibility of photographic superimposition onto postmortem dental images

(d) fingerprints

(e) unique skin and superficial body features, such as birthmarks, moles, tattoos, and scars

(f) medical records that detail physical characteristics, bone and soft tissue injuries, anomalies and pathology

(g) medical radiographs that display unique radiographic features, for example, the shape and form of the paranasal sinuses, the trabecular patterns in bone, the presence of pathology, fractures and anomalies or deformities

(h) the presence of medical, surgical or orthopaedic implants

(i) hair matching

(j) DNA matching with antemortem samples from the missing person or close relatives

(k) clothing; jewellery or other cultural artefacts known to belong to the missing person.

The methods of identification known to have been used in the cases of fatal crocodile attack reported in this paper are summarised in Table 3.

The commonest method of victim identification was by facial recognition of the unconsumed remains (eight cases: 2, 4, 6, 12–14, 17–18). This method of identification was still possible because the unconsumed remains were recovered within 3 days of the attack, and in most cases facial decomposition had not yet advanced sufficiently to completely destroy recognisable facial features. One victim (Case 1) was identified by facial recognition of the ingested head (after 2 days).

In Case 9 the face of the victim had already decomposed beyond recognition 2 days after the attack. In this case, the victim was identified by photosuperimposition of an antemortem photograph of the face of the smiling victim onto the exposed dentition in the decomposed skull.

Table 3
Summary of Identification Methods Applied to Case Material

Case no.	Identification method	Unconsumed remains	Ingested remains
1	Facial recognition		+
2	Facial recognition	+	
3	Unknown	+	
4	Facial recognition	+	
5	Hair match		+
6	Facial recognition	+	
7	Fingerprints from ingested remains		+
8	Medical records of a surgical scar; victim's clothing and watch	+	
9	Dental photo superimposition	+	
10	Medical X-ray matching with X-rays of the unconsumed remains	+	
11	Unknown	+	
12	Facial recognition	+	
13	Facial recognition	+	
14	Facial recognition	+	
15	No remains recovered but attack witnessed by friends		
16	No remains recovered but attack witnessed by wife		
17	Facial recognition	+	
18	Facial recognition	+	

Case 8 involved the recovery of a headless body, and identification was established from medical records of a surgical scar matching a scar on the victim, and from the victim's clothing and watch.

In Case 7, both unconsumed and ingested remains were recovered. Victim identification was by means of fingerprints recovered from degloved digital skin that had separated from the ingested upper limb remains. The lowest vertebra of the ingested thoraco-lumbar spine (L4) adjacent to the transection site, matched with the upper vertebra of the lumbosacral spine (L5) present in the unconsumed remains.

Case 10 was identified by matching X-ray characteristics of an unconsumed proximal femur with antemortem medical X-rays of the pelvis of the suspected victim that also included the proximal femora. The distal leg fractures on the unconsumed lower limb remains matched closely the proximal fracture sites on the ingested lower leg and foot remains recovered from the stomach of the crocodile.

Case 5 consisted mainly of ingested long bones from the upper and lower limbs of the victim, some cartilage, fingernails and a hairball. Although recognisable as human bones from an adolescent or adult, few other identifying characteristics could be ascertained from the limb bones. Instead, human head and pubic hair that was present on the surface of the gastric hairball (that was mainly of pig origin), was found to be consistent with antemortem hair recovered from the toiletries and bathroom of the suspected victim.

In two cases (Case 3 and Case 11) the identification method is not available, although unconsumed remains were recovered. These two cases involved Aboriginal victims. In one case only a torso was recovered (Case 3), while in the other the lower half of a transected body was all that was recovered (Case 11).

Two victims (Case 15 and Case 16) were seen by witnesses to be attacked by a crocodile but no remains were recovered.

DNA Survival in Crocodile Ingested Remains

The DNA profile of crocodile ingested human soft tissue samples is potentially available for identification of human remains but due to the rapid and severe degradation by digestive enzymes, soft tissue DNA is likely to be available only for a relatively short length of time after ingestion.

The compact cortical bone of ingested limb long bones has been demonstrated to last for more than 25 days (Case 5), presenting the possibility of bone DNA survival for a longer period of time after ingestion. To test this hypothesis preliminary compact bone DNA survival times were carried out by one of my postgraduate students (Walsh, 1994) on small samples of cadaveric compact bone.

Walsh (1994) used genomic and mitochondrial PCR-based DNA typing techniques applied to the analysis of human long bone samples digested by *Crocodylus porosus* for varying periods up to 10 days. Using the HLA-DQA1 locus, as a genomic marker, he produced valid results up to and including the 5th day of digestion. However, amplification from the bone sample retrieved after 10 days digestion was unsuccessful.

PCR amplification of the entire mtDNA control region was successful for all samples digested for up to 10 days. Sequence analysis of the first hypervariable segment demonstrated no loss of fidelity in any of the samples. HLA-DQA1 genotypes and mtDNA sequences were compared between reference samples and digested bone tissue for each time marker used.

In view of the above preliminary observations, it would be considered worthwhile obtaining both soft tissue and/or cortical bone samples from suspected crocodile ingested human remains for possible DNA identification when other methods of definitive identification are unavailable.

Acknowledgments

I wish to acknowledge the following as sources of information and/or images for this chapter: Dr Ian Wilkie (pathologist Queensland Health Department); Dr Kevin Lee (pathologist Northern Territory Health Department; Dr John Hilton (pathologist Western Australia Health Department); Northern Territory Coroner's Office; Queensland State Coroner's Office.

References

Burke, M. (1987). Eaten alive. *Australian Police Journal, 41*, 83–89.

Caldicott, D.G., Croser, D., Manolis, C., Webb, G., & Britton, A. (2005). Crocodile attack in Australia: an analysis of its incidence and review of the pathology and management of crocodilian attacks in general. *Wilderness and Environmental Medicine, 16*, 143–159.

Davidson, I., & Solomon, S. (1990). Was OH7 the victim of a crocodile attack? *Tempus, 2*, 197–206.

Edwards, H. (1998). *Crocodile attack in Australia*. Melbourne, Australia: JB Books.

Fisher, D. (1981). Crocodilian scatology, microvertebrate concentrations, and enamel-less teeth. *Paleobiology, 7*, 262–75.

Ford, D. (1994). *Digestion in the stomach of Crocodylus porosus and its effect on human cortical bone.* Unpublished batchelor of science (honours) thesis, Department of Anatomical Sciences, University of Queensland, Australia.

Kar, S.K., & Bustard, H.R. (1983). Saltwater crocodile attacks on man. *Biological Conservation, 25*, 377–382.

Mekisic, A.P., & Wardill, J.R. (1992). Crocodile attacks in the Northern Territory of Australia. *Medical Journal of Australia, 157,* 751–754.

Walsh, S. (1994). *The extraction, amplification and analysis of DNA from human bone following digestion by Saltwater Crocodile (Crocodylus porosus).* Unpublished batchelor of science (honours) thesis, Department of Anatomical Sciences, University of Queensland, Australia.

Webb, G.J.W. (1986). The status of saltwater crocodiles in Australia. *Search, 17,* 193–196.

Webb, G., & Manolis, C. (1989). *Australian crocodiles: A natural history.* Sydney, Australia: Reed Books.

Webb, G.J.W., Yerbury, M., & Onions, V. (1978). A record of *Crocodylus porosus* (Reptilia, Crocodylidae) attack. *Journal of Herpetology, 12,* 267–268.

Weldon, P. (2000). A study of the effects of crocodile digestion on human compact bone. Unpublished batchelor of science (honours) thesis, Department of Anatomical Sciences, the University of Queensland, Australia.

4

Legal, Ethical and Procedural Issues

17

CHAPTER

The Role of an International Law Enforcement Agency in the Identification of Deceased Persons and Remains

James Robertson

As recently as 5 years ago the answer to the question posed in the title of this chapter, 'the role of an international law enforcement agency in the identification of deceased persons and remains' would, at least in the case of the Australian Federal Police (AFP), have been an easy question to answer: almost no role!

Since the first Bali bombing in October 2002 the AFP has come of age in the world of disaster victim identification (DVI) through its involvement in a number of bombing incidents; through its overseas assistance to a number of countries in the South Pacific; and, through its role in responding to the December 2004 South-East Asian tsunami.

In this chapter I will consider the work of the AFP in the above incidents, our pathway of learning, and how we are trying to make a difference by building capacity with our regional colleagues and partners.

It would be presumptuous to say that the AFP experience is unique or that it is an international benchmark but there will be undoubted parallels with the experience of others and, I am certain, common themes.

The AFP, a National and an International Law Enforcement Agency

The AFP is a relatively young organisation. Formed in 1979 by bringing together the ACT Police, elements of Australian Customs and the Commonwealth Police, its initial functions included policing of the Australian Capital Territory (ACT), drug investigations, protection and guarding duties and a 'mixed bag' of whatever was required by the Commonwealth or Federal Government. The protection element was removed only a few years into the AFP's history, and by the early 1990s it was an organisation of about 2500 people of which about 700 were involved in policing the ACT.

Today the AFP has around 7000 people, with responsibilities for policing the ACT and major airports, and has a broader national and international law enforcement role (see Figure 17.1 for the AFP organisational structure).

A major focus for the AFP is our international role where the AFP works with law enforcement agencies in our regions, and worldwide, to combat transitional

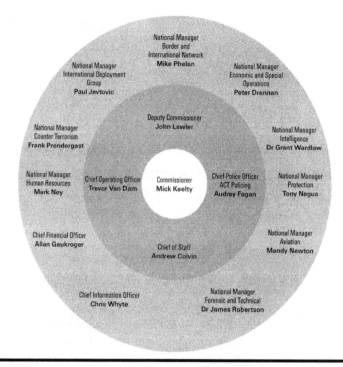

Figure 17.1
AFP organisational structure (Australian Federal Police Annual Report, 2005–006). Reproduced with permission from the Australian Federal Police.

crime, including terrorism. The AFP brings effect to its international obligations through its:

(a) international liaison officer network

(b) international deployment group (IDG)

(c) international training and capacity building

(d) community policing services in external Australian territories.

International Liaison Officer Network

The AFP has a range of international networks in place working with other agencies, as well as AFP International Liaison Officers located in 31 posts in 26 countries (see Figure 17.2 for location of current posts).

From our experience the success of any international deployment is highly dependent on the effectiveness of the AFP's Liaison Officer Network and the support of the Department of Foreign Affairs and Trade (DFAT).

In order to sustain a large-scale international deployment such as the Bali bombings or Tsunami response, the ongoing support of the Australian government for the mission is essential. This can only be achieved by the DFAT Head of Mission remaining confident that the activities of any Australian contingent remain in the national interest. In the case of the tsunami response in Thailand the Australian

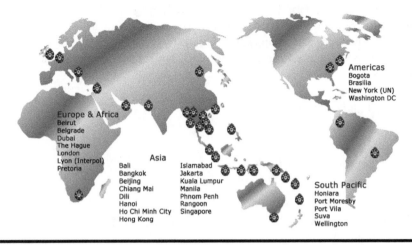

Figure 17.2
Current AFP international network: 86 AFP International Liaison Officers at 31 posts in 26 countries.
Reproduced with permission from the Australian Federal Police.

ambassador to Thailand, the Honourable Bill Patterson, played a critical role in providing exceptional leadership and support to the Australian-led mission. In the absence of this support there is no doubt that the mission could not have been sustained and the outcomes achieved.

Without the level of briefings and support provided by the AFP International Liaison Officers, the AFP DVI Commander in Thailand advised me that he could not have been effective. These members not only provided critical information regarding the political and cultural environment, but also had forged highly effective working relationships with key members of the Thai government and the Royal Thai Police. These relationships underpin any successful offshore mission.

International Deployment Group

The International Deployment Group, or IDG, was formed in early 2004 to manage the deployment of Australian police overseas. In August 2006, the IDG received additional funding of nearly $500M over 5 years to strengthen the AFP's capacity to respond to international crises.

The purpose of IDG is to work with overseas, neighbouring countries to contribute to international stability and security. This is achieved through (a) contributing to offshore law enforcement initiatives, and (b) participating in capacity development programs within the law and justice sector.

The IDG has managed the deployment of Australian and Pacific Island police offshore to multilateral law enforcement capacity building missions, bilateral law enforcement capacity building programs under the auspices of the Law Enforcement Cooperation Program, international monitoring missions, and international peace-keeping missions as civilian police with the United Nations.

The IDG consists of personnel from both sworn and enabling components of the AFP and police officers from the State and Territory police services, and from the countries of 12 Pacific Islands. The AFP currently has staff deployed in Cyprus, Jordan, Nauru, Solomon Islands, Sudan, Timor-Leste and Vanuatu.

A sense of the scope and complexity of this new role for the AFP can be seen from a list of the support teams established under IDG. The support teams include the following areas:

- Executive
- Capacity Building (LECP)
- Contracts and Logistics
- Corporate Services
- Foreign Police Liaison and Visits
- Forensics
- Intelligence
- Learning and Development
- Marketing and Media
- Missions
- Operations Response Team
- Pacific Islands Police Advisor
- Planning and Technical Support
- Specialist Operating Support Team
- Strategy, Monitoring and Governance
- Uniformed Protection
- Wellbeing Services.

The logistics required to support nearly 500 staff working overseas are considerable.

A Case Example

Soloman Islands: Regional Assistance Missions to the Solomon Islands (RAMSI)

In July 2003, RAMSI was established to restore law and order and to assist capacity development with the Solomon Island Police Force (SIPF).

RAMSI Participating Police Force (PPF) is in Phase 4 and 5 of the planned 10-phase engagement. Phase 1 involved direct intervention to stabilise the law and order environment of the Solomon Islands, while Phase 2 involved sustaining the outcomes of Phase 1. Phase 3 onwards is solely involved with the capacity building of the SIPF.

Since the arrival of RAMSI, in excess of 3700 weapons have been seized and over 7000 arrests have been made. The SIPF has commenced taking the lead in policing operations with the PPF in a support role. This is a solid indication of the success in capacity building the SIPF.

Today there are approximately 320 members deployed to the Solomon Islands from the AFP, Australian state police, New Zealand and 12 Pacific Island countries. This is part of a whole-of-government approach to maintain law and order, strengthen the criminal justice system and support peace building.

The AFP has deployed teams on two occasions to the Solomons to exhume in the order of 50 bodies from the Weatercoast area. This deployment included forensic pathologists, an anthropologist and other forensic personnel.

The PPF in mission play a great role in the capacity building of the SIPF, as well as actively engaging in various community projects, for example, recently the PPF Social Club facilitated the renovation of the Red Cross School in Honiara.

Capacity Building Initiatives

A significant component, perhaps in the long run *the* most significant component, of the AFP's contribution to our region is our capacity building program. Much of this is delivered through the Law Enforcement Cooperation Program (LECP).

As part of the IDG, the LECP team delivers capacity building projects to overseas law enforcement agencies on behalf of the wider AFP. Since 1998, almost $30M has been spent providing operational assistance, infrastructure, training, equipment and technical support.

Under the umbrella of the LECP, transnational crime fighting centres have been established with overseas law enforcement agencies in Indonesia, Thailand, Cambodia, Papua New Guinea, Tonga, Vanuatu, Samoa and Fiji. These countries provide a coordination point for gathering and sharing intelligence on transnational crimes, as well as running joint operations to dismantle organised crime groups.

Capacity Building: LECP Funded DVI Training in South-East Asia and the South Pacific

Following the 2002 Bali bombings and the 2004 tsunami Australia received a number of requests from regional neighbours for assistance in developing their DVI capabilities. This recognised the international dimension of mass casualty incidents and the expectation that identification of victims would meet international standards.

The AFP has developed a comprehensive program that incorporates training at various levels and the provision of DVI trailers/kits fully equipped to support a mass fatality incident of up to 200 deceased. To date the program has been delivered in Indonesia, Thailand, Singapore and the Philippines. Of note is the fact that the DVI kits have been used in actual incidents in Indonesia and the Philippines.

The program will be delivered in a further seven regional countries. On completion of this program the key outcomes will include:

(a) integration of a professional and capable DVI first response role into the existing organisational structures of recipient countries

(b) professional development of law enforcement personnel to take ownership of their own countries' future DVI first response roles

(c) delivery of 'best practice' training on DVI first response at management and practitioner level

(d) establishment of a uniform and consistent regional set of appropriate processes and protocols based on the Interpol Guidelines for a first response to a DVI incident

(e) establishment and provision of identical and interoperable resources to enable an effective regional first response to a major DVI incident

(f) establishment of a regional DVI network to encourage cooperation and enhance DVI capacity building.

International Training

In addition to the IDG related capacity building programs the AFP's International Training team provides a range of training programs to Australia's offshore, regional law enforcement agency partners.

Programs are customised to address the challenges and issues faced by each country or region, including the environment in which a program is conducted. A train-the-trainer component can also be incorporated into the program to assist participants in transferring their skills and knowledge to others.

To ensure that all aspects of the programs run smoothly, close liaison is undertaken with our AFP International Liaison Officer network. Training programs include Management of Serious Crime (MOSC), Criminal Intelligence, Investigations Management, Investigations, People Smuggling/Human Trafficking, Financial Investigation, Sexual Offences Investigation, Law Enforcement Intelligence, Law Enforcement Computer Software Systems, Surveillance, and Forensics.

As an example of the assistance provided to regional partners the following briefly summarises some of the AFP's work provided under its 'fighting terrorism at its source' program.

Fighting Terrorism at Its Source

Experience shows that one of the most effective ways to protect Australia from the threat of terrorism is to take the fight to the source, which is offshore.

Indonesia

The AFP's counter-terrorism team in Indonesia has helped the Indonesian National Police apprehend suspects of the terrorist attacks, including the Bali bombings and the Australian Embassy bombing in 2004.

The AFP is managing the implementation and development of the Jakarta Centre for Law Enforcement Cooperation (JCLEC). The Centre's key objective is to enhance the ability of regional law enforcement to deal with transnational crime with a primary focus on counter-terrorism skills.

Philippines

An AFP counter-terrorism team in the Philippines has helped investigate various terrorist incidents, including the Davao bombings in 2003, the Superferry 14 fire of February 2004, the General Santos City bombings of December 2004 and the multiple Valentine's Day bombings of February 14, 2005.

The AFP has also been involved in a multimillion dollar project to help law enforcement authorities in the Philippines develop capabilities in intelligence sharing, bomb investigation techniques, forensics and other areas of counter-terrorism.

Rapid Response

The AFP responds rapidly to requests for assistance from Asia–Pacific regional partners in areas such as disaster victim identification (DVI), crime scene forensics, post-bomb blast investigation, financial investigation, intelligence and technical support.

After the 2004 bombing of the Australian Embassy, the AFP had 30 members in Jakarta within 12 hours of a request from the Indonesian authorities.

Money Laundering

Money laundering is an important source of terrorism funding. Australia is a founding member of the 29-member Asia–Pacific Group (APG) on Money Laundering, formed in 1997 to help countries in the Asia–Pacific region enact laws that criminalise the laundering of the proceeds of crime, and dealing with mutual legal assistance, confiscation, forfeiture and extradition.

The APG also provides guidance for setting up systems to report and investigate suspicious transactions and for the establishment of financial intelligence units.

The AFP hosts Interpol or the International Criminal Police Organisation (ICPO) through the Australian National Central Bureau (NCB). We also host Australia's National Missing Persons Coordination Centre (NMPCC) that is funded by the Australian government. Its mission is to coordinate and promote a national integrated approach to reduce the incidence and impact of missing persons.

The NMPCC works in partnership with law enforcement, Commonwealth and State government agencies, tracing organisations, and the community. A coordinated approach means that each agency's role is clearly articulated. This prevents duplication of effort and leads to effective referral, informed decision-making and better utilisation of resources for all agencies.

Whole-of-Government Response

In the event of an international mass casualty incident and depending on a formal request for assistance, the AFP will form part of a whole-of-government approach. This will usually see the establishment of an Interdepartmental Committee (IDC). In the case of the 2004 tsunami this was called the Australian Interdepartmental Emergency Taskforce (IDETF). IDETF coordinated the Australian response that included the distribution of government aid, medical, and reconstruction assistance. Important as it was, the law enforcement assistance in victim identification was only a small part of the Australian effort. For example, Australia provided over $12M to provide services, supplies and support to tsunami-affected countries, donated $23.5M to the UN to support its activities, and committed to a $1 billion Australia–Indonesia partnership for reconstruction and development. Australia was the largest contributor, per capita, to tsunami aid, with over $300M raised by the community.

The AFP is now seen as an important member of a whole-of-government response to disasters, natural or man made. The AFP works closely with other key agencies and, in particular, the Australian Defence Force (ADF), the Department of Foreign Affairs and Trade (DFAT), and Emergency Management Australia (EMA). In the last 5 years the AFP has developed very significant experience and resources that it can deliver quickly as needed. Forensic support is delivered under the broader structure and we are able to deploy with staff and equipment within a matter of hours. The major advantage offered by the AFP is the ability to work cooperatively and in practical terms, seamlessly, with other agencies and to provide the type of logistics support that enables us to work in almost any environment. Of course, the AFP is not unique and other countries will have similar approaches and will have developed their own solutions. Nonetheless Australia, perhaps because of its size, has been able to develop a highly integrated whole-of-government approach in which law enforcement is accepted and recognised as a key contributor.

Interpol and the Australasian DVI Committee (ADVIC)

The starting point to explaining how the AFP contributes to DVI is to explain the structures that support DVI in Australia. First, as previously stated, the AFP is the Interpol hub for Australia. The Interpol website has a comprehensive section on DVI covering disaster handling procedures, identification, victim identification, elimination tables and international cooperation.

Interpol has also established a Standing Committee on Disaster Victim Identification, which has developed internationally agreed DVI forms to assist in ensuring comprehensive information is collected to ensure the transmission of identification data between member countries. The Interpol guide aims to promote good practice while recognising the guidelines may need to be adapted to conform to national or regional laws and regulations or to religious or organisational practice. The guide provides a wealth of quite detailed and practical advice. Of particular relevance to the role of the AFP is the section on international cooperation. Interpol recognises that the identification of victims and investigation on the cause of the incident will generally be within the jurisdiction of the country in which the disaster occurred, but may directly affect nationals or residents of other countries (Interpol Guidelines). Interpol has developed a number of recommendations aimed at ensuring (a) smooth and efficient cooperation, either through Interpol or directly between member countries, in the identification of victims; and (b) the basic human rights of victims and next-of-kin with regard to accurate identification whenever possible, irrespective of the origin of the deceased.

Appendix A gives details of the international identification standard, including the responsibilities of the Interpol General Secretariat and of member countries. As the host of the Australian National Central Bureau (NCB) the AFP has responsibilities to facilitate and promote adherence to these guidelines. Operating in a foreign jurisdiction also raises a plethora of potential legal issues. These range from the legal authority under which staff may participate, legal indemnities and, specifically in relation to DVI, regulations and laws relating to body transfer. The Interpol Guidelines include three relevant appendices on International Regulations for Body Transport 1937, Council of Europe: Agreement on the Transfer of Corpses 1973 and Pan American and World Health Organisations: International Transportation of Human Remains F66. Forensic specialists cannot be expected to be particularly knowledgeable in such matters. In the AFP, our legal group provides or sources legal advice that underpins our operations. Often we swear in non AFP staff as special members to afford them the protective umbrella of the AFP and the Commonwealth.

As a member country of Interpol, Australia is required to establish a Disaster Victim Identification Commission, which it has done through the establishment of the Australian Disaster Victim Identification Committee (ADVIC). ADVIC includes representatives of all Australian police services, New Zealand Police and scientific advisors representing forensic identification sciences. This committee has a reporting line to Police Commissioners and ultimately to the Australian Police Ministers Council (APMC). Through working groups, and at State and Territory jurisdictional level, ADVIC implements Interpol-consistent strategies and plans. ADVIC has also developed and promulgated a Strategic Plan that can be found at Appendix B. It also delivers training at the practitioner level and coordinates multi-agency exercises. The

DVI community in Australia is served well by this approach as it has built highly productive working relationships across both State and National boundaries.

The Australian Disaster Victim Identification Committee is also a critical forum for establishing the nature of a multiagency response to a mass fatality incident in Australia or Internationally. This is brought into effect through the ADVIC DVI Activation and Response Plan. The plan identifies the lead agencies for command, control and coordination of these incidents. Under this plan the AFP is the lead DVI agency in any instances where an Australian DVI response is requested by a foreign nation.

For an incident in Australia the relevant State coroner maintains control of human remains and has overall responsibility for the identification process. Responsibility for implementing the DVI plan remains at jurisdictional level and the role of the AFP, effectively as the ACT jurisdiction, would be to assist when requested by a responsible jurisdiction. Typically, the following personnel may be required to respond to an incident:

- DVI teams including a DVI Commander
- crime scene investigators
- fingerprint experts
- members of missing persons unit
- medical and dental experts
- technical investigators
- other support staff, including those from emergency services, nongovernment organisations and funeral services.

Forensic and Technical

The AFP's Forensic and Technical group provides a very broad range of scientific and technical services in support of the national and international roles of the AFP as previously described. The diversity of the role of the AFP translates into diverse functions for the Forensic and Technical group. This discussion will focus on forensic aspects; however, in terms of the AFP's broader role in supporting major and complex incidents a key factor is the ability to place, in the field, a broader range of logistics and other support. Two examples will illustrate this point.

In the AFP's response to the first Bali bombing in 2001 a critically important, early requirement was to establish secure communications. In situations such as Bali, or indeed the 2004 tsunami, existing communications systems will fail or are overwhelmed by everyone using mobile phones. There may also be issues of technical incompatibility of systems and security of communications. In terrorism situations there may also be a need to provide a layer of physical protection and security. In the AFP deployment to the Solomon Islands (and in subsequent recent deployments in Timor-Leste and Tonga) the initial response was by the Australian Defence Force (ADF). Only when the environment was secured did the AFP deploy. This is not to say that forensic staff are wholly immune from a degree of risk; hence our staff receive defensive skills training and situational awareness. Increasingly the areas into which forensic staff will deploy, in support of victim identification, will carry significant security risks (this issue is also raised by Anson and Trimble, Chapter 5, with respect to forensic investigation in Iraq).

Through experience gained in the last 5 years the AFP has built up considerable competence in concepts of operations, logistics support and specialist equipment to enable specialists to perform their roles effectively and safely.

As important as deployment in the field, either domestic or international, is the coordination at home base. For any significant incident to which the AFP responds, an Incident Coordination Centre (ICC) is established.

Standard practice in the AFP is to also set up a Forensic Major Incident Room (FMIR). The precise role played by the FMIR will depend on the circumstances of a particular incident but in all incidents it is a critical part of responding and ongoing coordination. Key roles include identification of forensic staff for deployment, specialist equipment, information management, exhibit management and liaison. Our experiences have shown that it is impossible to sustain any long-term deployment without the support of the FMIR.

The AFP's Role in Disaster Victim Identification (DVI)

As the AFP does not have staff to fulfill all of the above personnel categories, invariably this means we act in a management and coordination role to bring together appropriate teams. In smaller incidents, such as the recovery of bodies in the Solomon Islands, the AFP provided all personnel except for specialists such as forensic pathologists and forensic anthropologists. Recognising our ongoing need to have forensic pathology and other specialist support, we have entered into a Memorandum of Understanding (MOU) with the Victorian Institute of Forensic Medicine (VIFM) through which it is our intention to work with VIFM in further developing available capacity in these critical areas. We are particularly interested in enhancing forensic anthropology as a discipline. In larger and more complex incidents, such as Bali or the 2004 tsunami, clearly the AFP had neither all of the specialists areas or nor the capacity to cover incidents of this magnitude for prolonged periods of time. Hence, working with and through the ADVIC, the AFP provided the logistics and coordinated staff from across Australia to form Australian DVI teams. It is worth stressing once again that for every individual who is deployed overseas there is often a much greater number of individuals providing the wide-ranging tasks necessary to support the DVI team in the field.

Our experience over recent years has shown us that no one jurisdiction can stand alone in the event of a significant mass casualty incident. The nature of the work means that teams should only operate for limited times. Our experience also shows that this has to be balanced against rotating teams too quickly. In larger incidents where processing the scene can take months, the impact on human resources can be difficult to sustain. Australia is in the fortunate position that, as a result of our involvement in the 2002 Bali bombing and the 2004 tsunami response, we have a large number of very experienced practitioners who have worked together in the heat of real incidents. Australian contingents have also formed excellent relationships with DVI teams from other countries. Obviously ADVIC includes New Zealand, and our two countries worked very closely together in Thailand following the 2004 tsunami.

However, our experience in this incident showed us that even with the Interpol guidelines *actual* practices can still vary considerably. The challenge in coordinating personnel from nearly 40 countries who sent people to Thailand fell on the AFP. The request to first send staff to Thailand, and then to fill the key role of Joint Chief of Staff, were based on the strength of the AFP's relationship with Thai authorities built up over time through our Liaison Officer network. The initial AFP team included experts in all aspects of specialist DVI tasks along with other essential support staff. Because of our experience in Bali we had developed a forensic rapid response capability and at least arrived in country with some initial supplies. This was critical in enabling us to provide limited, immediate practical assistance. Australia quickly contracted an external private company, Kenyons, to assist with the vast logistics and supply demands that we quickly realised would be needed.

This first team, led by the AFP's Federal Agent Karl Kent, included members of several Australian State and Territory Police Services. Throughout the next year, all Australian Police services continued to support the AFP-led Australian team. Australia was also fortunate in having coordinated forensic odontology and pathology groups who provided a constant supply of these skill sets. Australian personnel occupied several key roles in the early establishment of the structures that supported the international contingent. Karl Kent was the first to occupy one of the two Joint Chiefs of Staff positions along with Colonel Jon Ponprasert of the Royal Thai Police. Federal Agent Michael Travers was the initial Commander of Site 1 at Wat Yang Yao and Inspector Jeff Ernery of the NSW Police the first Commander of the Information Management Centre (later renamed the Thai Tsunami Victim Identification Centre, TTVIC). Critical to the early success of the international effort was the establishment of an international group that acted in an advisory capacity to the Joint Chiefs of Staff. It has to be remembered that the international contingent was in Thailand to support the Thais. The Interpol DVI guide includes consideration of issues such as religion and culture and the need to respect member countries' laws and customs. The management of international relationships is critical and this necessarily involves considerable patience, discussion, consultation and diplomatic skills. I think it fair to say that these skills were displayed by all three AFP members who performed the role of Joint Chiefs of Staff: Karl Kent, Julian Slater and Hermann Metz.

Detective Inspector Peter Baines of the New South Wales Police has commented that he was 'constantly impressed with how the AFP handled international diplomacy … it was clear that they had a lot of experience working in international environments'; see Baines (2006) for an excellent personal perspective of the Thai aspects of the 2004 tsunami).

The DVI response to assist Thailand following the 2004 tsunami can only be viewed as a highly credible international success story. For a number of understandable reasons some bodies remain unidentified but almost all foreigners were identified. The value of the AFP as an international law enforcement agency was clear for all to see and at all levels Australia can be proud of the role it played. Of course, in situations as complex as this, it is important to review how well existing arrangements, practices and procedures hold up in the heat of a real incident. Reviews are important provided real lessons are learnt. At the international level, the Interpol DVI steering committee has commenced implementation of changes as a result of the Thai tsunami experience and is in the process of organising a lesson's learnt exercise involving senior personnel and key personnel from each of the five main stages of the DVI process. The outcomes of this process will no doubt form the basis for further development of the Interpol DVI guidelines. At least member countries of Interpol may consider what changes and improvements might assist even more efficient international support in the event of a future major mass fatality incident.

Two very useful publications from the United States are also worth some attention in considering best practice in mass fatality incidents. The United States National Institute of Justice (NIJ) report from 2005 on *Mass Fatality Incidents: A Guide for Human Forensic Identification,* produced by the Technical Working Group for Mass Fatality Forensic Identification (TWG-MFFI), is designed to assist in creating new mass fatality plans or reviewing existing plans. Notably this report has a short section on forensic anthropology that is reproduced as Appendix C.

The second major NIJ report is a 2006 report on *Lessons Learned From 9/11: DNA Identification in Mass Fatality Incidents.* This report is designed to augment the early NIJ report on mass fatality incidents and focuses specifically on issues around identifying deceased persons through DNA analysis.

The relative contribution of fingerprints, odontology and DNA to the identification of deceased persons in mass fatality incidents will depend on the circumstances of the incidents. It is important to consider the nature of the DVI incident when considering the role and extent DNA will be used in the identification process. The importance of DNA analysis increases in incidents where severe body disruption has occurred, where other antemortem data is not readily available, as in the case of young persons, and where the DVI is conducted in conjunction to a criminal investigation. In the tsunami DNA played a less significant role where antemortem data was available, when compared to the Bali bombings of 2002. Generally, in acts of terrorism, DNA will play a major role in identification of body parts.

Our international experience tells us that it is critical that the correct questions, often the hard questions, are asked at the earliest possible time. This is not facile as there are often considerable practical, diplomatic and political pressures on decision makers. A useful checklist from the NIJ DNA report is produced at Appendix D that, if followed, would be particularly useful. Uncomfortable as the question may be, a critical question in an international incident involving fatalities from many countries, is 'who pays' for DNA identification? The answer to this question may have a greater influence than matters of scientific or technical interest. Another critical question that needs to be confronted is whether or not every person or every recovered body part (or fragment) should be identified? A third critical question is 'assuming funding, can the laboratory do the work?' The NIJ report contains useful information to assist a laboratory to estimate the potential analytical workload and, hence, assess in a realistic way their capacity to meet the challenge. From an AFP perspective almost all DNA testing in the 2002 Bali bombing, which included 202 deceased and many hundreds of body fragments, was carried out in house. This was only achieved with the assistance of scientists from interstate laboratories and by working 7 days a week and with two shifts per day. It effectively shut down all normal laboratory work for several months. With the 2004 tsunami the AFP did not play a significant role in DNA testing. Although DNA played a minor role in the tsunami identifications, the answers to the three questions posed here could have resulted in more efficient, and earlier, outcomes.

If placed in the position of having the responsibility to coordinate and/or manage an incident, an important role is to ask the difficult questions with a view to also driving the best approach to whatever the issue. In an international context this is not an easy task and one has to accept that numerous factors, other than scientific knowledge of best practice, will come to bare in a final decision.

Family Coordination and Liaison

Police are well versed in their role in support of the relatives of deceased persons and invariably will have units, often missing persons units, and staff who specialise in providing information and support to relatives. The importance of this really cannot be over stressed. In an international mass fatality incident the challenge is even greater as there will be relatives who will wish to go to the country in search of their loved one. The former aspect is well covered in Australia through State and Territory police. A specific role for the AFP relates to the latter aspects, that of dealing with relatives who choose to travel to the affected country. The AFP has an extensive Family Liaison Officer (FLO) network who are deployed with the specialist teams. The role played by FLO's is vital and hugely important, especially overseas where layered on the tragic circumstances being confronted by a relative, will be unfamiliarity with the environment, laws and practices.

Interpol guidelines identify the benefits of having FLO's to include:

- ensuring the gathering of antemortem information without delay
- urgent and accurate completion of Interpol DVI forms
- that the gathering of any physical exhibits that could aid identification are gathered in an appropriate manner that would stand up to forensic scrutiny at home and abroad
- that all relevant statements are taken from the family with regards to lifestyle and history
- that at all times the family are furnished with timely, accurate and honest information about the investigation/recovery operation
- safely navigating the family through the workings of the justice system in order to prevent revictimisation
- arranging viewing by families of loved ones
- visits to the scene
- information regarding support agencies is supplied to families
- record all dealings with the family, thus ensuring that there is no duplication of requests made to the family that could affect the family's confidence in the procedure
- consulting about any police media strategy.

The Interpol guidelines provide useful detail on how to establish and train a FLO network and on their roles and responsibilities.

Media Relations

The media have an insatiable appetite for information, and will demand numbers and detail. It is beyond the scope of this chapter to deal with this topic in any detail. However, another way that an international policing agency can add value is through having media specialists with the operational team. Senior members of DVI teams need to develop media skills as they will still need to be the front person for interviews. The media team can, however, coordinate, facilitate and manage the sometimes (often!) unrealistic demands of the media. In mass fatality incidents the media will always focus on numbers, how many fatalities, how many people have been identified and so on. As far as possible, numbers should only be issued from one source so as to avoid any confusion or debate as to accuracy. This source should be the media spokesperson working on agreed numbers authorised by the DVI commander.

Conclusions

The circumstances in which a law enforcement agency may be called to play its part in the identification of deceased persons and remains are many and varied. In today's world, for the AFP, they could be anything from bones discovered in a shallow grave, to mass victim graves, to a terrorist bombing, to a natural disaster. The role of the AFP, and for that matter any law enforcement agency with an international role, will be as varied as the circumstances. A guiding principle should be to add value. This may be simply by liaising and facilitating through our international liaison network, by delivering training to enhance capability, or through more direct forms of support. Whatever role is played by the AFP there are two things that are obvious, we can only work with the cooperation and acceptance of countries involved and we cannot do it on our own. We must work as part of a team whether this is at a whole of government level or a technical level.

What the AFP is trying to do in a very practical way is to be a partner with whom others are comfortable to work and a partner who can offer real assistance. As Australia's international law enforcement agency we have a role to provide leadership where appropriate. The IDG and our international liaison network are prime examples. These are all critically important when we find ourselves called on to identify deceased persons as without these networks we simply would not have been asked to play lead roles. Our continued success will be judged on our ability to be intelligent and mature partners respecting the political and cultural environments in which we operate. It will also depend on delivering real outcomes such as the DVI training program to our regional neighbours. Forensic and DVI support is a multi-facetted and complex business and the AFP has developed an excellent operating framework capable of rapidly deploying physical resources supported by a logistics infrastructure. Our key strength is out ability to bring together people and resources to meet the most demanding challenges. We are continuing to further develop our concept of operations, to establish even stronger relationships with key supporters and partners and looking to support our colleagues in the business of DVI.

Acknowledgments

I wish to acknowledge the valued input of my AFP colleagues FA Karl Kent, Mr Hermann Metz and Mr Paul Reedy in the preparation of this chapter.

References

Australian Government Emergency Management Australia (2005). *Australasian disaster victim identification*. Available at http://www.ema.gov.au

Baines, P. (2006). Tsunami — A Police Prospective', *Australian Police Journal, 59*, 54–66.

Department of Justice, National Institute of Justice. (2005). Mass fatality incidents: A guide for human forensic identification. Available at http://www.ojp.usdoj.gov/nij

Department of Justice, National Institute of Justice. (2006). Lessons learned from 9/11: DNA identification in mass fatality incidents. Available at http://www.ojp.usdoj.gov

Appendix A

Interpol Statement on International Cooperation

6.1 Introduction

The growth in international travel that has occurred in recent years will undoubtedly continue, and this will considerably increase the likelihood of foreign nationals being involved in disasters whether they be natural, caused by man or caused by failures in technology. Land, sea and air transport are undoubtedly the sectors where the risks are greatest but, whatever the cause of the disaster, there will almost certainly be an ensuing need to identify victims and an expectation that this will be done in each and every case. The identification of victims and investigation of the cause of the incident will generally be within the jurisdiction of the country in which the disaster occurred, but may directly affect nationals or residents of other countries and be affected by the legal systems of those countries.

In the case of aircraft disasters, for example, the country in which the aircraft was registered will become involved, as will the country where it was manufactured. As a result ICAO Contracting States have agreed on certain minimum standards and procedures in respect of technical investigations, and these are accepted by all the countries and agencies concerned. Additional recommended procedures are also included in various international agreements. If these agreements did not exist, each country with an interest in the case would have to reinvestigate the incident to its own required standard.

However, no such international standards or agreements currently exist in respect of the identification of disaster victims. One consequence of this can be doubt in one country about the conclusions reached in another country. Such doubts are often unfounded, but it must be acknowledged that, on occasions, there have been incorrect or no identifications as a result of using unsatisfactory methods. Distrust may also arise if insufficient documentary evidence is made available after the event as proof of identification. Some countries have therefore felt obliged to carry out — or perhaps duplicate — the identification processes, using their own systems and resources; that could have been avoided had agreed standards been in force.

The identification of a foreign victim cannot always be achieved without the co-operation of the authorities of that person's home country. Information about a missing person is essential but, if the person's own country's authorities do not have confidence and trust, they may withhold information and retain material for their own later use. There have been extreme cases where all material has been withheld. This will clearly seriously hamper the identification process: citizens of foreign countries involved in a disaster may remain unidentified, and the accurate identification of other victims may also be compromised.

6.2 Liaison Between Member Countries

The following recommendations endeavour to ensure:
- smooth and efficient cooperation, either through Interpol or directly between member countries, in the identification of victims
- the basic human rights of victims and next-of-kin with regard to accurate identification whenever possible, irrespective of the origin of the deceased

6.3 International Identification Standard

6.3.1 Responsibilities of the Interpol General Secretariat

It is recommended that the General Secretariat, under the authority of the General Assembly, should:

1   maintain a Standing Committee on Disaster Victim Identification responsible for:
    - recommending measures for improving identification procedures and international cooperation in the identification processes
    - recommending improvements to, and the updating of, the Interpol Disaster Victim Identification Forms and Guide, as experience is gained and new techniques are discovered
    - updating and circulating recommendations on methods, procedures and Disaster Victim Identification documentation to member countries
2   encourage member countries to accept and apply the Standing Committee's recommendations
3   remind member countries of Resolution AGN/65/RES/13 (Appendix D) when dealing with incidents involving foreign nationals
4   ask for reports on the identification processes that took place after all known disasters in member countries
5   publish annual reports on disasters and keeps computerised records of such information to be made available — on diskette or by other means — to all member countries on request.

6.3.2 Responsibilities of Member Countries

In preparation for circumstances where disaster victim identification might be required, each member country is advised to take the following steps:

1   establish a Disaster Victim Identification Liaison Team affiliated to its National Central Bureau (NCB) and comprising a police officer, a forensic pathologist and forensic odontologists whose names should be circulated to all member countries on a list kept up to date by the General Secretariat. The members of this team should:
    - be familiar with the Interpol disaster victim identification procedures, forms and recommendations
    - be responsible for all contact, via Interpol if necessary, with the NCB of a country in which a disaster has occurred
    - be responsible for providing antemortem information on the Interpol form in an Interpol language, and for transmission of the form to the relevant country's Disaster Victim Identification Team
    - be responsible for the transmission of all identification evidence to the country concerned
    - ensure that, if a disaster occurs, their own regional and national authorities are informed of the procedures described in the Interpol Disaster Victim Identification Guide, including these recommendations.

2 establish a multidisciplinary Disaster Victim Identification Team (police officers, forensic pathologist, forensic odontologist, and so on) to:
- advise and assist the local police when a body or bodies are found that cannot rapidly be identified by someone who knew the missing person or persons and when circumstances suggest that identification may be difficult
- assist with disaster victim identification operations in another country.

6.3.2.1 If a disaster occurs on their territory, member countries should take the following action:
- immediately assume responsibility for identification
- notify all other countries whose citizens may be involved via Interpol
- obtain antemortem details on the Interpol Disaster Victim Identification Forms
- accept assistance from disaster victim identification personnel from countries whose citizens are involved
- make permanent evidential records of disaster victim identification material and data, and offer other countries' disaster victim identification personnel an opportunity to examine such records and material
- offer assisting Disaster Victim Identification Teams the opportunity to give their opinions on the identification of their citizens
- allow assisting Disaster Victim Identification Teams to examine physical evidence pertaining to the identification of their fellow citizens
- record all identification evidence on Interpol Disaster Victim Identification forms.

It is also strongly recommended that they:
- invite disaster victim identification personnel from other countries whose citizens are known to be involved, or if the task of identification is likely to be particularly difficult
- allow assisting disaster victim identification personnel to visit and examine the incident site
- allow appropriate visiting disaster victim identification experts to take part in or witness postmortem examinations and subsequent data comparison
- ask assisting disaster victim identification personnel to sign identification documents
- provide opportunities for disaster victim identification personnel from other countries to attend as observers, in order to gain experience.

6.3.2.2 Member countries whose citizens are missing in a disaster should:
- promptly answer all requests for information and assistance from the country on whose territory the incident has occurred
- immediately notify the relevant country when their nationals are reported as potentially involved
- rapidly provide full antemortem information on their missing citizens, including fingerprints, DNA samples, X-rays, dental records, etc., on Interpol forms and in an Interpol language
- provide disaster victim identification expert assistance and equipment if requested
- keep copies of any documents sent to another country
- sign the identification documents completed by the country in which the incident has occurred, seeking permission to do so if necessary.

6.4 Conclusion

Victims of disasters may not all be citizens of the country in which the disaster occurs. Whenever foreign nationals are or may be involved, the country dealing with identification should rapidly establish and then maintain close cooperation with the home countries of potential victims. It is preferable for a liaison officer from each of the countries involved to be attached to the disaster victim identification operation, for liaison purposes and to ensure that information is shared.

If a large number of victims are from a foreign country in which there is an established Victim Identification Commission, greater assistance from that country (in terms of expertise and equipment) could be sought. Although an expert group from a foreign country will normally work under the authority of the country inviting it to participate, there have been incidents in which the country dealing with the disaster did not possess the required expertise and resources. There have been cases where some or all responsibility for identification has been delegated to the foreign group.

There are no international agreements on cooperation, or the delegation of responsibility for disaster victim identification. Member countries are therefore advised to explore the possibility of one or more of their identification experts travelling immediately to the country in which an incident has occurred when their citizens are or may be victims. This would necessitate keeping a list of such experts with particulars of personal data, passport numbers and expiry dates, vaccinations and expiry dates, and photographs to facilitate visa applications. For each key person, alternatives should be listed in case that person is not available at the critical time. All those on the list must be prepared to travel at very short notice, and the important questions of personal insurance and remuneration on such occasions must be agreed on beforehand.

It may be possible for identification experts to be granted temporary diplomatic status on such occasions or, in the case of a commercial aircraft accident, be affiliated to a technical investigation commission for which international regulations already exist (viz. the ICAO Standards and Recommended Practices, Annex 13 to the Chicago Convention on International Civil Aviation).

Finally, the formation of one or more Interpol-approved International Identification Commissions may be considered the best way of assisting a member country, or other organizations such as the United Nations, whenever expertise and resources for handling victim identification are scarce or where impartiality is necessary.

The above information can be found at http://www.interpol.int/default.asp

Appendix B

Australasian Disaster Victim Identification Committee

Strategic Plan 2002–2005 and Terms of Reference

Mission
Excellence in the provision of Disaster Victim Identification for the community.

Goal 1
Develop, promote, coordinate and review quality management and International best practice in DVI throughout Australia and New Zealand.

Strategies:

- maintain national guidelines in line with INTERPOL standards
- promote and support the maintenance of jurisdictional policies and procedures in accordance with the national guidelines
- develop appropriate subplans for a DVI response to specific types of incidents, such as chemical, biological or radiological (CBR)
- ensure that all practitioners receive an agreed minimum standard of training
- develop systematic evaluations of DVI operations
- develop standards to ensure the competence of all practitioners is regularly monitored
- develop guidelines for the occupational health, safety and welfare of DVI practitioners
- ensure appropriate representation at international DVI meetings.

Goal 2
Develop, coordinate and conduct education and professional development programs in DVI.

Strategies:

- continued development and implantation of national DVI competency standards
- develop training programs for the separate phases of the DVI process
- facilitate the development, co-ordination and delivery of relevant workshops and seminars
- facilitate the development and implementation of DVI exercises for national use
- ensure appropriate representation and/or participation in jurisdictional and national DVI exercises.

Goal 3
Provide advice and assistance for the preparedness and coordination of DVI through-out Australia and New Zealand.

Strategies:

- identify resource implications associated with DVI responses and the individual capacity of each jurisdiction to manage the range of DVI incidents.

- foster partnerships between the individual disciplines involved in the DVI process to ensure effective and coordinated incident response
- identify relevant stakeholders/agencies and develop strategic alliances
- ensure appropriate partnerships are developed to provide assistance and support to families of victims
- maintain a register of DVI practitioners
- provide a focus for response and input into international DVI issues
- develop national information technology capabilities for DVI
- provide continuing national forum to enhance national DVI capabilities
- Identify research opportunities and support research programs within DVI.

Goal 4
Develop the DVI capacity and capability to prepare for and respond to multi-casualty terrorist incidents.

Strategies:
- identify potential terrorist incidents, that could impact on DVI
- support the development of networks for advice on threat assessment
- develop interagency protocols and agreements with affected emergency response agencies
- develop operational standards for DVI incident response
- identify and recommend appropriate research and development facilities or opportunities
- identify equipment specification requirements
- facilitate the development of jurisdictional capability assessments
- identify training equipment
- provide input into relevant training standards and programs.

Goal 5
Provide greater exposure of DVI to government, the community and police command.

Strategies:
- increase the awareness of the roles and functions of DVI to other emergency services by actively supporting participation in emergency response exercises
- enhance the awareness of DVI to relevant organisations and bodies by developing DVI information packages
- maintain cross-cultural partnerships with community leaders
- raise the awareness of the individual operational capabilities of each jurisdiction and their respective ability to deal with large scale DVI incidents.

Goal 6
Develop a DVI capability to support the South West Pacific Region in the event of a mass casualty incident.

Strategies:
- liaise with government and nongovernment agencies regarding protocols and provision of support.

- develop formal contact and reporting arrangements
- develop protocols for the provision of administrative and logistical support
- formulate national call out procedures.

Terms of Reference

Aim: To facilitate the achievement of professionalism and best practice in Disaster Victim Identification (DVI) throughout Australia and New Zealand.

Reason for establishment:
- on evaluating the DVI management of a number of multi-casualty incidents that had occurred within Australia it was identified that there was an overall lack of uniformity in approach and that there were differences in the levels of response and application of the DVI processes between the respective states/territories
- to develop national DVI guidelines and procedures that will facilitate a uniform approach to large scale incidents beyond the capacity of any one jurisdiction
- to raise the level of DVI practises within Australia to international standards.

Benefits of continuation:
- to provide a forum for the review of both international and national incidents for ongoing DVI development
- to maintain liaison between DVI commanders and other key emergency services personnel
- to provide opportunity for mutual support between Australia and New Zealand in DVI planning and response
- to develop and maintain liaison between Australia and New Zealand and other international DVI representatives
- to develop procedures in response to emerging and unrecognised DVI issues. (e.g., current research and development into chemical, biological and radiological (CBR) incidents)
- to provide the opportunity for Australian and New Zealand delegates to meet annually to discuss and resolve issues of regional importance
- to ensure that Australia and New Zealand maintain their status as world leaders in the area of DVI management.

Reporting lines:
- each state/territory/country has a senior police officer as the DVI commander responsible for the management of DVI incidents occurring within the respective jurisdiction
- the Australian DVI Committee comprises the jurisdictional DVI commanders and representatives from the other DVI disciplines, including forensic pathologists, forensic odontologists, forensic technicians and specialist police groups
- the Chairman of the Australasian DVI Committee reports to the Officer in Charge of the Conference of Commissioners of Police of Australasia and the South West Pacific Region.

Relationships with other agencies: The Australian DVI Committee has direct association with:

- state/territory and New Zealand DVI Committees
- Emergency Management Australia
- National Institute of Forensic Science
- INTERPOL Standing Committee on DVI
- Australasian Coroner's Society
- Australasia and South West Pacific Region Police
- Commissioners Conference
- ADF/NZDF

Timelines: Ongoing.

Funding arrangements: The Australasian DVI Committee is funded by annual contributions from the police services of Australia and New Zealand. The funding allocations are based on relative strengths of employees. The funds are held and maintained by the Chairman of the Australasian DVI Committee.

Membership: The membership of the Australasian DVI Committee comprises the eight Australian States and Territories and New Zealand DVI Commanders and a representative from one of the other DVI disciplines from each jurisdiction.

External relationships:

- airline industry
- other transport authorities
- funeral industry
- health departments/public hospitals
- defence forces
- Department of Foreign Affairs and Trade (Aus)
- Ministry of FAI (NZ)
- consulates
- INTERPOL
- other appropriate agencies as need arises.

The above information can be found at http://www.ema.gov.au

Appendix C

Identification of Human Remains — Forensic Anthropology

I. Role of the Forensic Anthropologist

Principle

The forensic anthropologist assists in the recovery and identification remains following a mass fatality incident.

A forensic anthropologist has specialised training, education and experience in the recovery, sorting and analysis of human and nonhuman remains, especially those that are burned, commingled, and traumatically fragmented.

Procedure

In a mass fatality incident, the forensic anthropologist assists in the recovery, sorting, analysis and identification of remains. Specifically, with regard to the identification of human remains, the forensic anthropologist is expected to:

- provide information concerning the biological characteristics (e.g., age at death, sex, race and stature) of the deceased
- assist the medical examiner/coroner in determining the circumstances surrounding the death of the individual.

Summary

The forensic anthropologist is expected to assist with the recovery, analysis and identification of the remains.

II. Initial Evaluation

Principle

The specifics of the mass fatality incident determine the relative state of preservation and degree of fragmentation of the remains.

Procedure

The forensic anthropologist is expected to:

- evaluate and document the condition of the remains, including: complete remains, fragmented remains, burned remains, decomposed remains, commingled remains and any combination of the above
- separate obviously commingled remains to calculate the minimum number of individuals, while ensuring continuity of the established numbering system
- analyse the remains to determine sex, age at death, stature and other distinguishing characteristics
- assist in determining the need for additional analysis by other forensic identification disciplines (e.g., radiology, odontology)
- maintain a log of incomplete remains to facilitate future reassociation
- document, remove and save nonhuman and/or nonbiological materials for proper disposal.

Summary

The forensic anthropologist assesses the condition of the remains and assists in analyses.

III. Forensic Anthropological Analysis

Principle

The forensic anthropologist is expected to analyse the remains, depending on their condition, using various methods to determine biological attributes (e.g., age, sex, race, stature and idiosyncrasies). Even very small skeletal fragments may be useful in both personal identification and determining of the circumstances surrounding death.

Procedure

The forensic anthropologist is expected to evaluate, when possible, the following: sex, age at death, race, stature, antemortem pathological conditions (e.g., diseases or healed fractures), anomalies/abnormalities (including surgical hardware and prosthetic devices), perimortem trauma.

Summary

The forensic anthropologist is expected to use skeletal features to develop a biological profile.

IV. Additional Forensic Procedures

Principle

The forensic anthropologist is expected to assist in other procedures and use additional information from other forensic identification specialists in the analysis of remains.

Procedure

The forensic anthropologist is expected to assist with the following:

- obtaining DNA samples from soft tissue and bone
- taking and interpreting radiographs/X-rays
- interpreting trauma (with the medical examiner/coroner)
- obtaining and isolating dental evidence
- comparing antemortem and postmortem records.

Summary

The multidisciplinary approach to the identification process is vital to the successful response to and outcome of a mass fatality incident.

Source: Mass Fatality Incidents: A Guide for Human Forensic Identification. Publication of the United States. Department of Justice, National Institute of Justice, June 2005. (Complete report available at http://www.ojp.usdoj.gov/nij)

Appendix D
Is the Laboratory Prepared to Handle a Mass Fatality?

Number of victims _____

Number of victim samples _____

Number of personal items _____

Number of kin _____

Whom will the laboratory be reporting to?

Who is responsible for funding the DNA identification effort?

How will the victim samples be collected and tracked?

How will the samples get to the laboratory?

How many family reference collection kits are immediately available? What modifications to the kits may need to be made?

Are there written instructions for kin reference sample collection?

How will the personal reference samples be coordinated locally, nationally, and internationally?

How will the personal reference samples and elimination samples be schedules and collected?

Is there an adequate accessioning area to receive all samples?

Are there procedures to handle incomplete of missing data?

Is there a laboratory information management system (LIMS) in place to track cases, including victim and reference samples?

Can cases be combined or separated in the LIMS?

How will a victim be defined (as a case)?

Is there adequate staffing for each of the following?
- collection
- accessioning
- extraction
- amplification
- analysis
- interpretation
- reporting
- quality control
- family relations
- media relations
- new personnel.

Is there sufficient space for the victim and reference samples? Are the areas separate?

Will the testing be done in house or will some of the samples be outsourced?

If samples will be outsourced, are contracts in place that can be modified?

What modifications need to be made specific to mass fatality? For example, how will the data be reported?

Will an advisory group be needed to provide technical support and to assist the laboratory in making major decisions?

Are there adequate extraction procedures and robotics to handle the volume? Do the parameters need to be changed for victim samples?

Can additional reagents be purchased from the same lot number already used by the laboratory?

Can the mass fatality identification effort be handled without purchasing additional equipment? Does the laboratory have the capacity?

If the lab does not have the capacity, are there procedures and policies in place to acquire equipment and consumables rapidly?

How will the generated profiles be stored?

How will matching take place?

Is there a mechanism to review the supporting metadata for accuracy?

Is there a checklist in place?

How will reports be generated?

How will reports be issued?

How will remains and personal items be returned to the families? How will this be documented?

Does the laboratory have the financial resources to handle the identification effort?

Can the laboratory handle a backlog of its normal casework while it works on the identification effort? If so, how big can the backlog get?

Does the laboratory have kinship analysis software?

Is there a policy to handle the situation in which the generis relationship is not consistent with the biological relationship reported by the family?

Does the laboratory have a relationship with a bioethicist?

Other _____

Source: Lessons Learned From 9/11: DNA Identification in Mass Fatality Incidents. United States Department of Justice, National Institute of Justice, September 2006. (Complete report available at http://www.ojp.usdoj.gov)

Forensic Nanotechnology, Biosecurity and Medical Professionalism: Improving the Australian Health Care System's Response to Terrorist Bombings

Thomas Alured Faunce

This chapter explores how medical professionalism in forensic bioterrorist investigations may be influenced by the enhanced surveillance, detection and data storage capacities offered by nanotechnology. It draws on the author's experience treating patients injured in the 2002 Bali bombings.

It is now well accepted that health professionals involved in forensic investigations may experience conflict of interest problems with moral, ethical, legal and human rights dimensions. Physicians acquiring information, for example, about crimes from patients may have to breach ethical and legal obligations of confidentiality in disclosing that information to justice authorities (British Medical Association, 2001). The professional obligations of physicians involved in forensic investigations extend to the collation of evidence and provision of testimony within an adversarial legal system (Freckelton, 2006). Many of these duties have the potential to create dilemmas for a physician's sense of professionalism, which is generally characterised by an emphasis on public service, rather than profit-earning, by an occupation with State-recognised special skill.

Physicians treating terrorist suspects or involved in investigating allegations of massacres, may be assisted in resolving any resultant conflict of interest dilemmas by reference not only to basic principles of medical ethics, but to relevant United Nations guidelines (United Nations, 1982; United Nations, 1995). International humanitarian law is another important source of professional norms by which physicians can calibrate legislation or other obligations to the state requiring their involvement in such areas. It is an aggregation of customary and treaty-based principles and rules concerned with the treatment of wounded, civilians and prisoners in war, and overlapping with many areas of medical ethics (United Nations, 1949). Of particular importance are the *Universal Declaration of Human Rights* (UDHR; United Nations, 1948), the *International Covenant on Civil and Political Rights* (ICCPR; (United Nations, 1966a), and the

International Covenant on Economic, Cultural and Social Rights (ICESCR; United Nations, 1966b). Article 7 of the *ICCPR*, as well as prohibiting torture or cruel, unusual or degrading treatment or punishment also provides that 'no one shall be subjected without his free consent to medical or scientific experimentation'. Vitally important is the influence of nongovernmental organisations (NGOs) such as *Physicians for Human Rights and Medecins Sans Frontiers* and *International Physicians for Prevention of War* (Hannibal & Lawrence, 1996). Such NGOs emphasise the role of physicians as promoters for the regime of international human rights developing, not in a legalistic way from consent of sovereign states, but as the outcome of an attitudinal global community of principle with the power to change democratic functioning in the age of electronic mass communication (Grossman, 1995; Lowe, 1988–1989).

Forensic Interest in Nanotechnology

Nanotechnology involves the engineering design, fabrication, application and regulation of products at atomic, molecular or macromolecular levels of approximately 1 nanometer to 100 nanometers; a nanometer constituting one-billionth of a metre (United States FDA, 2006). 'Bottom Up' nanomanufacturing uses methods such as atomic condensation and chemical vapour deposition to self-assemble nanostructures under control of reactant or physical restrictions. 'Top-Down' nanoassembly techniques rely on pattern transfer to a nanosubstrate from bulk materials, by means of, for example, focused ion-beam milling (Freeman, Luther-Davies, & Madden, 2006) electron-beam lithography and nanoimprint lithography (Belotti, Galli, Bajoni, Andreani, Guizzetti et al., 2004). Nanostructures have much greater strength, stability and surface area per unit mass than standard materials. Those below 10 nm possess quantum effects where size may control, for example, conductivity or the specific wavelength of emitted light (Sone, Fujita, Ochiai, Manako, Matsui et al., 1999).

Applications of nanotechnology are likely to enhance forensic capabilities in almost every area, including enhanced surveillance capabilities and capacity to detect toxicological compounds and forensic evidence in tissue, materials and soil.

The United States Department of Justice (DOJ) National Institute of Justice (NIJ) has a program to develop a nanotechnology device that will be integrated into the current crime laboratory processes and protocols to analyse forensic DNA samples (Roco, 2006).

As another example, forensic analysis of gun-shot residue will benefit from nanotechnology-facilitated detection of the related elemental and crystallographic signatures of nanoparticles created by nonequilibrium thermodynamic processes. This should reduce the amount of residue required for analysis and the need for its relative lack of contamination (Reynolds & Hart, 2004).

Biosecurity, Nanotechnology and Medical Professionalism

Detecting, preventing and punishing bioterrorism is a national research priority in most developed nations, including Australia (Smallwood, Merianos, & Matthews, 2002). Bioterrorist threats could involve aerosol attacks on individuals or crowds, 'dirty' bombs and targeted contamination food sources (Alberts, 2005) such as botulinum in milk (Wein & Liu, 2005), or release of pathogenic organisms or biotoxins in the water supply (Nuzzo, 2006). Such threats might also exploit unexpectedly virulent scientific discoveries such as mousepox IL-4 (Jackson et al., 2001), or medical publication of the full genetic sequence of a highly lethal strain of influenza virus, such as caused the Spanish influenza pandemic in the winter of 1918–1919 (Taubenberger et al., 2005; Tumpey et al., 2005).

Atlantic Storm was a simulated bioterrorism exercise based on the deliberate release of smallpox viruses in various European and North American cities. It revealed many nations had inadequate vaccine stockpiles and plans, while highlighting the need to develop innovative technologies (including nanotechnology) capable of allowing health workers to rapidly diagnose such an atypical infection and effectively communicate its details to public health authorities (Hamilton & Smith, 2006).

Ethical and legal regulatory interventions against such bioterrorism may involve research project biosecurity review systems and internationally binding rules on data publication and laboratory biosecurity, as well as a standing biosecurity board (Atlas, Campbell, Cozzarelli, Curfman, Enquist et al., 2003; Royal Society, 2004). Many are concerned, however, that such a system might inhibit that sharing of data that is vital for collegiality in the international medical and scientific communities (United States National Academy of Sciences, 2004).

Nanotechnology offers the prospect that biosecurity in the future may be critically dependent on billions of widespread invisible sensors, integrated into clothing, buildings, vehicles and natural objects, collating unprecedented amounts of data for capacious nanodata storage units in a form of 'ambient intelligence'. Skin-implanted nanosize radio frequency ID (RFID) tags, for instance, could control access to biosecure premises. Nanofluidics may provide rapid analysis of biological samples (such as blood, semen and saliva) by forcing them through nanosized channels etched onto a microchip (Thomas, 2006).

The United States DOJ and NIJ have a program to develop a wearable, low-cost nanotechnology device that overcomes limitations with the existing biologic detection method based on vapour exposure of an immobilised enzyme surface, and aims to provide health workers, among others, with early warning of exposure to unanticipated chemical and biological hazards (Roco, 2006).

The Forensic Science Centre at Lawrence Livermore National Laboratory in the United States is developing nanostructured materials for applications to forensics and homeland security. These include silica-based nanomaterials, molecular imprinted polymers, and silicon platforms, for the collection, concentration and detection of chemical weapons or other related compounds (Reynolds & Hart, 2004)

A major concern for physicians involved in such forensic use of nanotechnology for biosecurity purposes is likely to be safety for themselves and their patients. Engineered nanoparticles (ENPs) may present unique health risks when used in medical and forensic applications (Faunce, 2007). They are highly reactive and mobile within the human body and there are currently no effective methods to monitor ENP exposure risks in patients or healthcare workers (Department of Employment and Workplace Relations, 2005). Health risks of nanostructures cannot be predicted a priori from their bulk equivalent. ENPs in isolated cell experiments have caused DNA damage. Short-term animal exposure to ENPs has produced dose-dependent inflammatory responses and pulmonary fibrosis. Crucial chronic in vivo exposure studies (in particular of reproductive toxicity) have yet to be published. Such (limited) animal studies as do exist, raise serious concerns about preferential accumulation in, and inhibition of, mito-chondrial function and the fact that nanostructures may become unstable in bio-logical settings and release elemental metals (Faunce, 2007).

In such a nanosurveillance-dominated society, doctors may play crucial roles in controlling the privacy and confidentiality of patient information as well as in the detection and prevention of injury from bioterrorism. States negotiating under the *Biological and Toxin Weapons Convention* (BTWC) recently empha-sised the need for codes of conduct for scientists and public health physicians to counter future bioterrorist threats, partly by warning of the professional perils involved in deliberate or inadvertent release of information and substances (United Nations, 2005). How such nanotechnology developments are likely to impact on medical professionalism issues in the biosecurity context may be further illustrated by a reconsideration of the medical treatment of the 2002 Bali bombing victims.

Nanotechnology and Improving the Australian Health Care System's Response to Terrorist Bombing

Analysis of casualties from terrorist bombings shows that the majority of survivors, generally those furthest from the blast and presenting earliest to hospital, suffer only minor, noncritical injuries; for example, minor penetrating trauma, tinnitus, psychological stress, and simple fractures (Leibovici, Gofrit, Stein, Shapira, Noga et al., 1996). These injuries are often to the face, hands and arms; probably showing the protective effects of clothing (Brismar & Bergenwald, 1982; Golan, Golan, Alder, Sternberg, Zagher et al., 1982). Only approximately 10% to 20% of survivors require admission to an intensive care unit (Frykberg, 2002). This situation, however, is likely to change as terrorists incorporate radioactive and biological hazards into such bombs.

The traditional teaching about terrorist bomb injuries classifies as 'primary' those deriving from the blast wave itself (Freund, Kopolovic, & Durst, 1980). 'Secondary' injuries are described as arising relatively immediately from shrapnel, structural debris or heat propelled by the blast wave. 'Tertiary' injuries are caused by the patient's immediate displacement against solid objects or from building collapse or fire. Building collapse is a deliberate terrorist aim to maximise casual-ties from a bomb blast. Most mortality from the Oklahoma City bombing in 1995 and from the World Trade Centre attack in 2001, for example, arose from tertiary injuries caused by building collapse and fire (Mallonee, Shariat, Stennies, Waxweiler, Hogan et al., 1996).

A fourth category of terrorist bomb injury, however, could arise from the terror-ists' deliberate intention to create secondary hazards for victims, rescuers or medical staff. Techniques include a second bomb attached to a mock or pseudovictim, or par-ticularly relevant in this context, additional use of radiation or biologic vectors.

On October 12, 2002, the author was on duty in Melbourne as a senior registrar at one of the largest intensive care units in Australia. On that day, a bomb containing approximately 500 mg g^{-1} TNT and 80 cm to 120 cm above the ground, exploded near the northern wall of a bar in Kuta, Bali. The first patient later received by our unit, a fit 28-year-old male, was standing in the main walkway approximately 15 m to 20 m away from this blast. Approximately 5 minutes later a larger bomb, constructed from 50 kg to 150 kg chlorate and ammonium nitrate located in a van outside the nearby Sari Club, was also detonated by remote control. The second and third patients admitted to our unit, a 52-year-old male and a 36-year-old female, were approximately 5 m to 10 m from this blast (Faunce, 2003a)

The first patient extricated himself from the burning and collapsed building. His primary, secondary and tertiary injuries were partial and full thickness burns to 40% of his body (neck, back, arms and legs), shrapnel wounds to the buttocks, multiple 1 cm to 2 cm lacerations and bilateral perforated tympanic membranes. He underwent debridement and removal of shrapnel and suturing of multiple lacerations under general anaesthetic at the Sanglah Central General Hospital in Denpasar, Bali, being further assessed by a team of Australian medical specialists on the tarmac. He was transported by RAAF Hercules aircraft to Darwin and at Darwin Hospital was resuscitated in the general ward, before being transferred to our ICU via an RAAF Hercules aircraft then helicopter.

The second patient had been 5 m to 10 m from the blast at the Sari Club. The details of his initial removal from the building and treatment at the scene or in Bali were largely unknown. He was diagnosed as suffering from the secondary injury of 44% burns to the head, neck, face and back, as well as the right and left arm. He underwent an escharotomy to the back of the right and left leg and the left arm in Bali. The patient was transferred via fixed wing aircraft from Bali to the Royal Darwin Hospital ICU, then to our unit.

The third patient had been standing close to the explosion and suffered significant primary blast injury and secondary 33% full thickness burns. The blast or associated shrapnel severely traumatised her left lower limb. She was also diagnosed to have suffered rupture of the globe of the right eye, a fracture of the right iliac wing and subluxation right ankle. She was intubated at Denpasar Hospital. Her haemoglobin level there was recorded as 4.0 g dl^{-1} and she was transfused 4 units of packed cells. She received an escharotomy of both limbs via the Australian field retrieval service. At Royal Darwin Hospital the patient was noted to have secondary shrapnel wounds in her abdomen. A left above-knee amputation was performed and a fasciotomy of the left leg. She was evacuated via fixed wing aircraft and helicopter to our ICU.

The motivation for these bombings remains controversial, but probably related to the involvement of Australian military forces in Afghanistan and Iraq. As a senior intensive care registrar in one of Australia's largest ICUs, I was unaware of any plan for handling such terrorist bombing injuries and, in particular, believe there were no guidelines at that time requiring assessment of bioterrorist threats in this situation (Faunce, 2003b). How would the use of nanotechnology in biosurveillance change the hospital management of such patients?

First, the patients would have been subjected to nanotechnology screening for bioterrorist chemical and viral vectors before being brought into the ICU. Second, nanosize radio frequency ID (RFID) tags would have controlled and documented access of staff and relatives to these biosecure premises. Nanofluidics would have provided rapid analysis of biological samples from the patients. Nanotechnology diagnostics would more rapidly detect pleural effusions, rib fractures, ruptured organs and blood vessels and shrapnel. The resultant chest drains would be coated with nanoparticles to reduce risk of infection. Split skin grafting and wound debridement would be facilitated by nanotechnology sensors able to detect and remove minute shrapnel and debris particles. Nanotherapeutics (for example nanomanufactured artificial red blood cells) may provide better treatments for septicaemia and multiorgan failure.

The three patients discussed here all developed complex gram negative infections due to atypical organisms. The dominant organism was *acinetobacter*, but of a type not previously seen in our unit. What if it had been a form of the 1918 influenza virus, or smallpox? Would not the presence of nanosensors on the clothing of the treating health professionals have protected them and assisted treatment of the patient?

Hepatitis (HBV/HCV) and HIV serology were obtained in all three patients by the infectious disease staff, after discussion with the patient's family. Such samples were taken from the other two patients and were designed to monitor contamination during the possibly chaotic resuscitation in Bali. Nanofluidics would have facilitated rapid analysis of such biological samples. Nanocomputing would have assisted rapid compilation of a large amount of information about the nature of the injuries, the associated risks and best responses thereto.

This widespread use of nanotechnology in such a setting would raise significant issues for health professionals about balancing patient and staff confidentiality and privacy with the requirements of public health disaster plans and quarantine laws (Rubinson et al., 2005).

Use of nanotechnology in critical care biosurveillance is likely to make staff and patients feel more secure and do their jobs better in such pressure, tense and often fear-filled situations. Among the critically injured after such a terrorist attack, approximately one third will die within the first 2 weeks of treatment (Frykberg, Tepas, & Alexander, 1989; Hadden, Rutherford, & Merrett, 1978). Most ICUs now have systems of individual peer support and group debriefing, often augmented by the services of consultation-liaison-psychiatry, for staff suffering unique physical, cognitive, emotional or behavioural symptoms as the result of exposure to a mass casualty terrorist event (Gidron, 2002). Surviving patients and staff may experience long-term post traumatic stress disorder (Lee, Isaac, & Janca, 2002).

All three patients from the 2002 Bali bombings were given hyperbaric oxygen treatment, two chiefly for cerebral gas embolism and the third to speed recovery from burns. The use of hyperbaric oxygen in burns treatment remains controversial, the chief factor being accessibility and the hazards of transfer (Brannen et al., 1997). Theoretically, high pressure oxygen, while preserving oxygen delivery through massively enhanced plasma partial pressures, may reduce postcapillary leak by vasoconstriction, enhance white blood cell function and promote activation of fibroblasts and elaboration of collagen (Neizgoda et al., 1997). Its impact, however, on pathogenic organisms and biotoxins (and their monitoring by nanotechnology) is an area that urgently needs to be researched.

In Australia, the Federal government may use biosecurity-linked nanotechnology to implement sweeping control and surveillance powers relevant to such health care institutions under legislation based on the constitutional quarantine power (s51(ix)). Disaster plans based on modelling of such biosecurity threats may require constraints over hospital staff that conflict, for example, not only with the Australian constitutional prohibition on 'civil conscription' of 'medical services' (s51(xxiiiA)) but fundamental norms of medical ethics and international human rights. The successful implementation of such plans may actually depend on how carefully they have been integrated with basic standards and principles of medical professionalism.

Conclusions

The secondary targeting of hospitals by bioterrorist agents may be part of a tactic to disable disaster response plans. Nanotechnology allows medical professionals to much more effectively assess, warn and protect the public in relation to such bioterrorist threats. Implementation of a forensic protocol requiring use of nanotechnology sensors to rapidly and effectively detect biohazardous substances associated with such patients, is also likely to facilitate forensic processes associated with the formal justice system.

References

Alberts, B. (2005) Modeling attacks on the food supply. *Proceedings of the National Academy of Sciences USA, 102,* 9737–9738

Atlas, R., Campbell, P., Cozzarelli, N.R., Curfman, G., Enquist, L., Fink, G. et al. (2003). Statement on scientific publication and security, *Science, 299,* 1149.

Belotti, M., Galli, M., Bajoni, D., Andreani, L.C., Guizzetti, G., Decanini, D. et al. (2004). Investigation of SOI photonic crystals fabricated by both electron-beam lithography and nanoimprint lithography. *Microelectronic Engineering, 73–74,* 405–411.

Brannen, A.L., Still, J., Haynes, M., Orlet, H., Rosenblum, F., Law, E., & Thompson, W.O. (1997). A randomised prospective trial of hyperbaric oxygen in a referral burn centre population. *The American Surgeon, 63,* 205–208.

Brismar, B., & Bergenwald, L. (1982). The terrorist bomb explosion in Bologna, Italy 1980: An analysis of the effects and injuries sustained. *Journal of Trauma, 22,* 216–220.

British Medical Association. (Eds.) (2001). The forensic doctor. In British Medical Association (Ed.), *The medical profession and human rights: Handbook for a changing agenda* (pp. 130–161). London: Zed Books.

Brower, V. (2006). Is nanotechnology ready for primetime? *Journal of the Natural Cancer Institute, 98,* 9–11.

Department of Employment and Workplace Relations (DEWR). (2005). *Australian Government: Submission to senate inquiry into workplace exposure to toxic dusts and nanoparticles.* Canberra: Author.

Faunce, T.A. (2003a, May). *The Bali disaster: principles of management for Australian intensive care.* Paper presented at the Australian and New Zealand Anaesthesia and Intensive Care Scientific Meeting, Hobart, Tasmania.

Faunce, T.A. (2003b, March 24). Hospitals are not protected from bioterrorism. *Canberra Times*, p. 11.

Faunce, T. (2007.) Nanotechnology in global medicine and human biosecurity: private interests, policy dilemmas and the calibration of public health law. *Journal of Law, Medicine and Ethics, 35*(4), 629–642.

Freckelton, I. (2006). Doctors and forensic expertise. In I. Freckelton & K. Petersen (Eds.), *Disputes and dilemmas in health law* (pp. 406–435). Sydney, Australia: Federation Press.

Freeman, D., Luther-Davies, B., & Madden, S. (2006, July). *Real-time drift correction of a focused ion beam milling system.* Abstract of oral presentation, Australian Research Council Nanotechnology Network International Conference on Nanoscience and Naotechnology, Brisbane, Australia.

Freund, U., Kopolovic, J., & Durst, A. (1980). Compressed air emboli of the aortas and renal artery in blast injury, *Injury, 12*, 37.

Frykberg, E.R. (2002). Medical management of disasters and mass casualties from terrorist bombings: how can we cope? *Journal of Trauma, 53*, 201–212.

Frykberg, E.R., Tepas, J.J., & Alexander, R.H. (1989). The 1983 Beirut airport terrorist bombing: Injury patterns and implications for disaster management. *The American Surgeon, 55*, 134–141.

Gidron, Y. (2002). Posttraumatic stress disorder after terrorist attacks: A review. *Journal of Nervous and Mental Disease, 190*, 118–121.

Golan, J., Golan, E., Alder, J., Sternberg, N., Zagher, U., Rosenberg, B. et al. (1982). Plastic surgery and civilian casualties due to 'terrorist' activities. *Annals of Plastic Surgery, 8*, 359–362.

Grossman, L.K. (1995). *The electronic republic: Reshaping democracy in the information age.* New York: Viking.

Gunn, J., Yang, A., Palmbach, T., Dongguang, W., & Sinha, S. (2006). Nano-forensics-nanoparticles in gun-shot-residues emerging technologies. *Nanoelectronics, 2006 IEEE Conference,* 269–272.

Hadden, W.A., Rutherford, W.H., & Merrett, J.D. (1978). The injuries of terrorist bombing: A study of 1532 consecutive patients. *British Journal of Surgery, 655*, 25–531.

Hamilton, D.S., & Smith, B.T. (2006). Atlantic storm. *EMBO Reports, 7*, 4–9.

Hannibal, K., & R. Lawrence. (1996). The health professional as human rights promoter: Ten years of Physicians for Human Rights (USA). *Health and Human Rights, 2(1)*, 110–127.

Institute of Occupational Medicine for the Health and Safety Executive. (2004). *Nanoparticles: An occupational hygiene review.* Retrieved August 14, 2006, from http://www.hse.gov.uk

Jackson, R.J., Ramsay, A.J., Christensen, C.D., Beaton, S., Hall, D.F., & Ramshaw, I.A. (2001). Expression of mouse interleukin-4 by a recombinant ectromelia virus suppresses cytolytic lymphocyte responses and overcomes genetic resistance to mousepox. *Journal of Virology, 75*, 1205–1210.

Lee, A., Isaac, M., & Janca, A. (2002). Post-traumatic stress disorder and terrorism. *Current opinion in psychiatry, 15*, 633–637.

Leibovici, D., Gofrit, O.N., Stein, M., Shapira, S.C., Noga, Y., Heruti, R.J. et al. (1996). Blast injuries: Bus versus open-air bombings. A comparative study of injuries in survivors of open-air versus confined space explosions. *Journal of Trauma, 41*, 1030–1035.

Lowe, V. (1988–1989). The role of equity in international law. *Australian Yearbook of International Law, 12*, 54–81.

Mallonee, S., Shariat, S., Stennies, G., Waxweiler, R., Hogan, D., & Jordan, F. (1996). Physical injuries and fatalities resulting from the Oklahoma City bombing. *Journal of the American Medical Association, 276*, 382–387.

Niezgoda, J.A., Cianci, P., Folden, B.W., Ortega, R.L., Slade, J.B., & Storrow, A.B. (1997). The effect of hyperbaric oxygen therapy on a burn wound model in human volunteers. *Plastic and Reconstructive Surgery, 99*, 1620–1625.

Nuzzo, J.B. (2006). The biological threat to US water supplies: Toward a national water security policy. *Biosecurity and Bioterrorism, 4*, 147–159.

Reynolds, J.G., & Hart, B.R. (2004). Nanomaterials and their application to defense and homeland security. *Journal of Metals, 56*, 36–39.

Roco, M.C. (2006). *National nanotechnology investment in the FY 2003 Budget Request by the President*. National Science and Technology Council's subcommittee on Nanoscale Science, Engineering and Technology (NSET). Retrieved August 28, 2006, from http://www. nano.gov/2003budget.html

Royal Society. (2004). *The individual and collective roles scientists can play in strengthening international treaties*. London: The Royal Society.

Rubinson, L., Nuzzo, J.B., Talmor, D.S., O'Toole, T., Kramer, B.R., & Inglesby, T.V. (2005). Augmentation of hospital critical care capacity after bioterrosist attacks or epidemics: Recommendations of the Working Group on Emergency Mass Critical Care. *Journal of the American Medical Association, 33*, E1–E13.

Smallwood, R.A., Merianos, A., & Matthews, J.D. (2002). Bioterrorism in Australia. *Medical Journal of Australia, 176*, 251–253.

Sone, J., Fujita, J., Ochiai, Y., Manako, S., Matsui, S., Nomura, E. et al. (1999). Nanofabrication toward sub-10 nm and its application to novel nanodevices. *Nanotechnology, 10*, 135–141.

Taubenberger, J.K., Reid, A.H., Lourens, R.M., Wang, R., Jin, G., & Fanning, T.G. (2005). Characterization of the 1918 influenza virus polymerase genes. *Nature, 437*, 889–893

Thomas. J. (2006). Nanotechnology and surveillance. Little Brother is watching you. *Chain Reaction, 97*, 29.

Tumpey, T.M., Basler, C.F., Aguilar, P.V., Zeng, H., Solorzano, A., Swayne, D.E. et al. (2005). Characterization of the reconstructed 1918 Spanish influenza pandemic virus. *Science, 310*, 77–80.

United Nations. (1948). *Universal declaration of human rights*. Adopted 10 Dec. 1948. (GA Res 217A (III). UN Doc A/810 (1948) 71)

United Nations. (1949). *Convention for the amelioration of the condition of the wounded and sick in armed forces in the field* (UNTS 1949; 75: 31). *Convention for the amelioration of the condition of the wounded, sick and shipwrecked members of armed forces at sea* (UNTS 1949, 75, 85). *Convention relative to the treatment of prisoners of war* (UNTS 1949; 75: 135). *Convention relative to the protection of civilian persons in time of war* (UNTS 1949, 75, 287). *Additional protocol I 1977*.

United Nations. (1966a). *International covenant on civil and political rights*. Adopted 16 Dec 1966, entry into force 23 March 1976. (GA Res 2200A (XXI). UN GAOR Supp (No 16) 52. UN Doc A/6316 (1966). 999 UNTS 17), reprinted in ?*International Legal Materials 1967, 6*, 368.

United Nations. (1966b). *International covenant on economic, cultural and social rights*. Adopted 16 Dec 1966, entry into force 3 Jan. 1976. (GA Res 2200A(XXI). UN Doc A/6316 (1966). 993 UNTS 3), reprinted in *International Legal Materials 1966, 6*, 360.

United Nations. (1982). *Principles of medical ethics relevant to the role of health personnel, particularly physicians, in the protection of prisoners and detainees against torture and other cruel, inhuman or degrading treatment or punishment*. (GA Res 37/194, 18 Dec. 1982)

United Nations. (1995). *Guidelines for the conduct of United Nations inquiries into allegations of massacres 1995*. DPI/1710-1 UN Office of Legal Affairs.

United Nations. (2005). *States parties to biological weapons convention conclude meeting after discussing scientific codes of conduct*. Press release DC05044E, 9 Dec. New York: United Nations.

United States FDA. (2006). United States Food and Drug Administration. *Regulation of nanotechnology*. Retrieved August 19, 2006, from http://www.fda.gov/nanotechnology/regulation.html

United States National Academy of Sciences. (2004). *Biotechnology research in an age of terrorism*. Washington, DC: National Academies Press.

Wein, L.M., & Liu, Y. (2005). Analyzing a bioterror attack on the food supply: The case of botulinum toxin in milk. *Proceedings of the National Academy of Sciences USA, 102,* 9984–9989.

Institutions and the Health of Prisoners and Detainees

Christine Phillips

There are currently nine million persons in prisons around the world, with three countries — China, Russia and the United States — accounting for almost half the world's prison population (Walmsley, 2006). Penal practices in Australia reflect an international trend towards higher rates of imprisonment. Between 1995 and 2005, the imprisonment rate in Australia rose from 129 per 100,000 to 163 per 100,000. The largest increase in imprisonment in Australia has occurred among Indigenous Australians, whose imprisonment rate over the same period rose from 1335 to 2021 per 100,000 (Australian Bureau of Statistics, 2005).

People deprived of their liberty by the state may be subjected to two types of failure of protection. *Failures of commission* are events such as torture, in which detainees are physically or psychologically assaulted with the assent of the state. *Failures of omission* occur when the physical health and safety of detainees are damaged through failure to construct protective measures or adequate health care.

This chapter explores the physical impact of imprisonment on the imprisoned, and outlines the legal sanctions and ethical guidelines that may or may not allow physical harm to come to those detained by the state.

International Law and the Health and Safety of Detainees

Protection from torture is codified in a number of international instruments: the Convention Against Torture and Other Cruel, Inhuman and Degrading Treatment or Punishment (UNCAT), and the third and fourth Geneva Conventions. Each of these conventions is located within the framework of the Universal Declaration of Human Rights (1948), which declared protection from torture, and other cruel, inhuman or degrading treatment or punishment, to be an essential human right.

Torture was defined under UNCAT as:

> any act by which severe pain or suffering, whether physical or mental, is intentionally inflicted on a person for such purposes as obtaining from him or a third person information or a confession, punishing him for an act he or a third person has committed or is suspected of having committed, or intimidating or coercing him or a third person, or for any reason based on discrimination of any kind, when such pain or suffering is inflicted by or at the instigation of or with the consent or acquiescence of a public official or other person acting in an official capacity (Article 1).

'Cruel, inhuman or degrading treatment or punishment' is defined as acts of a severe nature that do not amount to torture. Most of the proscriptions against torture in UNCAT also apply to cruel, inhuman or degrading treatment or punishment. One exception to this rule is the proscription against refoulement (removal of a person to a state where they may be placed in danger). While ratifying states may not undertake refoulement for the purposes of torture, no such proscription exists in relation to cruel, inhuman or degrading punishment. This means it may be possible for a ratifying state to practise refoulement provided the treatment meted to the person was not severe enough to constitute torture.

By May 2006, 141 countries had become parties to the Convention, and therefore accepted it as a binding legal obligation. A further 74 countries have signed the Convention (Office of the High Commissioner for Human Rights, 2006).

The third Geneva Convention (GCIII) covers the treatment of prisoners of war in an international armed conflict. Article 17 states that:

> No physical or mental torture, nor any other form of
> coercion, may be inflicted on prisoners of war to secure
> from them information of any kind whatever. Prisoners
> of war who refuse to answer may not be threatened,
> insulted or exposed to unpleasant or disadvantageous
> treatment of any kind.

The fourth Geneva Convention (GCIV) covers the rights to physical safety of civilians in war. GCIV states that civilians in an armed conflict are usually 'Protected Persons'. Protected persons have the right to protection from 'murder, torture, corporal punishments, mutilation and medical or scientific experiments, but also to any other measures of brutality whether applied by noncombatant or military agents' (Article 32). This is not a universal protection. Exempted are individuals who are 'definitely suspected of or engaged in activities hostile to the security of the State', although GCIV states that 'such persons shall nevertheless be treated with humanity.' In addition, citizens of countries that have not signed GCIV, or citizens of countries that continue to have normal diplomatic representations with the country that holds them, are not protected under GCIV. In practice, this means that most citizens of neutral countries in a war zone cannot claim protection under GCIV.

Torture: A Failure of Commission

Coercive torture is undertaken generally for the purpose of gaining confessions or information about the activities of others. The paradigms of coercive torture are the Spanish and French inquisitorial courts of the 14th and 15th centuries. These courts sanctioned torture (at a time when the legal system also used torture) to gain confessions, although these confessions were invalid if they could not be repeated without torture (Peters, 1988). In the 20th century, coercive torture became part of the instruments of political inquisitors from many regimes (Conroy, 2001). In many ways torture has benefited from a globalised economy. Technological innovations such as electro-shock devices, which can cause severe pain without leaving permanent marks on the body, can be readily disseminated to interested countries, as can training in torture techniques. Amnesty International (2003) estimated that electro-shock devices, first developed in the 1970s, had been used for torture in over 87 countries between 1990 and 2003.

Although torture is regarded as a serious breach of human rights, the case for coercive torture is periodically revisited, often when the state perceives itself under threat. The 'ticking time-bomb' scenario is a well-known hypothetical used to underpin an argument for torture in extreme circumstances (see Box this page). The argument for torture in this scenario is premised on the assumption that torture is an effective and efficient inquisitorial method, an assumption that has been called into question (Rumsey, 2006).

Retributive torture is torture carried out for punishment. Forms of corporal punishment included in criminal codes around the world include stoning, limb or digit amputation, flagellation, branding and enucleation of the eye. From a human rights perspective, both corporal and capital punishment can be viewed as examples of cruel and inhuman punishment or torture. Arguments for corporal and capital punishment assert that these activities do not constitute torture as there is provision under UNCAT for exemption for 'pain and suffering that occurs arising from, inherent in, or incidental to lawful sanctions'. In a response to this position, the Special Rapporteur on torture to the UN Commission on Human Rights (1997) argued that 'lawful sanctions' refers to those principles and practices accepted by the international community; if internationally accepted norms about lawful practice are not taken into account, this would mean that unjust practices could always be deemed lawful on the basis that they were authorised through procedurally legitimate channels.

After the revelation of the work undertaken by Josef Mengele in Auschwitz, the medical profession clarified the ethical responsibilities of doctors in relation to persons in detention. The World Medical Association, in its Declaration of Tokyo (1975), expressly forbids doctors from participating in coercive or retributive torture. Despite this, doctors and health workers have participated in torture, or have failed to adequately advocate for those who are likely to have been tortured. The death of Steve Biko under interrogation in South Africa (Silove, 1990; Woods, 1991)

The Ticking Timebomb Argument

Somewhere in a crowded city, a time-bomb is primed to explode. Hundreds, possibly thousands, of people may be injured. Authorities hold in custody a person who they believe may be able to identify the location of the bomb, but the suspect says he cannot provide information. Are the authorities justified in torturing the suspect?

An argument for torture
In this very rare circumstance, if the authorities were certain they had the correct suspect, it would be hypocritical not to undertake torture in this circumstance, as it would be a preventive activity (Steinhoff 2006).

An argument against torture
Coercive torture may waste time if false or misleading answers are given in order to stop the torture. The dubious utility of this strategy is outweighed by the larger implications of overriding the prohibition against torture (Bufacchi and Arrigo 2006).

---

is an example of institutionalised failure of three doctors to intervene and prevent the death of someone who was clearly being tortured (see Box this page). In the United States there has been unease around the use of confidential medical information and the assistance of psychiatrists in crafting behavioural interrogation for detainees in Guantanamo Bay (Bloche & Marks, 2005).

Failures of Omission: Health and Safety in Prisons

Prisons are not safe places. Prisoners are more likely to be murdered or to commit suicide in prison (Butler & Karamina, 2005: 17). Sexual assault, especially for young men, is also very common. One of the few studies addressing prison rape in New South Wales found that one quarter of prisoners surveyed between the ages of 18 and 25 years had been sexually assaulted, with 9% being sexually assaulted at least weekly (Heilpern, 1998).

The cause of violence in prisons is probably multifactorial. Since around 47% of inmates of Australian prisons have committed violent crimes, prisons may act as concentrators of people who have experience in using violence as a strategy, or who may be prone to impulsive acts of violence (Butler & Karamina, 2005). In addition, prisons are themselves stressful, crowded places that run on systems of reward and punishment, and may trigger reactive violence from inmates.

Prevention of violent assault in prisons is complex; there are few examples in the prison literature of programs with successful outcomes (Butler & Karamina, 2005: 20). The Royal Commission into Aboriginal Deaths in Custody (1991) was convened to study the extremely high numbers of suicides by Aboriginal people in custody, and made a number of findings about suicide response by custodial institutions in general. Many suicides in Australian prisons have occurred as a result of

---

The Death of Steve Biko

Steve Biko, a political leader in the South African black consciousness movement, was taken into custody on the August 18, 1976, in Port Elizabeth. On the September 12 he died in detention, a day after being transferred to Pretoria, Transvaal. He was reported to have died while on a hunger strike. A postmortem revealed that Biko had died of severe brain injury and bleeding as a result of a blow to the head.

In the 5 days before Biko died, he was examined by four doctors, all of whom noted signs and symptoms of severe brain injury. At the request of a police officer, one of the doctors filed several reports that Biko had no abnormality, at the request of a police officer, supporting the police diagnosis that he was malingering. Another doctor gave permission for Biko to be transported 750 miles, unattended, naked and manacled, in the back of a motor vehicle. At the inquest one doctor stated that he was unaware that he could override the decisions made by the responsible prison officer. The case highlighted the compromises made by doctors in the employ of the prison, and the lack of direction provided by the major medical organisations in South Africa on ethical practice in the apartheid era (Silove 1990, Woods 1991).

---

failure to recognise indications of suicidal intent, and poor monitoring of inmates once they were recognised to be distressed. Prevention programs around the country have tended to focus on better systems for monitoring, rather than on primary prevention of suicide.

The most common health conditions among prisoners are substance abuse and mental illness. About half of Australian prisoners have a history of injecting drug use, and about half of those prisoners who have injected drugs in the past will manage to do so in prison (Crofts, 1997). Women are more likely to have a history of injecting, with 73% of women in one survey reporting prior injecting drug use (Butler & Milner, 2003). Approximately one third of prisoners in Victoria and New South Wales have been exposed to hepatitis C and to hepatitis B, indicating that prisons can act as powerful sites of transmission for blood-borne viruses (Butler et al., 1997; Crofts, 1997), either through sharing needles or through sex. Smoking has become normalised in prisons, with 72% of NSW prisoners being regular smokers in a survey in 2000, a rate three times higher than the smoking rate in the general community (Awofeso, Testaz, Wyper, & Morris, 2001). The rates of HIV (Butler, Allnutt, Cain, Owens, & Muller, 2005) and tuberculosis infection (Butler & Milner, 2003: 75) in Australian prisons remain low. Concerns about the spread of hepatitis C and B have led to a robust public debate about the place of needle-supply programs and condoms in prisons.

Surveys of inmates in Australia have repeatedly demonstrated high rates of depression and anxiety among inmates. In a questionnaire distributed among correctional institutions in New South Wales, 43% had at least one major psychiatric diagnosis (Butler, Boonwaat, & Hailstone, 2005). Among female inmates, rates are of psychiatric illness were particularly high (61%, compared with 39% for male inmates). Nine per cent of all inmates reported symptoms consistent with psychosis. The high rates of major mental illnesses reported among inmates have been exacerbated by the increasing role of forensic services as the place to detain unstable mentally ill patients, who are not supported sufficiently in the community.

In general, then, prisoners are in poorer health than the general community. This reflects, in part, the fact that many prisoners have preexisting health conditions, often arising from substance abuse, mental illness and poor primary health care. However, prisons themselves can have direct negative impacts on health, through providing an environment in which prisoners are exposed to physical and sexual violence, through enabling the spread of blood borne viruses, and through exacerbation of mental illness.

Protecting the Health and Safety of Detained Persons

From a human rights perspective, there are three types of protection possible for detained persons. The first, primary prevention, focuses on mechanisms that prevent people entering detention systems. Such an approach in Australia would recognise the great disparity between imprisonment rates for Indigenous and non-Indigenous Australians. In 2006, Aboriginal people were 12 times as likely as non-Aboriginal people to be imprisoned (Australian Bureau of Statistics). In the years since the Royal Commission into Aboriginal Deaths in Custody, custodial rates for Indigenous Australians have continued to increase, by up to 12% per year. High rates of incarceration make prison, and all its attendant risks, part of the normal experience for some Aboriginal communities; in themselves they may contribute to ongoing patterns of violent behaviour that lead to incarceration. Strategies to decrease incarceration such as circle sentencing, and the abolition of mandatory sentencing legislation, are part of a diverse program needed to decrease incarceration for indigenous Australians.

The second type of protective strategy concerns institutionalised norms. The United Kingdom has begun to address the implications of the Human Rights Act for prisons (Coyle, 2003). In Australia, only the Australian Capital Territory has a Human Rights Act, and it is also engaged in the process of developing a framework for building a prison that recognises human rights at its core. Ethical guidelines for health care workers are also built on human rights principles (United Nations, 1990). The guidelines for prisons assert the principle of equivalence, that is, that prisoners are entitled to the same level of health care that they could access outside. For people with multiple, often complex health problems, this demands a comprehensive health care system, able to take the opportunity to improve the health of inmates. The guidelines also underline the independence of health care workers, and the expectation that their first responsibility is to their patient, not the institution.

A drawback of institutionalised norms is that the normalising process can work both ways. Torture, or other forms of cruel and inhuman treatment, can also be normalised. When their conduct was reviewed by the South African Medical and Dental Council (SAMDC), the doctors in the Biko case were found to have committed no clear mistakes. The reluctance of the SAMDC to sanction the doctors suggests that the SAMDC had become institutionally incapable of taking a stand against a prevailing political climate that accepted torture of detainees (Silove, 1990).

The third type of protective strategy is provided through oversighting mechanisms. Australian prisons have provision for an official visitor, whose function is to hear and investigate prisoner complaints in some states, and in others to provide independent advice on the operation of the prison. As a signatory to the Optional Protocol of UNCAT, Australia also undertakes to provide regular reports on our compliance with the Convention, and the strategies for meeting it set out in the Protocol. Appeals may also be made by individuals to the Committee Against Torture in respect of claims under UNCAT, such as potential refoulement. The International Committee of the Red Cross (ICRC) has an official role under the Geneva Conventions in monitoring the physical safety of detainees. The effectiveness of this depends on the quality of the access given to the ICRC. In apartheid era South Africa, the ICRC was given access to high profile prisoners like Nelson Mandela, but not to detainees under interrogation or awaiting trial (Forsythe, 1993).

Conclusions

Prisons and other places of detention pose risks for the health and physical safety of prisoners. Whether or not a community is willing to accept these risks on behalf of its detained population tells us something about the role of prisoners themselves in the polity, and the relative importance of rehabilitation or retribution in the prison system. The most extreme intentional failure of protection, torture, has been part of the legal and investigative system for much of human history. Electroshock devices are an example of innovative technologies that originated in the medical field, but have found a role in torture around the world. Failure of protection also occurs when we undertake large-scale imprisonment of any population, when we fail to adequately protect the health and safety of detainees, and when we do not provide adequate oversight of the institutions in which people are detained. The mechanisms we have in place to protect and monitor freedom from torture and cruel and inhuman treatment are fragile. They will only succeed if the community agrees that deprivation of liberty is sufficient punishment for its transgressors, and that torture has no place in interrogation.

References

Amnesty International. (2003). *The pain merchants: Security equipment and its use in torture and other ill treatment*. London: Amnesty International.

Australian Bureau of Statistics. (2005). *Prisoners in Australia 4517.0*. Canberra, Australia: Commonwealth of Australia:

Awofeso, A., Testaz, R., Wyper, S., & Morris, S. (2001). Smoking prevalence in NSW correctional facilities. *Tobacco Control, 10*, 84–85.

Bloche, M.G., & Marks, J.H. (2005). Doctors and interrogators at Guantanamo Bay. *New England Journal of Medicine, 353*, 6–8.

Bufacchi, V., & Arrigo, J.M. (2006). Torture, terrorism and the state: A refutation of the ticking-bomb argument. *Journal of Applied Philosophy, 23*, 355–373.

Butler, T.G., Dolan, K.A., Ferson, M.J., McGuinness, L.M., Brown, P.R., & Robertson, P.W. (1997). Hepatitis B and C in New South Wales prisons: Prevalence and risk factors. *Medical Journal of Australia, 166*, 127.

Butler, T., & Milner, L. (2003). *The 2001 NSW Inmate Health Survey*. Sydney, Australia: Corrections Health Service.

Butler, T., & Kariminia, A. (2005). Prison violence: Perspectives and epidemiology. *NSW Public Health Bulletin, 17*, 17–20.

Butler, T., Allnutt, S., Cain, D., Owens, D., & Muller, C. (2005). Mental disorder in the New South Wales prisoner population. *Australian and New Zealand Journal of Psychiatry, 39*, 407–413.

Butler, T., Boonwaat, L., & Hailstone, S. (2005). *National prison entrants' bloodborne virus survey, 2004*. University of NSW: Centre for Health Research in Criminal Justice and National Centre in HIV Epidemiology and Clinical Research.

Conroy, J. (2001). *Unspeakable acts, ordinary people: The dynamics of torture*. Berkeley, CA: University of California Press.

Convention Against Torture and Other Cruel, Inhuman and Degrading Treatment or Punishment. (1987). G.A. res. 39/46, [annex, 39 U.N. GAOR Supp. (No. 51) at 197, U.N. Doc. A/39/51 (1984)] entered into force June 26, 1987.

Coyle, A. (2003). *A human rights approach to prison management*. London: International Prison Studies Centre, King's College.

Crofts, N. (1997). A cruel and unusual punishment. *Medical Journal of Australia, 166*, 116.

Forsythe, D.P. (1993). Choices more ethical than legal: The International Committee of the Red Cross and Human Rights. *Ethics and International Affairs, 7*, 139–140.

Geneva Convention relative to the treatment of prisoners of war. (1950). 75 U.N.T.S. 135, entered into force Oct. 21, 1950.

Geneva Convention relative to the Protection of Civilian Persons in Time of War. (1950). 75 U.N.T.S. 287, entered into force Oct. 21, 1950.

Heilpern, D. (1988). *Fear or favour: Sexual assault of young prisoners*. Lismore, Australia: Southern Cross University Press.

Office of the High Commissioner for Human Rights. (2006). Ratifications and reservations. Convention against Torture, and Cruel, Inhuman or Degrading Treatment or Punishment. Retrieved February 25, 2008, from http://www.ohchr.org/english/countries/ratification/9.htm

Peters, E. (1988). *Inquisition*. New York: The Free Press.

Report of the Special Rapporteur on Torture to UN Commission on Human Rights. (1997). E/CN.4/1997/7, January 10, 1997, paras 4–11.

Rumney, P.N.S. (2006). Is coercive interrogation of terrorist suspects effective? A response to Bagaric and Clark. *University of San Francisco Law Review, 40*, 479–513.

Royal Commission into Aboriginal Deaths in Custody. (1991). Recommendations. In *National Report, Vol. 5, Commonwealth of Australia, 1991*. Canberra, Australia: Australian Government Publishing Service.

Silove, D. (1990). Doctors and the State: Lessons from the Biko Case. *Social Science and Medicine, 30*, 417–429.

Steinhoff, U. (2006). Torture — The case for Dirty Harry and against Alan Dershowitz. *Journal of Applied Philosophy, 23*, 337–353.

Woods, D. (1991). *Biko* (3rd ed.). New York: Henry Holt and Co.

World Medical Association. (1975). *Declaration of Tokyo*. Adopted by the World Medical Association, Toyko, Japan. October 1975.

Universal Declaration of Human Rights. (1948). G.A. res. 217A (III), U.N. Doc A/810 at 71 (1948).

United Nations. (1990). Basic principles for the treatment of prisoners. General Assembly resolution 45/111, 14 December 1990.

Walmsley, R. (2005). *World prison population list* (7th ed.). London: International Prison Studies Centre, King's College.

CHAPTER

Expert Witness in a Courtroom: Australian Experience

Maciej Henneberg

I have practised forensic anthropology since 1976 and appeared as an expert witness in courts in Poland, Texas (United States), South Africa and Australia. My last 10 years of expert witness practice have been spent in Australia, hence what follows is based largely on this recent experience of my appearances in courts of law in South Australia, New South Wales, Queensland and Northern Territory and assisting with some cases in Western Australia and in the Australian Capital Territory. Although each Australian state and territory has separate laws, all these legal systems are similar in their general structures and practices. On an international plane, differences among legal systems are greater, and yet basic underlying principles of all those systems are the same: justice based on evidence that seeks to establish the truth regarding particular events and persons.

The role of an expert witness, as for any other witness, is to assist the court in reaching the verdict by providing evidence. Unlike other witnesses who are only allowed to make statements regarding the facts of a case, an expert witness is also allowed to state an opinion. This opinion is accepted by a court of law as part of evidence to be considered in formulating a judgment. The opinion of an expert witness can be accepted as evidence only if the following conditions are met: (a) the field of knowledge of a witness is outside of common experience of most people and it is recognised as a specialised field of knowledge, (b) the witness is qualified in this field (has sufficient knowledge and skills), (c) members of the jury cannot be expected to have sufficient knowledge to draw their own conclusions (Plueckhahn & Cordner 1991).

Legal Systems

Although an expert witness is simply concerned about stating facts and expressing professional opinion, it is useful to understand where and how in the legal system this opinion will be used. It is also useful to understand specific legal terminology and the rights and obligations of the parties in legal proceedings. Legal systems use two sources of law: (a) common law, and (b) statutes. The common law is that established by legal practice, especially during proceedings in various courts of law where judges, barristers and juries have argued and assessed what human actions are right or wrong using logic and concepts operating within a society. Proceedings of each case were recorded and judgments and reasoning of those cases are used as precedents in judging subsequent cases. The statutes are specific laws made by legislative bodies such as parliaments. They can recognise, amend or abrogate common law or establish new laws. Statutes may be short acts of parliament addressing a specific situation, such as euthanasia, or large documents covering an extensive area of human activities. Criminal codes are an example of statute law that covers all the law relating to criminal offences, incorporating common law and consolidating earlier statutes. Statutes also provide for establishment of subordinate legislation, such as regulations and statutory rules that allow adjustment of general rules of an act to specific situations that may change from time to time or from place to place. This subordinate legislation can only clarify a statute. It is made within the authority given by the statute to, for example, a minister of the government.

In practice, law is divided into the civil law and the criminal law, although in many cases both civil injustice and criminal offence may result from the same action; for example, severe bodily injury. As a general rule, civil law deals with disputes between private persons or legal entities, while criminal law deals with offences against the society as represented by the state or some higher political organisation (e.g., a union). Thus civil law deals with recognition and satisfaction of rights while the criminal law identifies and punishes wrongs.

Rights may be violated either when general rules of conduct are not observed or when specific rules established by a contract are not followed. Breaches of the generally recognised rules of conduct are called 'torts'. Their examples are trespass, defamation, or negligence. Civil law does not aim to deter people from unlawful actions by simple punishment of the wrongdoer, but rather seeks a compensation for the affected. This, of course, deters people from wrongdoing because it is the wrongdoer who will have to compensate the affected. Civil cases are brought to a court of law by persons who feel the wrong was done to them — called plaintiffs — against supposed wrongdoers, who are called defendants. The objective of the proceedings is to establish whether the wrong was done and what would be a fair compensation for it (commonly called 'damages'). The standard of proof required in the civil law is 'on balance of probabilities'. An expert witness, by reporting facts and offering opinions, contributes to establishing probabilities of various acts or situations.

In the criminal law, concern is with regulating behaviours in the society by punishing certain acts that are called offences. An omission may also be considered an offence. The criminal law prescribes what must not be done. Punishment of a particular criminal offence is supposed to act as a deterrent, so that in the future members of a society will avoid committing an offence. There are various forms of punishment: imprisonment, fine, restriction of personal freedom (e.g., home detention, community service) or supervision, such as probation or good behaviour bond. Cases are brought before courts by public prosecution (police, directors of public prosecutions), and the guilt of the accused must be proven beyond reasonable doubt. This requirement must be considered by an expert witness giving evidence in criminal cases. Only well-established facts and opinions based on sound and proven knowledge should be presented. Parties to a criminal case are called prosecution and defence, while the defendant is called the accused.

Courts of Law

The origin of the courts of law historically comes from the need for adjudication of various behaviours in a society by its rulers. A prince, a tyrant or an elected official held court, to which subjects or citizens could bring their disputes for settlement. Offenders of public rules were also brought to the court for punishment. Plaintiffs and defendants or accused were sometimes allowed to have other persons presenting or defending their cases. These individuals were considered counsels. As societies grew larger and the business of their government became more complex, the function of adjudication became separated from that of executive government by appointment of respected members of the society as judges. Judges were vested with certain powers normally held by the head of state. These judges held court, to which plaintiffs and public officers presented cases for judgment, sometimes supported by their counsels, while defendants argued against complaints, assisted by their counsels. Judges could ask for help of assessors or of a jury comprised of representative members of a community. Since judges held powers conferred on them from higher levels of the hierarchy of governance, their decisions could be questioned by the parties appealing to the higher authority — either the court of the higher standing or the head of state. This basic structure of judicial system is still current. Details vary. A major variation is that of the prerogatives of the judge.

Inquisitorial and Adversarial Systems

In inquisitorial legal systems derived from the Roman law the judge investigates circumstances of the case, supervising gathering of evidence by the police, and questions witnesses while prosecution and defence counsels help the judge in those tasks. Expert witnesses are called by the court. They are independent of prosecution and defence. They can provide evidence in writing and are not necessarily required to give oral evidence in the court. These systems prevail in continental Europe and countries that derived their models of governance from those of continental Europe.

In the adversarial systems derived from Great Britain, the judge plays the role of an umpire, while cases are argued by the prosecution and defence, who call and question witnesses and on whom rests the burden of proof of the case. Police and prosecution gather all evidence and present it to a magistrate (lower court judge) for either judgment or committal to the trial by a higher court. In this system, the judge will decide points of procedure and of law, and if a jury is present, give legal directions to the jury, but he does not conduct questioning of witnesses. All admissible evidence must be presented firsthand during an open trial. This is required to fully familiarise the judge and the jury with the entire evidence and to enable detailed scrutiny of this evidence. Thus, the expert witness must appear in the court and give oral evidence that is subject to cross-examination and re-examination. At the end of the contest between the opposing parties the jury decides issues of fact. If a jury is not present, as happens in civil cases and in some criminal cases, the judge will decide issues of fact.

Types of Courts

In Australia the first (lower) level of courts are the courts of summary jurisdiction. These exercise jurisdiction over less serious matters and are located in nearly every city or shire. They are usually presided over by professional magistrates trained in law. They are commonly known as 'magistrates' courts'. Their purpose is to deal with cases in a summary fashion, that is, simply and quickly. Besides making judgments in less serious cases, such as some civil disputes of property claims or debts, or criminal offences of petty theft and the like, magistrates' courts conduct committal hearings in cases of serious criminal offences such as armed robbery or murder. These are preliminary hearings aimed at establishing whether there is enough evidence of probable guilt presented by prosecution to warrant a trial by the higher court. No decision of guilt is made, but the decision may be made to hold accused in custody or to grant a bail.

The courts of intermediate level are usually called District Courts. They are presided over by a judge who is an experienced lawyer, and criminal trials are as a rule conducted in the presence of the jury. With regard to criminal cases, these courts deal with nearly all offences, with the exception of the most serious ones like a murder.

Supreme courts of states and territories have jurisdiction that concerns all cases (unlimited jurisdiction). Judges of these courts are appointed from among experienced trial lawyers (barristers). The chief judge of the supreme court is the Chief Justice. The supreme courts also act as courts of appeal. Appeals are heard by the Full Court that consists of at least three judges.

Federal courts decide on matters arising under laws related mostly to civil matters common for the entire Commonwealth. The High Court of Australia is the highest legal authority in the Commonwealth. It acts as an appellate court in cases previously considered by supreme courts of states and territories.

Children's courts deal with criminal cases in which children are accused. If a guilty verdict is made by such a court its main concern is not with simple punishment, but with ordering such custody of the accused that is likely to result in rehabilitation.

Coroner's courts of each state or territory are of a special kind. They do not hear disputes between parties, but hold inquiries into causes of those deaths that occurred in abnormal circumstances and are thus suspicious. Procedures of these courts are similar to those of courts of summary jurisdiction.

In addition to the courts described above there is a variety of courts and tribunals that deal with special cases, such as family courts, or industrial tribunals. These, however, by their nature are unlikely to require the help of archaeologists or biological anthropologists. The majority of cases in which such experts play a role are criminal cases. Thus the rest of this chapter will be devoted to this kind of cases.

The Role of an Expert Witness in Criminal Cases

The role of an expert witness called by a prosecution usually begins when an expert is approached by the police or by the office of public prosecutions. Defence lawyers may also engage expert witnesses. This, however, usually occurs only after the evidence gathered by prosecution is presented to the defendant. In criminal cases this is typically at the time of the committal hearing in the court of summary jurisdiction.

The expert witness is usually engaged by the defence to provide independent opinion about the facts already examined by witnesses of the prosecution, but novel facts may be discovered and interpreted by defence witnesses. There is no difference in obligations and rights of experts called by prosecution and by the defence. They all must help the court to discover the truth.

When being called by a party in the Australian adversarial legal system, an expert witness may feel that their role is to support the case of the prosecution or the defence. This, however, is incorrect, because the foremost duty of an expert witness is to assist the court by providing truthful statement of facts and objective opinion based on the best professional knowledge. Like all witnesses, experts testify under oath (if religious) or affirmation (if nonreligious) and are liable to prosecution for perjury when lying; their testimony is subject to cross-examination and scrutiny by witnesses called by the opposing party. The role of an expert witness is regulated in Australia by appropriate rules modified from time to time and by the codes of conduct (e.g., NSW Schedule 7 'Expert Witness Code of Conduct' to the Uniform Civil Procedure Rules, 2005) and Practice Directions (e.g., Federal Court of Australia, 1998, Supreme Court of South Australia, 2002). These modifications are necessary as knowledge in various areas of expertise progresses and operations of legal systems are refined. Depending on their area of expertise and on the evolution of social systems, morals, ethics and performance of legal practices, precise roles and responsibilities of expert witnesses evolve and opinions as to their conduct are debated (e.g., Freckelton, Reddy, & Selby, 1999; McAbee & Freeman, 2005; Plueckhahn & Cordner, 1991). The need for objective, truthful expert opinion remains, however, unchanged.

Experts should not engage in advocacy. They should only present facts and opinions within their area of expertise. Thus, in my practice I ask specifically not to be informed about all details of a case. I only want to have information directly related to my task. Although work of an expert witness is by its nature objective, emotions play a role in it as in any other human activities. Hence, information extraneous to the task may colour expert witness' thinking, especially in those instances where physical evidence is fragmentary and allows a fair degree of latitude in making a decision. For instance, when examining poorly preserved skeletal remains that lack some clues for reliable diagnosis of sex, the information that the remains come from a 'soldier's grave' may produce a tendency to assess sex as male. I do not suggest that experts will consciously bias their statements to achieve a predetermined result in court, I simply state the reality of human thinking; we want to make a categorical decision rather than to admit to uncertainty. I am automatically suspicious of expert witness reports that do not contain a statement regarding the probability with which they reached their conclusion. My reports always end with a statement: 'I identified remains presented for my examination as so-and-so with XX% probability due to the …'. Police or lawyers who engage experts do not like such statements by expert witnesses because courts of law base their decisions in criminal cases on evidence that is 'beyond reasonable doubt'. Therefore, pressure is sometimes put on an expert to omit the statement of probability, or to modify it so as to produce impression of certainty. Although it may help in a particular case to yield to such pressure, in the long run experts who make incorrect statements regarding certainty of their opinions will be discredited.

The majority of work that archaeologists, anthropologists, or medical scientists do for forensic cases concentrates on the recovery and analysis of evidence in the field and in the laboratory. Very often, the report describing results of these works is all that is required of an expert. Evidence of that report may be accepted by both parties and the accused may either admit to the conclusions of the report, or plead guilty based on what was described in a report. This ends the role of an expert witness in a case.

If, however, for whatever reason, evidence of an expert is required in the court of law, the expert will have to move from the familiar world of fieldwork and laboratory to the unfamiliar world of legal proceedings. This world, that evolved over centuries to provide the fairest possible judgment of potentially punishable human actions, is different from the world of everyday experience and of the work environment of archaeologists and anthropologists. It is characterised by ritualised procedures and strict reliance on spoken word. Although it aims to take account of soberly stated facts only and to literally apply the law, it is full of emotions that may and do influence the course of cases presented. Expert witness entering this world must adjust to its specific culture in order to be helpful to the process of justice. During all stages of his work, an expert witness must be conscious of this and aim to provide the best evidence that will help the court to formulate a judgment based on truth. This requires not only truthful statement of facts and opinions to the best knowledge of an expert, but also formulation of submissions in a way that will result in their correct and objective use.

The work of an expert witness starts with engagement by a party. Parties identify expert witnesses based on what is known about their professional standing and former experience. Formal registration as a forensic expert, though helpful in being recognised as such, is not necessary, because the parties seek to choose a person who has the best expertise relevant to the case and who will thus be able to provide maximum assistance to the court irrespective of formal qualifications. Anyone can be called as an expert witness, provided the court will recognise his/her expertise as relevant. This is reflected in the requirement of providing a statement regarding the expert's education and professional experience at the beginning of any witness report irrespective of whether the witness is or is not formally registered as such. Experts' qualifications will also be discussed in a courtroom prior to asking for statements in the case. Evidence of expert witnesses will be admitted on grounds of their qualifications being assessed as appropriate and relevant to the task, and lying outside of common knowledge that members of the jury would be able to use in formulating their judgment.

Steps in the Work of an Expert Witness
Examination of the Evidence and Writing of the Report
The work starts with being approached by a party. At this stage the expert witness must explain to the party what his/her specific expertise is and thus state whether he/she is an appropriate person for the task. Lawyers and police sometimes are confused as to the kind of expertise a particular witness can offer. Explanation of the witness's abilities must be completely truthful and honest. Witnesses who undertake to provide opinions beyond their knowledge and abilities may be discredited during

cross-examinations, while the court will not be correctly appraised of the facts of cases and their interpretation. This may cause a miscarriage of justice.

Once the witness's ability to undertake specific tasks for the party is established and the witness agrees to undertake them any exhibits (objects), information relevant to the tasks, and appropriate resources to conduct fieldwork and analyses should be provided. Witnesses have every right to demand that all relevant information be provided and ask for appropriate resources to discover, examine and assess this information. It is preferable that only information relevant to witness's task should be provided. In their work, witnesses should not venture beyond their areas of expertise and should use only well-established methods that can be independently shown as reliable. One should avoid any information extraneous to the task that may bias feelings and thus judgment of the witness. The witness is free to, and strongly advised to, consult the most recent literature, use the best possible equipment and consult with colleagues. Such consultations must be conducted in such a manner that will not breach confidentiality of the case. Although eventually all the admissible information that witness will provide will become available to the open court, at the initial stages of the case breaches of confidentiality may jeopardise the process of justice. Any discussion of the case with the third party must be approved by the party that engaged the witness.

Younger professionals, quite naturally, may have a tendency to be proud to be asked to provide their expertise and may thus feel the urge to boast about this fact. This must be avoided. Details of the case should not even be discussed with partners or family members. These rules hold until the final verdict in the case is reached. It is especially difficult to abstain from discussing high profile cases where journalists wait outside of the courtroom for emerging witnesses and try to ask them questions, and yet it must be done.

In the performance of their tasks the witness must preserve independence to arrive at an objective opinion. The witness takes instructions from the engaging party, but these are valid only with regard to the law and availability of factual information. Witnesses may not bias their observations and opinions to suit the expectations of the party. When a witness finds something that does not support the party's arguments, there may be a tendency to omit this finding from the final report. This is incorrect and must not be done. Witnesses must reveal the whole truth to the best of their abilities.

At the conclusion of a task, a witness provides a written report. In the case of the police, the report is usually made on a prescribed form and must contain certain statements in its initial part. Exact requirements in this regard vary from jurisdiction to jurisdiction. In general, a statement of qualifications is required. This should include academic and professional formal degrees/diplomas/fellowships, appointments, publications and forensic experience. Usually one concise paragraph suffices. In New South Wales a statement that the expert is familiar with a particular Code of Practice is also required. The written report will be studied by the opposing party. Presentation of the expert's report to the accused and his/her lawyers often results in a decision to admit to the circumstances described in the report, or to a guilty plea. This ends the expert's role in the case. If the plea of not guilty is entered, the case goes to trial where expert witness will have to give oral evidence.

Pretrial Conference

When several experts are engaged, especially by both parties, it is advisable to hold a pretrial conference to iron out all details on which there is an agreement between the experts. Such a conference also serves to clarify specialist statements and terminology for the lawyers. All this saves time during actual court proceedings and minimises confusion that may occur during the hearing. I have participated in conferences with the prosecution and the defence even when I was a single expert witness. During a conference, witnesses must be conscious that anything they say can be used by the opposing party. Thus witnesses must be very clear in their statements and limit them only to those matters on which they have absolute clarity within their areas of expertise.

Court procedures require that all information must be provided orally during a formal sitting of the court. Experts are free to supplement their oral statements with exhibits that may have a form of graphs, photos, moving images, recordings and specific objects, if appropriate. A demonstration of movements or situational interplay may also be allowed. All illustrations are retained by the court as exhibits. Only exhibits judged by the court as admissible can be presented. They must, of course, be prepared before the court hearing.

Expert Appearance in the Court of Law

I will limit myself here to the description of proceedings in criminal cases and use the first hearing in the lower court as a general model. Differences between the magistrates' court and higher courts, relevant to witness appearance and interaction with the courts will be highlighted.

In criminal cases the first hearing takes place in the magistrates' court (a court of summary jurisdiction). In serious cases the aim of this hearing is not to establish guilt but to find out whether there is sufficient cause to commit a case to trial in the higher court. At the committal hearing admissibility of witnesses and of their evidence is established. In legal proceedings there are strict rules of evidence. These are too complex to describe here; lawyers of both parties and the presiding judge will explain and apply them as necessary in a particular case. One of the basic rules of evidence is that against the hearsay. This means that witnesses are not allowed to tell what they heard from other people, but only state what they established or observed themselves. There are exceptions to this rule. They apply when an expert witness consulted work of others to arrive at an opinion. For example stating that 'in my opinion there was an extensive blunt trauma to the parietal bones because the edges of broken bones displayed characteristics described by … as typical for blunt trauma' is acceptable. It is unacceptable, however, to say 'I think the sex of this person was male because Dr XX told me so while I had no opportunity to examine the skeleton'.

The first thing to be considered regarding a particular witness is admissibility of his/her evidence in terms of qualifications, type of evidence to be given and methods used. This part of the hearing takes place in closed court, with only the magistrate/judge and parties are present. As a general rule the witness must have generally recognisable academic/professional qualifications, appropriate experience and use well-established methods. Experience as an expert witness may also be taken into account. If a witness gave evidence before other courts in similar cases, it is more likely that evidence to be given in a new case will be considered admissible. It is unlikely that the magistrate will accept as admissible results of analysis that used a method specifically developed for this case by an expert. Such a method, even if the best one, is considered unproven and difficult to assess by other experts because it has not been published, nor used by others. Once, appearing before magistrate as a witness for the prosecution who identified a bank robber by his auricle (external ear), I had my evidence considered inadmissible because there were no standards of ear morphology variation available for Australians.

The physical layout of the magistrates' court and the general rules of witness behaviour are similar in various jurisdictions and not much different from those of higher courts. The main difference is that no jury is present. The courtroom has a dais opposite the main entrance. On the dais there sits the magistrate, or presiding judge. Facing the dais, approximately in the middle of the room, there are tables and chairs for prosecution and defence legal teams. Behind them, filling space to the entrance there are seats for the public. On the sides of the room, between the dais and the lawyer's tables there are a witness stand, a dock for the accused and (in case of higher courts) seats for the jury. Immediately below the dais there are tables and seats for sheriffs, clerks and judge assistants. Anyone entering or leaving the court in session must bow towards the dais. All present must stand when the presiding judicial officer enters or leaves the room.

Legal teams of prosecution and defence typically consist of a barrister who asks questions and makes statements, a solicitor who assists the barrister with details of the case and, sometimes, junior assistants who perform a variety of legal and clerical tasks. In minor cases in the magistrates' courts prosecution may be presented by the police officer rather than by a barrister. Expert witnesses may sit with the legal team of the party that engaged them.

In most cases, in the interests of objectivity, witnesses are not allowed to be present in the courtroom during examination of other witnesses. They are required to be available to the court throughout the entire length of the proceedings and thus witnesses will usually wait to be called, or recalled, outside the courtroom. Witnesses should not communicate with other witnesses, nor discuss the case with anyone else at this stage. A witness may be excused from further presence after completing the testimony, but the court has the right to recall the witness. In Australia, where distances between cities are large, it is possible to give evidence by means of a video-conference rather than require physical presence of a witness in the court. A telephone link is also acceptable in some instances. The court asks expert witness to be present under subpoena (meaning under the threat of penalty if this order is not followed). Thus the expert must attend the court.

Under normal circumstances it is understood that experts are busy with many tasks and the parties will endeavour to make such arrangements for the witness presence in the court that minimise any inconvenience to the witness. The court is amenable to accommodate special requests of the parties in this regard. It happened to me that having appeared in the court in Sydney, travelling there from Adelaide, it turned out that my presence was required for a period much longer than originally expected. I had a very important meeting scheduled in Adelaide falling in that period. The prosecution, who engaged me in this case, organised for me a 1-day return trip to Adelaide to enable me to attend the meeting. Next day I was back in court in Sydney. An expert witness is entitled to be financially compensated for travel related to the court appearance and for time spend in court.

On being called to the stand, the expert witness enters the courtroom, bows towards the dais and proceeds to the witness stand. There the officer of the court will administer the oath (on the Bible) or an affirmation (if the witness is nonreligious). Following this the witness may sit down. The examination starts from the prosecution leading the evidence-in-chief. It opens with statements regarding witness' qualifications. Answers should be given clearly and precisely. This is usually an easy part of the proceedings because the witness worked on the case, wrote a report and in court is just repeating contents of the report in answer to questions of the prosecution. The magistrate or the judge may intervene and ask the witness additional questions or rule on admissibility of certain statements. The witness should address the magistrate as 'Your Worship' and the judge 'Your Honour'. In these days of declining formality, magistrates will not protest if addressed 'Your Honour'. Instructions of the judge must be strictly followed. If a witness is not certain whether some action is permissible he/she should ask the judge: 'Your Honour, may I approach the exhibit on the posterboard and indicate the shape of ...?' Although the entire evidence must be given orally, experts may bring copies of their reports and ask leave to refresh their memories from their notes.

Following the evidence-in-chief the defence leads the cross-examination. This part is more difficult because the defence barrister may try to undermine witness qualifications, credibility and reliability of factual statements and opinions. One has to be cautious and brief in answering these questions. The defence sometimes uses a tactic of making a statement and then asking 'Do you agree?' A very clear answer is required and in most cases it will be 'I disagree'. No need to explain further unless a witness has an obvious factual statement to the contrary. Defence may use a number of other tactics that are too detailed to be discussed here (Kassin, Williams, & Saunders, 1990). The best policy is to be meticulously truthful and direct in giving answers at this stage. On the completion of the cross-examination, the prosecution is able to re-examine the witness. Following re-examination, the witness is excused, leaves the stand and in most cases exits the courtroom, bowing towards the dais.

If the committal hearing decides to commit case to trial the full hearing of each witness will take place in the district court or in the supreme court. Since courts require to hear afresh the entire evidence in an oral form, it will be necessary for the witness to repeat all statements already made in the magistrates' court. In most criminal cases at this level a jury is present. Questioning of the witness by both parties is aimed to elicit a full opinion rather than just concentrate on its admissibility. The witness must be conscious that it is the jury who will make the judgment. This requires very clear formulation of answers in plain language and need for simple, yet correct, explanations of professional terminology. Despite the solemn nature of court proceedings, it happens that the jury will laugh as a result of a certain witness' statements or answers. The laughter is usually an excellent indicator that the jury fully understood what the witness wanted to say. Making the jury laugh should not be avoided, but is certainly not an obligatory part of the witness' performance.

The involvement of an expert witness usually ends with the completion of the evidence given by this witness, though the witness may be recalled to be further questioned on various points. After the court has reached its verdict and passed a sentence, the case may be appealed by a party. If leave to appeal is granted, the expert witness may be recalled by the appellate court. This does not happen often, but experts must be aware that their involvement does not end with the verdict of the court. It is essential to keep all the documentation of each case since appeals may drag on for years, and special appeals may lead to re-examination of some cases decades after they have started. In those appeals, evidence of expert witnesses may be required, or challenged.

Ethical Conduct

It is absolutely necessary to adhere strictly to all legal requirements and the requirements of professional ethics at all stages of the case. Objectivity, good professional knowledge, and validation of one's results by colleagues (a peer review) are the best policy. Under no circumstances should expert witnesses venture beyond the area of their expertise, nor knowingly pass opinions based on incomplete or outdated professional knowledge and methods. It is easy for experts to fall into the trap of thinking too highly of themselves, especially after 'wining' a few cases. This produces the attitude 'trust me, I am a doctor' and inevitably leads to overstepping the limits of expertise. Most commonly it takes a form of issuing judgments rather than objective professional opinions. Such conduct is unethical and may be subject to challenge by professional bodies. Although expert witnesses can legitimately charge fees for their services, financial gain should not motivate their opinions. It is the basic rule of professional conduct to separate provision of services from collection of payment. Witnesses should discuss their compensation with the engaging party at the very outset of their involvement, state that the fee will not be dependent on the result of their investigations, and charge the fee only on completion of their role in the case. Those of us who are employees of public institutions should leave the issue of compensation to be arranged by relevant officers of these institutions. In my practice, I do not charge fees for my analysis of facts and formulation of an opinion. As an employee of a public university I feel that this is a part of my duties. In this way I am also completely independent in formulation of my opinions. My travel expenses, and time spent away from my normal place of work while working on the case or appearing in court, are paid for by the engaging party.

Personal integrity, professional excellence, objectivity, independence and truthfulness are the best policy in the work of expert witnesses.

References

Federal Court of Australia. (1998). Practice direction: Guidelines for expert witnesses in proceedings in the Federal Court of Australia, 15 September 1998.

Freckelton, I., Reddy, P., & Selby, H. (1999). *Australian Judicial Perspectives on Expert Evidence: An Empirical Study*. Melbourne, Australia: Australian Institute for Judicial Administration.

Kassin, S.M., Williams, L.N., & Saunders, C.L. (1990). Dirty tricks of cross-examination: The influence of conjectural evidence on the jury. *Law and Human Behavior, 14*, 373–384.

McAbee, G.N., & Freeman, J.M. (2006). Expert medical testimony: Responsibilities of medical societies. *Neurology, 65*, 337.

Supreme Court of South Australia. (2002). SCR 38.01 A. *Practice Direction 46 A.*

Plueckhahn, V.D., & Cordner, S.M. (1991). *Ethics, legal medicine and forensic pathology* (2nd ed.). Melbourne, Australia: Melbourne University Press.

Contributors

Tim Anson completed a PhD in biological anthropology in 2004 at the University of Adelaide. Tim's studied 80 skeletons archaeologically recovered from the St. Mary's Church Free Ground cemetery in suburban Adelaide. He used the principles of biological anthropology to build a life profile for European pioneers of early South Australia. In February 2005 Tim joined the Iraq Mass Graves Team in Baghdad to begin 2 years of forensic investigation. As part of a team of biological anthropologists and archaeologists, he assisted in the forensic analysis of over 300 skeletons, the remains of men, women and children purged by a repressive regime. Tim now lives in Adelaide and works at the University of Adelaide.

Richard Barwick is a former reader in zoology at the Australian National University who has gravitated to palaeontology in his 'retirement'. He currently researches Devonian fossil fish from sites around the world. He is a Visiting Fellow in the Research School of Earth Sciences. As a graphic illustrator for over 50 years he has published over 60 works in many fields ranging from postage stamp designs to journal and book covers, and many extensively illustrated scientific papers. His hobbies include saltwater fishing and occasional silversmithing.

Hallie R. Buckley, PhD, Senior Lecturer, Department of Anatomy and Structural Biology, School of Medical Sciences, University of Otago. Dr Buckley's expertise is in the field of bioarchaeology, the excavation and analysis of human skeletal remains from archaeological sites. She is specifically interested in health and disease in the prehistoric Pacific Islands. Buckley also acts as a consultant for the NZ Police in forensic cases involving skeletonised human remains.

Ian R. Dadour received his PhD in zoology specialising in acoustics and population genetics of grasshoppers. This was followed by a series of postdoctoral fellowships and an 8-year position with the Western Australian Department of Agriculture. As Officer in Charge of the biological control of bushflies by dung beetle program, this association with flies became the catalyst for a research life involving forensic entomology. Currently, he is Director of the Centre for Forensic Science and a Registered Forensic Practitioner. He is the State's Honorary Forensic Entomologist and as an expert witness in the science of entomology has appeared in courts in Western Australia, Northern Territory, Queensland and New South Wales. He has organised a number of forensic entomology workshops around Australia, which include the investigation of decomposition of bodies buried and on the surface, and is now part of the team involved in teaching the Human Remains Recovery School for the Federal Bureau of Investigation Evidence Response Teams.

Denise Donlon is curator of the Shellshear Museum of Physical Anthropology and senior lecturer in the Discipline of Anatomy and Histology, University of Sydney. She has a PhD in physical anthropology and a BA(Hons) in archaeology. She coordinates courses in comparative primate anatomy and forensic osteology and supervises postgraduate students. Research interests include forensic anthropology of the Sydney region, dental and postcranial skeletal variation and Australian Aboriginal burial archaeology. She is a consultant to the NSW Department of Forensic Medicine and a member of the RAAF Specialist Reserves.

Thomas A. Faunce, Associate Professor, BA/LLB(hons) BMed PhD, has a joint position in the College of Law and Medical School at the Australian National University. He is Project Director of two Australian Research Council Grants investigating (1) the impact of trade agreements on medicines policy, and (2) regulation of nanomedicine. He was a consultant for the UNESCO Global database on Health Law and Biomedicine.

Shari Forbes is an Assistant Professor and Director of the Forensic Science program at the University of Ontario Institute of Technology. Dr Forbes received both her BSc (Hons) in Applied Chemistry–Forensic Science and PhD from the University of Technology Sydney, Australia. Her research is focused around the processes of decomposition, particularly in burial environments, and employs a multidisciplinary approach involving forensic chemistry, taphonomy, and archaeology. The significance of the research is the potential to assist forensic and human rights investigations involving clandestine grave sites.

Michelle Harvey completed her undergraduate studies (BSc/BA) in entomology and Chinese, and on graduation was motivated to apply her entomological interests to benefit society. Discovering the developing area of forensic entomology, she completed a Master of Forensic Science and PhD at the University of Western Australia specialising in the molecular systematics of forensically significant blowflies. During her studies, she studied in both South Africa and the United States, gaining practical experience in casework and decomposition studies. She is currently Senior Lecturer in Forensic Biology, based in the School of Biological Sciences at the University of Portsmouth in the United Kingdom.

Ian Hanson, MSc, is Senior Lecturer in Forensic Archaeology with the Centre of Forensic Sciences, and the Centre for Anthropology, Archaeology and Heritage at Bournemouth University, United Kingdom, leading forensic masters programs in archaeology and anthropology. He has worked as a professional archaeologist across the Middle East, in the United Kingdom, United States and Europe. His experience on international investigations and excavations has taken him to Bosnia, Croatia, Central America, Africa and the Middle East, serving as a consultant for various agencies including the United Nations, International Criminal Tribunal for the Former Yugoslavia, Fundacion de Anthropologia Forense de Guatemala, Kenyon International and the police.

Maciej Henneberg, PhD DSc, is a Foundation Wood Jones Professor of Anthropological and Comparative Anatomy at the University of Adelaide. He also holds a title of Professor of Biology, awarded by the President of the Republic of Poland. Since 1973 his research included skeletal identification and identification of living people from anatomical features. He has conducted fieldwork at ancient burial grounds in Poland, Italy, Texas and South Africa. He appeared as an expert witness in courts in Australia, South Africa, the United States, and Poland. He has published six books/monographs and over 230 papers/book chapters. He is currently the President of the American Dermatoglyphic Association.

Rebecca Kinaston is a PhD student from the Department of Anatomy and Structural Biology at the University of Otago. Her current research involves stable isotope analysis of South-East Asian remains, while her master's research was on remains from the Pacific.

Tom Knight, BA MLitt MA, is currently undertaking his doctorate in archaeology at the Australian National University in Canberra. He has worked as a consultant archaeologist in New South Wales, Victoria and the Northern Territory. His present research is focused on the prehistoric Aboriginal ritual use of the natural landscape in the montane zone of southern New South Wales.

Judith Littleton is an associate professor in biological anthropology at the University of Auckland. She has worked since 1994 on the recording and analysis of Aboriginal burials in western New South Wales as well as undertaking, at the request of local iwi and authorities identification of human remains from New Zealand contexts.

Marc Oxenham, PhD, has a joint position in archaeology and biological anthropology in the Department of Archaeology and Anthropology, Australian National University. His main research interest centres on reconstructions of past human health, disease and behaviour using ancient skeletonised remains; while one of his chief teaching foci is the development and promotion of forensic archaeological and anthropological skills in forensic investigations of serious crime and natural disasters. To this end Marc has established the first Master of Arts (forensic anthropology) in an Australian university institution. When not excavating in Vietnam and the Philippines he assists the police and other government bodies with the identification of skeletonised material.

Donald Pate is an Associate Professor in the Department of Archaeology at Flinders University in Adelaide, South Australia. He completed graduate and post-doctoral studies in archaeological chemistry at Brown and Harvard Universities. Post-doctoral research included an Australian Institute of Aboriginal and Torres Strait Islander Studies fellowship at the Australian National University. Donald commenced archaeological research in Australia in 1983 and has been employed at Flinders University since 1990. Pate was a member of the Australian Archaeological Association Executive and editor of its journal *Australian Archaeology* from 1999 to 2006.

Christine Phillips, MBBS BMedSc MA MPH DipEd FRACGP, is a general practitioner, and Senior Lecturer in Social Foundations of Medicine at the Australian National University Medical School. Her clinical work has encompassed prisoner health, drug and alcohol medicine, and refugee health. Between 2001 and 2005 she served as the medical member of the ACT Corrections Health Board. She is currently senior medical officer at Companion House Medical Service, a health service for refugee survivors of torture and trauma.

David Ranson is a forensic pathologist involved extensively in medical law. David is the Deputy Director of the Victorian Institute of Forensic Medicine, a Clinical Associate Professor in the Department of Forensic Medicine at Monash University and the Director of the National Coroners' Information System in Australia. He is an associate in the Faculty of Law at Monash University and a Senior Fellow in the Faculty of Medicine, Dentistry and Health Sciences at the University of Melbourne. David graduated in medicine in 1980 and graduated in law in 1987. He is a Fellow of the Royal College of Pathologists of Australasia, a Fellow of the Royal College of Pathologists of Great Britain, a Fellow of the Australian College of Legal Medicine and a Fellow of the Faculty of Forensic and Legal Medicine of the Royal College of Physicians (UK). David has contributed to a number of international disaster investigation deployments including the investigation of mass graves in Kosovo and the identification of Tsunami victims in Thailand.

James Robertson, PhD, has led the AFP's forensic group since 1989. He moved to Australia from the United Kingdom in the mid-1980s, having been a lecturer in forensic science at the University of Strathclyde from 1976. He has wide-ranging interests in the forensic sciences, is an active researcher, has published extensively, has edited several books and was the long-standing editor of the Taylor and Francis series on the forensic sciences. He holds adjunct and courtesy professorial appointments at three universities and was recently made an Honorary Doctor of the University of Canberra. He holds the Australian Public Service medal for services to law enforcement and forensic science. His group played a significant role in disaster victim identification in the Bali bombings and in the 2004 south Asia tsunami.

Carl N. Stephan, BHlthSc HBHlthSc PhD GCertHEd, is an anatomist and biological anthropologist. His PhD researched and improved facial approximation methods and he has since published in excess of 25 full-length scientific articles relating to craniofacial identification. He has reviewed numerous papers for leading forensic science and physical anthropology journals and has provided expertise in local, national and international forensic investigations (including mass graves). Carl holds academic experience from two 'Group of Eight' Australian Universities and currently works as a lecturer in the School of Biomedical Sciences at The University of Queensland, Australia.

Jane A. Taylor, OAM BDS BScDent(Hons) MScDent GCertPTT FICD, has been a practising forensic odontologist for nearly 20 years. She was Director of the Forensic Odontology Unit at the University of Adelaide from 2000 until relocating to New South Wales in 2004. Her Masters thesis investigated distortion in cranio-facial video superimposition. Jane is a Past President of the Australian Society of Forensic Odontology, and the SA Branch of the Australian and New Zealand Forensic Science Society. She is currently a Senior Lecturer in Oral Health at The University of Newcastle, Australia.

Ronn G. Taylor, AssocDipAppSci (Dental Technology) RMIT FAISDT, has held the position of forensic sculptor to the Victorian Institute of Forensic Medicine for the past 20 years. He specialises in facial approximation, bite-mark impression and the duplication of skeletal remains. He has nearly 40 years of experience in teaching dental anatomy and manufacturing facial and dental prosthesis at the Royal Dental Hospital of Melbourne, Peter MacCallum Cancer Hospital and the School of Dental Science, The University of Melbourne. Ronn is currently the Laboratory Manager and Senior Dental Prosthetist in the School of Dental Science at The University of Melbourne, Australia.

Mark Tibbett, Associate Professor, is director of the Centre for Land Rehabilitation at the University of Western Australia. As a soil microbiologist with a long-standing interest in decomposition processes in terrestrial ecosystems, his interests in forensic taphonomy arose from research into organic nutrient patch dynamics in soils; the principles of which he has applied to forensic science. He has worked in many of the world's ecoregions including tropical, Mediterranean, temperate, boreal, and polar ecosystems. He has published 70 peer reviewed papers, and has recently co-edited a book on the latest advances in soils and forensic taphonomy.

Michael K. Trimble, PhD, is Chief of the Curation and Archives Analysis Branch US Army Engineer District, St Louis, and Director of the Corps of Engineers' Mandatory Center of Expertise for the Curation and Management of Archaeological Collections. He has led major curatorial efforts on Kennewick Man, The African Burial Ground, and Navy collections from the South West Pacific. Michael served as the Program Director of the Mass Graves Investigation Team, Iraq, and was responsible for planning, preparing, and leading a 22-person international team that performed archaeological and forensic exhumations and analysis that supplied forensic evidence for the prosecution by the Iraqi High Tribunal of members of the former regime.

Michael Westaway is an archaeologist and biological anthropologist who has undertaken field work in South East Australia, Indonesia, India and Jordan. In the past Michael has been a government archaeologist with Aboriginal Affairs Victoria, where he had responsibility for investigating suspected Aboriginal skeletal remains for AAV and the State Coroner. Following this he was employed as a collection manager and biological anthropologist with the National Museum of Australia and was responsible for identifying the provenance of skeletal remains, liaising with the relevant Aboriginal community and documenting the remains prior to their repatri-ation. He is currently executive officer for the Willandra Lakes World Heritage Area where he is actively involved in research and conservation issues there.

Kelly Whittle, PGDipSci (Otago), has completed postgraduate studies in the Department of Anatomy & Structural Biology. Focussing on forensic science, her research encompassed several areas: the biomechanics of blunt force trauma, cranio-facial blunt force injury and blood spatter analysis. She is also particularly interested in biological anthropology and forensic osteology.

Walter Barry Wood, MBBS BSc, is Associate Professor of Human Anatomy and Forensic Anthropology at Bond University, Gold Coast, Queensland. From 1973 to 2001 he held the position of senior lecturer in anatomy at the University of Queensland. In 1990 he was appointed an adjunct professor of forensic anthropology at the University of Tennessee, United States. For over 30 years he has been a consultant in forensic anthropology for the Forensic Pathology section of the Queensland Health Department. He co-authored the chapter on 'Forensic Osteology' in the publication *Expert Evidence*, published by The Australian Law Book Company Ltd in 2003.

Richard Wright is Professor Emeritus of Anthropology at the University of Sydney. An archaeologist, in 1990 he turned his attention to forensic applications. For the 4 years from 1997 to 2000 he managed forensic work in Bosnia, as Chief Archaeologist for the UN's mission of discovering, exhuming and interpreting mass graves. He concentrated on the killing events that followed the fall of Srebrenica in 1995. A long-standing armchair interest has been the programming of solutions to multivariate problems in archaeology and physical anthropology.

CPSIA information can be obtained
at www.ICGtesting.com
Printed in the USA
BVHW01s1137040618
518151BV00008B/57/P

9 781875 378906